Endovascular Management of Neurovascular Pathology in Adults and Children

Editors

NEERAJ CHAUDHARY
JOSEPH J. GEMMETE

NEUROIMAGING CLINICS OF NORTH AMERICA

www.neuroimaging.theclinics.com

Consulting Editor
SURESH K. MUKHERJI

November 2013 • Volume 23 • Number 4

ELSEVIER

1600 John F. Kennedy Boulevard ● Suite 1800 ● Philadelphia, Pennsylvania, 19103-2899

http://www.neuroimaging.theclinics.com

NEUROIMAGING CLINICS OF NORTH AMERICA Volume 23, Number 4
November 2013 ISSN 1052-5149, ISBN 13: 978-0-323-24231-8

Editor: John Vassallo (j.vassallo@elsevier.com)
Developmental Editor: Yonah Korngold

Neuroimaging Clinics of North America (ISSN 1052-5149) is published quarterly by Elsevier Inc., 360 Park Avenue South, New York, NY 10010-1710. Months of issue are February, May, August, and November. Business and editorial offices: 1600 John F. Kennedy Blvd., Suite 1800, Philadelphia, PA 19103-2899. Business and editorial offices: 6277 Sea Harbor Drive, Orlando, FL 32887-4800. Periodicals postage paid at New York, NY, and additional mailing offices. Subscription prices are USD 360 per year for US individuals, USD 514 per year for US institutions, USD 180 per year for US students and residents, USD 415 per year for Canadian individuals, USD 655 per year for Canadian institutions, USD 525 per year for international individuals, USD 655 per year for international institutions and USD 260 per year for Canadian and foreign students and residents. To receive student/resident rate, orders must be accompanied by name of affiliated institution, date of term, and the *signature* of program/residency coordinator on institution letterhead. Orders will be billed at individual rate until proof of status is received. Foreign air speed delivery is included in all *Clinics* subscription prices. All prices are subject to change without notice. POSTMASTER: Send address changes to *Neuroimaging Clinics of North America*, Elsevier Health Sciences Division, Subscription Customer Service, 3251 Riverport Lane, Maryland Heights, MO 63043. Telephone: 1-800-654-2452 (U.S. and Canada); 314-447-8871 (outside U.S. and Canada). Fax: 314-447-8029. E-mail: journalscustomerservice-usa@elsevier.com (for print support); journalsonlinesupport-usa@elsevier.com (for online support).

Reprints. For copies of 100 or more of articles in this publication, please contact the Commercial Reprints Department, Elsevier Inc., 360 Park Avenue South, New York, NY 10010-1710. Tel.: 212-633-3874; Fax: 212-633-3820; E-mail: reprints@elsevier.com.

Neuroimaging Clinics of North America is covered by *Excerpta Medical/EMBASE,* the RSNA Index of Imaging Literature, *MEDLINE/PubMed (Index Medicus),* MEDLINE/MEDLARS, SciSearch, Research Alert, and Neuroscience Citation Index.

Printed and bound by CPI Group (UK) Ltd, Croydon, CR0 4YY

Transferred to digital print 2012

PROGRAM OBJECTIVE

The goal of Neuroimaging Clinics of North America is to keep practicing radiologists and radiology residents up to date with current clinical practice in radiology by providing timely articles reviewing the state of the art in patient care.

TARGET AUDIENCE

Practicing radiologists, radiology residents, and other healthcare professionals who utilize neuroimaging findings to provide patient care.

LEARNING OBJECTIVES

Upon completion of this activity, participants will be able to:

1. Review endovascular treatment of cerebral vasospasm, cerebral arteriovenous malformations, cerebral dural and pial arteriovenous fistulas, carotid occlusive disease, intracranial atherosclerotic disease, acute ischemic stroke, vascular anomalies, and adult spinal arteriovenous lesions.
2. Discuss intracranial endovascular balloon test occlusion and its indications, methods, and predictive value.
3. Recognize, diagnose and manage spontaneous cervical and cerebral arterial dissections.

ACCREDITATION

The Elsevier Office of Continuing Medical Education (EOCME) is accredited by the Accreditation Council for Continuing Medical Education (ACCME) to provide continuing medical education for physicians.

The EOCME designates this enduring material for a maximum of 15 *AMA PRA Category 1 Credit*(s)™. Physicians should claim only the credit commensurate with the extent of their participation in the activity.

All other health care professionals requesting continuing education credit for this enduring material will be issued a certificate of participation.

DISCLOSURE OF CONFLICTS OF INTEREST

The EOCME assesses conflict of interest with its instructors, faculty, planners, and other individuals who are in a position to control the content of CME activities. All relevant conflicts of interest that are identified are thoroughly vetted by EOCME for fair balance, scientific objectivity, and patient care recommendations. EOCME is committed to providing its learners with CME activities that promote improvements or quality in healthcare and not a specific proprietary business or a commercial interest.

The planning committee, staff, authors and editors listed below have identified no financial relationships or relationships to products or devices they or their spouse/life partner have with commercial interest related to the content of this CME activity:

Felipe C. Albuquerque, MD; Salah G. Aoun, MD; Bernard R. Bendok, MD, FACS, FAANS, FAHA; Mandy J. Binning, MD; Stefan Brew, MD, FRANZCR, FRCR; Nohra Chalouhi, MD; Neeraj Chaudhary, MD, MRCS, FRCR; Indran Davagnanam, MBBCh, FRCR; Aaron Dumont, MD; Tarek Y. El Ahmadieh, MD; Augusto Elias, DDS, MD; Jorge L. Eller, MD; Vijeya Ganesan, MB, ChB, MD, FRCP; Joseph J. Gemmete, MD, FSIR; Luis Fernando Gonzalez, MD; Pamela Hetherington; Brynne Hunter; Pascal Jabbour, MD; Steven J. Kasten, MD; Sandy Lavery; Christopher J. Lenart, MD; Cameron G. McDougall, MD; Jamal McClendon, Jr., MD; Jill McNair; Suresh K. Mukherji, MD, FACR; Sabareesh K. Natarajan, MD, MS; Aditya S. Pandey, MD; Lindsay Parnell; Rudy J. Rahme, MD; Ciro Randazzo, MD; Fergus Robertson, MRCP, FRCR; Robert Rosenwasser, MD; William Stetler, MD; Karthikeyan Subramaniam; Byron G. Thompson, MD; Stavropoula Tjoumakaris, MD; Ahmed K. Toma, MD, FRCS; Erol Veznedaroglu, MD.

The planning committee, staff, authors and editors listed below have identified financial relationships or relationships to products or devices they or their spouse/life partner have with commercial interest related to the content of this CME activity:

David Fiorella, MD, PhD has research grants from Siemens AG and MicroVention, Inc.; is a consultant/advisor for Covidien, ev3, Cordis Corporation, Nfocus Medical Inc., Micrus Endovascular Corporation; has royalties/patents from Codman & Shurtleff, Inc.; and has stock ownership in Vacular Simulations, LLC, TDC Technologies, and CVSL.

L. Nelson Hopkins, MD is a consultant/advisor for Boston Scientific, Cordis Corporation, Micrus Endovascular Corporation, Abbott Laboratories and Silk Road; is on Speakers Bureau for Abbott Laboratories; has an employment affiliation with Access Closure and Claret Medical Inc.; has stock ownership with Micrus Endovascular Corporation, Boston Scientific, Access Closure, Inc., Valor Medical and Claret Medical Inc.; spouse/partner has stock ownership with Toshiba Corporation.

Mohammad Yashar Sorena Kalani, MD, PhD has a research grant from the National Institutes of Health.

Elad I. Levy, MD has research grants from Codman & Shurtleff, Inc., ev3, Covidien, and Boston Scientific/Wingspan Stents; has stock ownership in Intratech Medical, Ltd.; and is a consultant/advisor for Codman & Shurtleff, Inc., ev3, Covidien, TheraSyn Sensors, Inc. and Blockade Medical LLC. He also received other financial support from ev3 and Abbott Laboratories for carotid stenting.

Cameron G. McDougall, MD is a consultant/advisor for Covidien, Terumo Medical Corporation and Cordis Corporation.

Kenneth V. Snyder, MD, PhD is on speakers bureau for EV3 Inc. and Toshiba Corporation; is a consultant/advisor for EV3 Inc., Toshiba Corporation, Medtronics Inc., EPI, Guidant Corporation, Micrus Endovascular Corporation, Zimmer, Boston Scientific, and Cordis Corporation; has stock ownership in Boston Scientific, Access Closure, Inc., and Niagra Gorge Medical; has research grants with Toshiba Corporation, EV3 Inc., Abbott Laboratories, Medtronics Inc., EPI, Guidant Corporation, Micrus Endovascular Corporation, Zimmer, Boston Scientific, and Cordis Corporation.

Adnan H. Siddiqui, MD, PhD has research grants from National Institutes of Health and the University of Buffalo; is on speakers bureau for Codman and Shurtleff, Inc.; has stock ownership in Hotspur, Intratech Medical, StimSox, Valor Medical, Inc., and Blockade Medical, LLC.; is a consultant/advisor for Codman and Shurtleff Inc., Covidien, Concentric Medical, Inc., GuidePoint Global Consulting, LLC., Penumbra Inc., Stryker, Pulsar Vascular and MicroVention, Inc.; also claims Honoraria from Abbott Laboratories and Penumbra Inc.

Erol Veznedaroglu, MD is a consultant/advisor for Codman & Shurtleff, Inc., Cordis Corporation, Microvention, Inc. and Micrus Endovascular Corporation.

UNAPPROVED/OFF-LABEL USE DISCLOSURE

The EOCME requires CME faculty to disclose to the participants:

1. When products or procedures being discussed are off-label, unlabelled, experimental, and/or investigational (not US Food and Drug Administration (FDA) approved); and
2. Any limitations on the information presented, such as data that are preliminary or that represent ongoing research, interim analyses, and/or unsupported opinions. Faculty may discuss information about pharmaceutical agents that is outside of FDA-approved labelling. This information is intended solely for CME and is not intended to promote off-label use of these medications. If you have any questions, contact the medical affairs department of the manufacturer for the most recent prescribing information.

TO ENROLL

To enroll in the *Neuroimaging Clinics of North America* Continuing Medical Education program, call customer service at 1-800-654-2452 or sign up online at http://www.theclinics.com/home/cme. The CME program is available to subscribers for an additional annual fee of $212 USD.

METHOD OF PARTICIPATION

In order to claim credit, participants must complete the following:

1. Complete enrolment as indicated above.
2. Read the activity.
3. Complete the CME Test and Evaluation. Participants must achieve a score of 70% on the test. All CME Tests and Evaluations must be completed online.

CME INQUIRIES/SPECIAL NEEDS

For all CME inquiries or special needs, please contact elsevierCME@elsevier.com.

NEUROIMAGING CLINICS OF NORTH AMERICA

RELATED INTEREST

Neurologic Clinics, Vol. 30, No. 1, February 2012
Neurologic Emergencies
Alireza Minagar, Alejandro A. Rabinstein, *Editors*

NOW AVAILABLE FOR YOUR iPhone and iPad

Contributors

CONSULTING EDITOR

SURESH K. MUKHERJI, MD, FACR
Currently, Professor and Chairman,
W.F. Patenge Endowed Chair, Department
of Radiology, Michigan State University, East
Lansing, Michigan; Formerly, Department of
Radiology, University of Michigan Health
System, Ann Arbor, Michigan

EDITORS

NEERAJ CHAUDHARY, MD, MRCS, FRCR
Assistant Professor, Departments of Radiology
and Neurosurgery, Division of
Neurointerventional Radiology, University of
Michigan Health System, Ann Arbor, Michigan

JOSEPH J. GEMMETE, MD, FSIR
Associate Professor, Departments of
Radiology, Neurosurgery, and Otolaryngology,
Division of Neurointerventional Radiology and
Skull Base Surgery, University of Michigan
Health System, Ann Arbor, Michigan

AUTHORS

FELIPE C. ALBUQUERQUE, MD
Division of Neurological Surgery, Barrow
Neurological Institute, St. Joseph's Hospital
and Medical Center, Phoenix, Arizona

SALAH G. AOUN, MD
Department of Neurological Surgery,
Northwestern University Feinberg School of
Medicine, Chicago, Illinois

**BERNARD R. BENDOK, MD, FACS, FAANS,
FAHA**
Associate Professor of Neurological Surgery
and Radiology, Department of Neurological
Surgery, Northwestern University Feinberg
School of Medicine, Chicago, Illinois

MANDY J. BINNING, MD
Stroke and Cerebrovascular Center of New
Jersey, Trenton, New Jersey

**STEFAN BREW, MBBS, MHB, MSc,
FRANZCR, FRCR**
Consultant, Lysholm Department of
Neuroradiology, National Hospital for Neurology
and Neurosurgery, University College London

Hospitals, Queen Square; Department of
Neuroradiology, Great Ormond Street Hospital
for Children, London, United Kingdom

NOHRA CHALOUHI, MD
Department of Neurosurgery, Jefferson
Hospital for Neuroscience, Thomas
Jefferson University Hospital, Philadelphia,
Pennsylvania

NEERAJ CHAUDHARY, MD, MRCS, FRCR
Assistant Professor, Departments of Radiology
and Neurosurgery, Division of
Neurointerventional Radiology, University of
Michigan Health System, Ann Arbor, Michigan

**INDRAN DAVAGNANAM, MD, MB BCh,
BAO, BMedSci, FRCR**
Consultant, Lysholm Department of
Neuroradiology, National Hospital for
Neurology and Neurosurgery, University
College London Hospitals, Queen Square;
Brain Repair and Rehabilitation Unit, Institute
of Neurology, University College London,
London, United Kingdom

AARON DUMONT, MD
Department of Neurosurgery, Jefferson
Hospital for Neuroscience, Thomas
Jefferson University Hospital, Philadelphia,
Pennsylvania

TAREK Y. EL AHMADIEH, MD
Department of Neurological Surgery,
Northwestern University Feinberg School of
Medicine, Chicago, Illinois

AUGUSTO E. ELIAS, DDS, MD
Neurointerventional Fellow, Division of
Interventional Neuroradiology, Department of
Radiology, University of Michigan Health
System, Ann Arbor, Michigan

JORGE L. ELLER, MD
Endovascular Neurosurgery Fellow,
Department of Neurosurgery, School of
Medicine and Biomedical Sciences, University
at Buffalo, State University of New York;
Department of Neurosurgery, Kaleida Health,
Buffalo, New York

DAVID FIORELLA, MD
Department of Neurological Surgery, Stony
Brook University Medial Center, Stony Brook,
New York

VIJEYA GANESAN, MD, FRCP
Consultant, Department of Pediatric
Neurology, Great Ormond Street Hospital for
Children, London, United Kingdom

JOSEPH J. GEMMETE, MD, FSIR
Associate Professor, Departments of
Radiology, Neurosurgery, and Otolaryngology,
Division of Neurointerventional Radiology and
Skull Base Surgery, University of Michigan
Health System, Ann Arbor, Michigan

LUIS FERNANDO GONZALEZ, MD
Department of Neurosurgery, Jefferson
Hospital for Neuroscience, Thomas Jefferson
University Hospital, Philadelphia, Pennsylvania

L. NELSON HOPKINS, MD
Chairman and Professor, Department of
Neurosurgery, Kaleida Health; President and
CEO, Jacobs Institute; Departments of

Neurosurgery and Radiology, Toshiba Stroke
Research Center, School of Medicine and
Biomedical Sciences, University at Buffalo,
State University of New York, Buffalo,
New York

PASCAL JABBOUR, MD
Department of Neurosurgery, Jefferson
Hospital for Neuroscience, Thomas Jefferson
University Hospital, Philadelphia, Pennsylvania

**MOHAMMAD YASHAR SORENA KALANI,
MD, PhD**
Division of Neurological Surgery, Barrow
Neurological Institute, St. Joseph's Hospital
and Medical Center, Phoenix, Arizona

STEVEN J. KASTEN, MD
Assistant Professor, Department of Plastic
Surgery, University of Michigan Health System,
Ann Arbor, Michigan

CHRISTOPHER J. LENART, MD
Stroke and Cerebrovascular Center of
New Jersey, Trenton, New Jersey

ELAD I. LEVY, MD
Professor, Department of Neurosurgery,
Kaleida Health; Departments of
Neurosurgery and Radiology, Toshiba Stroke
Research Center, School of Medicine and
Biomedical Sciences, University at Buffalo,
State University of New York, Buffalo,
New York

JAMAL MCCLENDON Jr, MD
Department of Neurological Surgery,
Northwestern University Feinberg School
of Medicine, Chicago, Illinois

CAMERON G. MCDOUGALL, MD
Division of Neurological Surgery, Barrow
Neurological Institute, St. Joseph's
Hospital and Medical Center, Phoenix,
Arizona

SABAREESH K. NATARAJAN, MD, MS
Clinical Assistant Instructor, Department of
Neurosurgery, School of Medicine and
Biomedical Sciences, University at Buffalo,
State University of New York; Department of
Neurosurgery, Kaleida Health, Buffalo,
New York

ADITYA S. PANDEY, MD
Assistant Professor, Division of Interventional Neuroradiology, Department of Radiology; Department of Neurosurgery, University of Michigan Health System, Ann Arbor, Michigan

RUDY J. RAHME, MD
Department of Neurological Surgery, Northwestern University Feinberg School of Medicine, Chicago, Illinois

CIRO RANDAZZO, MD
Department of Neurosurgery, Jefferson Hospital for Neuroscience, Thomas Jefferson University Hospital, Philadelphia, Pennsylvania

FERGUS ROBERTSON, MRCP, FRCR
Consultant, Department of Neuroradiology, National Hospital for Neurology and Neurosurgery, University College London Hospitals, London, United Kingdom

ROBERT ROSENWASSER, MD
Department of Neurosurgery, Jefferson Hospital for Neuroscience, Thomas Jefferson University Hospital, Philadelphia, Pennsylvania

ADNAN H. SIDDIQUI, MD, PhD
Associate Professor, Department of Neurosurgery, Kaleida Health; Departments of Neurosurgery and Radiology, Toshiba Stroke Research Center, School of Medicine and Biomedical Sciences, University at Buffalo, State University of New York, Buffalo, New York

KENNETH V. SNYDER, MD, PhD
Assistant Professor, Department of Neurosurgery, Kaleida Health; Department of Neurosurgery, Toshiba Stroke Research Center, School of Medicine and Biomedical Sciences, University at Buffalo, State University of New York, Buffalo, New York

WILLIAM STETLER, MD
Neurosurgery Resident, Department of Neurosurgery, University of Michigan Hospitals, Ann Arbor, Michigan

BYRON G. THOMPSON, MD
Professor, Departments of Neurosurgery and Radiology, University of Michigan Hospitals, Ann Arbor, Michigan

STAVROPOULA TJOUMAKARIS, MD
Department of Neurosurgery, Jefferson Hospital for Neuroscience, Thomas Jefferson University Hospital, Philadelphia, Pennsylvania

AHMED K. TOMA, MD, FRCS (Neurosurg)
Neurosurgery Resident, Victor Horsley Department of Neurosurgery, National Hospital for Neurology and Neurosurgery, University College London Hospitals, Queen Square, London, United Kingdom

EROL VEZNEDAROGLU, MD
Department of Neurosurgery, Capital Institute for Neurosciences; Stroke and Cerebrovascular Center of New Jersey, Trenton, New Jersey

Contents

Endovascular Methods for the Treatment of Intracranial Cerebral Aneurysms   563

Joseph J. Gemmete, Augusto Elias, Neeraj Chaudhary, and Aditya S. Pandey

> This article briefly discusses the clinical features, natural history, and epidemiology of intracranial cerebral aneurysms, along with current diagnostic imaging techniques for their detection. The main focus is on the basic techniques used in endovascular coiling of ruptured and nonruptured saccular intracranial cerebral aneurysms. After a discussion of each technique, a short review of the results of each form of treatment is given, concentrating on reported large case series. Specific complications related to the endovascular treatment of saccular intracranial aneurysms are then discussed.

Endovascular Treatment of Cerebral Vasospasm: Vasodilators and Angioplasty   593

Aditya S. Pandey, Augusto E. Elias, Neeraj Chaudhary, Byron G. Thompson, and Joseph J. Gemmete

> Cerebral vasospasm following aneurysmal subarachnoid hemorrhage (SAH) is a delayed, reversible narrowing of the intracranial vasculature that occurs most commonly 4 to 14 days after aneurysmal SAH and can lead to permanent ischemic injury. Angiographic spasm occurs in up to 70% of patients following SAH, and approximately half become symptomatic. Estimates of patients who are disabled by vasospasm, or die because of it, range from 5% to 9%, with vasospasm accounting for 12% to 17% of all fatalities or cases of disability after SAH. This article discusses the multiple medical and endovascular therapies used to prevent or treat vasospasm.

Endovascular Treatment of Cerebral Arteriovenous Malformations   605

Mohammad Yashar Sorena Kalani, Felipe C. Albuquerque, David Fiorella, and Cameron G. McDougall

> Treatment of arteriovenous malformations of the central nervous system requires a multidisciplinary approach with input from vascular neurosurgeons, endovascular interventionalists, and radiation oncologists. Treatment paradigms based on a thorough understanding of the natural history of the lesion and the cumulative risks of multimodality treatment maximize the likelihood of a positive outcome. This article outlines the role of endovascular embolization in the treatment of arteriovenous malformations with specific emphasis on decision making during treatment planning. Technical considerations when treating arteriovenous malformations are discussed, including the choice of embolic agents, potential intraprocedural and periprocedural complications, and postprocedural management of patients.

> Dural arteriovenous fistulas (DAVFs) are arteriovenous shunts from a dural arterial supply to a dural venous channel, typically supplied by pachymeningeal arteries and located near a major venous sinus. Pial arteriovenous fistulas (PAVFs) are composed of one or more arterial feeders draining into a single vein in the absence of an intervening nidus. Fistulas manifesting features of high risk for rupture should be treated aggressively, the spectrum of treatment varies from endovascular, surgical resection, and stereotactic radiosurgery. This article describes the natural history, clinical presentation, and treatment of dural and pial fistulas, with emphasis on endovascular treatment.

> Carotid occlusive disease is one of several etiologic factors for stroke. Of all strokes, an estimated 88% are ischemic in nature. Less than 20% of these are caused by atheroma in the carotid bifurcation. Traditionally, carotid artery stenosis has been treated with carotid endarterectomy (CEA); however, carotid artery balloon angioplasty and stent placement has enjoyed significant technological advances over the last decade and can now offer a comparable treatment alternative to CEA. In this review, the authors concentrate their discussion on the treatment of carotid atherosclerotic disease with particular attention on the endovascular treatment.

> Stroke is the third leading cause of death in the United States. Intracranial atherosclerotic disease plays a role in cerebrovascular accidents, with well-characterized modifiable and nonmodifiable risk factors. Surgical bypass has so far not proved to be superior to medical therapy. Both medical and endovascular therapies for intracranial atherosclerosis have evolved since the initial off-label use of cardiac devices for its treatment. Initial reports on the results of stent placement for symptomatic high-grade intracranial atherosclerotic disease were initially encouraging. However, debate remains as to the optimal treatment of symptomatic intracranial atherosclerotic disease.

> Arterial dissections of head and neck arteries were first identified pathologically in the 1950s, but not until the 1970s and the 1980s did they begin to be widely recognized as a clinical entity. Carotid and vertebral artery dissections account for only 2% of all ischemic strokes, but they account for approximately 20% of thromboembolic strokes in patients younger than 45 years. The cause of supra-aortic dissections can be either spontaneous or traumatic. This article addresses spontaneous cervical and cerebral artery dissections.

> Endovascular stroke therapy has revolutionized the management of patients with acute ischemic stroke in the last decade and has facilitated the development of

sophisticated stroke imaging techniques and a multitude of thrombectomy devices. This article reviews the scientific basis and current evidence available to support endovascular revascularization and provides brief technical details of the various methods of endovascular thrombectomy with case examples.

Abrupt interruption of the internal carotid artery without a balloon test occlusion (BTO) carries a 26% risk of cerebral infarction. BTO is a test used to decrease this risk by evaluating the efficacy of the collateral circulation. Clinical tolerance of parent vessel occlusion can be assessed by a BTO with several variables, including the clinical examination, angiographic assessment, stump pressure, induced hypotension, perfusion scanning, transcranial Doppler ultrasonography, and neurophysiologic monitoring. This review discusses the indications, methods, predictive value, and complications of BTO.

Vascular malformations are congenital lesions secondary to errors in the development of arteries, capillaries, veins, or lymphatics. Most of these lesions are sporadic; however, a certain percentage present with syndromes. This article discusses the clinical features, natural history, and epidemiology of these lesions, and the diagnostic imaging features of vascular anomalies of the head and neck are presented. The percutaneous/endovascular treatment of each of the vascular anomalies is described, and surgical and additional treatment options are discussed briefly. The clinical outcomes of the main forms of treatment and level of evidence are presented.

Spinal arteriovenous lesions (SAVLs) are rare disorders, the diagnosis of which can be established using various imaging modalities. To discern the various types of SAVL, spinal angiography of the entire neural axis is required. Surgery is the standard treatment of choice; however, ever advancing endovascular technology can provide a viable alternative. This article discusses the normal anatomy, arterial supply, and venous drainage of the spinal cord. The classification, pathophysiology, epidemiology, clinical presentation, natural history, and pathophysiology of SAVLs in adults are reviewed. Finally, endovascular treatment of these lesions is discussed.

Pediatric spinal arteriovenous shunts are rare and, in contrast to those in adults, are often congenital or associated with underlying genetic disorders. These are thought to be a more severe and complete phenotypic spectrum of all spinal arteriovenous shunts seen in the overall spinal shunt population. The pediatric presentation thus accounts for its association with significant morbidity and, in general, a more challenging treatment process compared with the adult presentation.

Intracranial arteriovenous shunts (AVSs) in children can be divided into pial arteriovenous malformations, vein of Galen malformations, and arteriovenous fistulae (AVF). Dural AVF and dural sinus malformations are rare entities within this group. The relative immaturity of the anatomy and physiology of the neonatal and infant brain results in the inability of the hydrovenous system to compensate in the face of such disorders. Thus, the clinical presentation reflects this difference in the underlying anatomy, physiology, and disorder between children and adults. In this article, we briefly review the presentation, natural history and management of these entities.

Childhood intracranial aneurysms differ from those in the adult population in incidence and gender prevalence, cause, location, and clinical presentation. Endovascular treatment of pediatric aneurysms is the suggested approach because it offers both reconstructive and deconstructive techniques and a better clinical outcome compared with surgery; however, the long-term durability of endovascular treatment is still questionable; therefore, long-term clinical and imaging follow-up is necessary. The clinical presentation, diagnosis, and treatment of intracranial aneurysms in children are discussed, and data from endovascular treatments are presented.

Acute ischemic stroke affects 3.3 of 100,000 children per year. The causes of AIS in children can be broadly divided into the following 6 categories: cardiac disease, sickle cell disease, moyamoya, arterial dissection, other arteriopathies, and other causes. Approximately 24% of the cases are classified as idiopathic. Magnetic resonance imaging (MRI) and cerebral angiography play an important role in determining the causes of an AIS in children. Medical approaches, including anticoagulation, anti-inflammatories, and antiplatelet therapies, surgical revascularization and endovascular approaches may have a role in the management of AIS in children.

Foreword

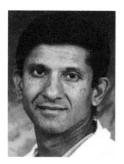

Suresh K. Mukherji, MD, FACR
Consulting Editor

In my 25+ years in Radiology, I would suggest some of the greatest advancements have been made in neurointerventional radiology (NIR). Drs Neeraj Chaudhary and Joe Gemmete are my colleagues and friends at the University of Michigan and have created an excellent state-of-the-art update of the advancements in neuroendovascular treatment of aneurysms, vascular malformations, and anomalies. The editors give a wonderful historical perspective of the advancements of NIR in their preface. On a personal note, I still remember cutting innumerable strands of silk to treat arteriovenous malformations during my fellowship, which despite what my teenage daughter tells me, was NOT that long ago! It is amazing to see how much the field has evolved over a relatively short period of time.

This issue covers both adult and pediatric neurointerventional topics. The issue begins by providing an overview of the current endovascular methods for treatment of intracranial aneurysms and is followed by a discussion of the endovascular treatment of cerebral vasospasm. Subsequent articles focus on a discussion of endovascular treatment options for cerebral arteriovenous malformations, cerebral dural and pial arteriovenous fistulas, carotid occlusive disease, intracranial atherosclerotic disease, cervical and cerebral arterial dissections,

acute ischemic stroke, vessel sacrifice, vascular anomalies, and adult spinal arteriovenous lesions. The final four articles in the pediatric section describe the endovascular management of cerebral aneurysms, acute ischemic stroke, spinal arteriovenous shunts, and the not so well understood cerebral arteriovenous shunts in children. I personally thank all of the article authors for their outstanding contributions to this fantastic issue.

I also commend Drs Chaudhary and Gemmete for emphasizing their collaborative efforts with the Department of Neurosurgery and specifically with Dr Aditya Pandey. We are fortunate to have a fully integrated service at the University of Michigan, thanks to the mutual respect and collaboration between the outstanding faculty members of two great departments. I am sure the readers will enjoy this issue and find the information useful in their daily practice.

Suresh K. Mukherji, MD, FACR
Department of Radiology
University of Michigan Health System
1500 East Medical Center
Ann Arbor, MI 48109-0030, USA

E-mail address:
mukherji@med.umich.edu

Neuroimag Clin N Am 23 (2013) xv
http://dx.doi.org/10.1016/j.nic.2013.07.002
1052-5149/13/$ – see front matter © 2013 Published by Elsevier Inc.

neuroimaging.theclinics.com

Preface

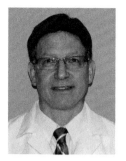

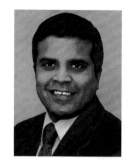

Joseph J. Gemmete, MD, FSIR   Neeraj Chaudhary, MD, MRCS, FRCR

Editors

In 1991, Dr Guglielmi and Dr Vinuela reported the use of a detachable coil for the treatment of a cerebral aneurysm in an animal model at UCLA. Since this time, endovascular technology has improved tremendously and the number of devices available for treatment of various neurovascular diseases has increased exponentially. Furthermore, the number of trained neurointerventionalists has multiplied, so that currently nearly every large size hospital in the United States has access to a trained physician. Likewise, the governing society during this time has grown and experienced considerable change as reflected in the name change from the American Society of Interventional Neuroradiology to the current name of the Society of Neurointerventional Surgery. This name change reflects the acknowledgment that radiologic imaging, neurosurgical, and neurologic expertise is necessary to become a proficient neurointerventionalist.

The first decade, toward the close of the 20th century, saw the establishment of coil embolization as the preferred treatment for ruptured cerebral aneurysms based on the ISAT trial. The beginning of the 21st century gave us improved aneurysm coil platforms, balloons and stents specially designed for intracranial use, mechanical thrombectomy devices for treatment of acute ischemic stroke, and liquid embolic agents for treatment of vascular tumors and brain vascular malformations. Recently, with the development of flow diverter stents for treatment of cerebral aneurysms, there is new hope that cerebral aneurysms treated from an endoluminal approach may

have similar recurrence rates to our neurosurgical colleagues. Advancements in technology, while striving to improve patient outcome, pose a separate set of unanswered questions. This is what makes our medical subspecialty so unique and stimulating.

Neurointerventional Radiology/Surgery encompasses all therapeutic interventions for diseases of the nervous system. Neurovascular diseases of the brain and spinal cord form a significant subset of patients that the neurointerventionalist can treat. We have collected fourteen articles in this issue that deal with the endovascular management of neurovascular pathology of the brain and spinal cord in adults and children. The editors want the readers to develop a detailed understanding of the underlying pathophysiology, clinical presentation, endovascular treatment, and outcomes based on the published literature.

The issue is divided into the adult and pediatric sections. The issue begins by providing an overview of the current endovascular methods for treatment of intracranial aneurysms. This is followed by a discussion of the endovascular treatment of cerebral vasospasm. Subsequent articles focus on a discussion of endovascular treatment options for cerebral arteriovenous malformations, cerebral dural and pial arteriovenous fistulas, carotid occlusive disease, intracranial atherosclerotic disease, cervical and cerebral arterial dissections, acute ischemic stroke, vessel sacrifice, vascular anomalies, and adult spinal arteriovenous lesions. The final four articles in the pediatric section describe the endovascular management of cerebral

Neuroimag Clin N Am 23 (2013) xvii–xviii
http://dx.doi.org/10.1016/j.nic.2013.07.001
1052-5149/13/$ – see front matter © 2013 Published by Elsevier Inc.

neuroimaging.theclinics.com

aneurysms, acute ischemic stroke, spinal arterio-venous shunts, and the not-so-well-understood cerebral arteriovenous shunts in children.

We would like to sincerely commend all the authors for their concerted efforts in completing this project. The authors have been handpicked based on their immense expertise in the field and significant contributions to our improved understanding of neurovascular disease. This could not have been possible without the collaborative efforts from our neurosurgery colleague and coauthor Dr Aditya Pandey. He was instrumental in garnering the experts from the neuroendovascular surgery community for this effort. We would also like to acknowledge the efforts of our coauthors from London, England for their contributions in the pediatric section. Dr Gemmete has put in a tremendous effort in coordinating all the various authors to keep to the deemed timeline. At our institution, we have a very collaborative atmosphere between Radiology and Neurosurgery that enables learning from each other. We feel this edition of the *Neuroimaging Clinics* provides an excellent update of the advancements in endovascular treatment of neurovascular pathology in adults and children. We hope that the readers will enjoy this issue and find the information useful in their daily practice.

Last but not the least we want to thank Dr Suresh Mukherji for his kind invitation and support to make this issue a reality. We also would like to thank Joanne Husovski, Sarah Barth, and Pamela Hetherington from Elsevier for all their patience, encouragement, and deadline reminders.

For my beautiful wife, Demi, and my loving daughters, Anna Maria and Zoe Athina: thank-you for your hugs, smiles, kisses, and support. I would also like to thank my parents, who stressed education.
—Joseph J. Gemmete, MD

To my loving wife, Pallavi, and my dear sons, Tushar and Rohit Chaudhary, who always bring a smile to my face. To my parents, without whose support all of this would not have been possible.
—Neeraj Chaudhary, MD

Joseph J. Gemmete, MD, FSIR
Departments of Radiology, Neurosurgery, and Otolaryngology
Division of Neurointerventional Radiology and Skull Base Surgery
University of Michigan Health System
UH B1D 328, 1500 E. Medical Center Drive SPC 5030
Ann Arbor, MI 48109, USA

Neeraj Chaudhary, MD, MRCS, FRCR
Departments of Radiology and Neurosurgery
Division of Neurointerventional Radiology
University of Michigan Health System
UH B1D 330A
1500 E. Medical Center Drive, SPC 5030
Ann Arbor, MI 48109, USA

E-mail addresses:
gemmete@med.umich.edu (J.J. Gemmete)
neerajc@med.umich.edu (N. Chaudhary)

Endovascular Methods for the Treatment of Intracranial Cerebral Aneurysms

Joseph J. Gemmete, MD, FSIR[a],*, Augusto E. Elias, DDS, MD[b],
Neeraj Chaudhary, MD, MRCS, FRCR[c], Aditya S. Pandey, MD[c]

KEYWORDS

- Intracranial cerebral aneurysm • Balloon remodeling • Flow diverters • Coiling of cerebral aneurysm
- Stent-assisted coiling of cerebral aneurysm • Onyx HD 500
- Complications from coiling of intracranial aneurysms

KEY POINTS

- The annual risk of aneurysm rupture, based on the International Study of Unruptured Intracranial Aneurysms, is 0.7% per year.
- The 30-day case fatality after subarachnoid hemorrhage (SAH) is 38%, and 10% to 20% of SAH survivors remain dependent.
- Cerebral aneurysms can be treated with simple coiling, balloon remodeling, stent-assisted coiling, Onyx HD 500, and flow diversion.
- The International Subarachnoid Trial showed an absolute risk reduction in death of 7.4% in patients presenting with SAH treated with endovascular coiling in comparison with surgical clip placement.
- A Barrow Institute study prospectively randomized 500 SAH patients to clipping versus coiling. At 1 year a modified Rankin Score of greater than 2 was observed in 33.7% of clipped patients, compared with 23% of patients with coils.
- The Pipeline Embolization Device in the Intracranial Treatment of Aneurysms trial treated 31 intracranial aneurysms with a mean aneurysm size of 11.5 mm and mean neck size of 5.8 mm. Follow-up angiography at 6 months demonstrated complete occlusion of the aneurysm in 93.3% of patients.

INTRODUCTION

Microsurgical clipping of intracranial aneurysms has been the historical definitive standard for the treatment of intracranial aneurysms.[1] Today's surgical techniques routinely achieve complete exclusion of the aneurysm from the circulation without compromise of the parent vessel or arterial perforators in a large number of patients. However, there are several risk factors that may put the patient at increased risk of morbidity and mortality, including aneurysm size and location, patient's age, and the medical condition of the patient.[2] In addition, according to the International Subarachnoid Trial (ISAT), patients with subarachnoid hemorrhage (SAH) fared better with endovascular coiling than those with surgical clipping.[3] To overcome some of the limitations of surgical clipping,

[a] Division of Interventional Neuroradiology and Cranial Base Surgery, Departments of Radiology, Neurosurgery, and Otolaryngology, University of Michigan Health System, UH B1D 328, 1500 East Medical Center Drive, Ann Arbor, MI 48109-5030, USA; [b] Division of Interventional Neuroradiology, Department of Radiology, University of Michigan Health System, 1500 East Medical Center Drive, Ann Arbor, MI 48109-5030, USA; [c] Division of Interventional Neuroradiology, Departments of Neurosurgery and Radiology, University of Michigan Health System, 1500 East Medical Center Drive, Ann Arbor, MI 48109-5030, USA
* Corresponding author.
E-mail address: gemmete@med.umich.edu

Neuroimag Clin N Am 23 (2013) 563–591
http://dx.doi.org/10.1016/j.nic.2013.03.007
1052-5149/13/$ – see front matter © 2013 Elsevier Inc. All rights reserved.

endovascular treatments have been developed, which have grown considerably in number over the last 15 years since the US Food and Drug Administration (FDA) approval of the Guglielmi detachable coil (GDC) in 1995.[4,5] This article briefly discusses the clinical features, natural history, and epidemiology of intracranial cerebral aneurysms, along with current diagnostic imaging techniques for their detection. The main focus is on the basic techniques used in endovascular coiling of ruptured and nonruptured saccular intracranial cerebral aneurysms. After a discussion of each technique, a short review of the results of each form of treatment is given, concentrating on reported large case series. Specific complications related to the endovascular treatment of saccular intracranial aneurysms are then discussed.[6,7]

CLINICAL FEATURES

Most intracranial aneurysms are asymptomatic and remain undetected until the time of rupture. Autopsy reports have shown that aneurysms are present in roughly 5% of the population.[8–10] SAH, a medical emergency, is the most common initial clinical presentation. It was the first symptom in 58% of patients in one series.[11] A history of the abrupt onset of a severe headache of atypical quality ("the worst headache of my life") is typical of SAH; this may be associated with brief loss of consciousness, a focal neurologic deficit, nausea and vomiting, or meningismus. However, SAH is frequently misdiagnosed. Nearly one-half of the patients present with a milder form of a headache 1 to 2 weeks before full rupture of the aneurysm.[12] A review of 111 patients referred to a tertiary care center for the management of unruptured aneurysms found that only 41% of the aneurysms produced symptoms.[13]

Common presentations of intracranial aneurysms in specific locations include the following.

Paraclinoid Aneurysms

Paraclinoid aneurysms, like other intracranial aneurysms, present with SAH.[14,15] The second most common form of presentation for aneurysms in this location is visual loss, which is usually unilateral from involvement of the ipsilateral optic nerve.[16] As an ophthalmic artery aneurysm grows, it usually impinges on the lateral aspect of the optic nerve. This process can produce a monocular superior nasal quadrantanopia, and in an aneurysm with significant mass effect of the nerve complete visual loss may be present. A much more unusual form of presentation is that of ischemic symptoms caused by embolization from a partially thrombosed aneurysm.[17] A majority of patients presenting with a paraclinoid aneurysm are women, and there is a high incidence of multiple aneurysms in patients with aneurysms in this region.[18,19] Posterior communicating aneurysms usually present with SAH or isolated third-nerve palsy. The third-nerve paresis is commonly painful and the pupil is usually involved. Anterior choroidal artery aneurysms can on occasion present with a third-nerve palsy.

Aneurysms of the Internal Carotid Artery Bifurcation

Aneurysms arising at the distal bifurcation of the internal carotid artery also commonly present with SAH. These aneurysms can produce a large intraparenchymal hematoma that may be mistaken for a hypertensive hemorrhage. The lesions may also cause signs and symptoms owing to a local mass effect.

Anterior Communicating Artery Aneurysms

Aneurysms in this location typically present with SAH. The initial hemorrhage may be minor, causing a severe headache without neurologic signs, or may be more extensive, causing a neurologic deficit. Given the intimate location of these aneurysms within the third ventricle and hypothalamus, local hemorrhage often causes changes in mental status including confusion, memory distortion, or even coma.[20] The aneurysm commonly ruptures into the third ventricle, often causing hydrocephalus. Involvement of the hypothalamic region can produce bradycardia, diabetes insipidus, inappropriate antidiuretic hormone secretion, and visual disturbances.[21] Rarely there is bleeding into the internal capsule, causing hemiparesis.

Middle Cerebral Artery Aneurysms

The most common presentation for patients with a middle cerebral artery aneurysm is SAH. The second most common is incidental detection of an asymptomatic aneurysm on computed tomography (CT) or magnetic resonance (MR) imaging. Large middle cerebral artery aneurysms can cause local mass effect on the temporal lobe, leading to a seizure. Transient ischemic attacks and cerebral infarction are uncommon with intracranial aneurysms, although they are more frequent in this location.[22] About 60% of patients with a middle cerebral artery aneurysm will have a transient loss of consciousness at the time of rupture. About one-third of patients will have a headache localized to the side of the aneurysm. Middle cerebral artery aneurysms are more likely than an aneurysm in any other location to present with an intraparenchymal hematoma.[23]

In addition, a patient with a ruptured middle cerebral artery aneurysm is more likely to have a subdural hematoma.

Basilar and Posterior Cerebral Artery Aneurysms

Patients with basilar and posterior cerebral artery aneurysms commonly present with SAH indistinguishable from SAH from other aneurysms. Occasionally large or giant aneurysms in this location will present with seizures, hydrocephalus, or signs of mass effect such as hemiparesis or third-nerve palsy.

Vertebrobasilar Junction Aneurysms

Aneurysms of the vertebrobasilar junction usually arise from the carina between the basilar artery and the dominant vertebral artery. Occasionally they occur in relation to a fenestration of the lower basilar artery.[24] The patient usually presents with SAH or signs of lower brainstem compression.

Posterior Inferior Cerebellar Artery Aneurysms

Aneurysms of the vertebral-posterior inferior cerebellar artery usually arise at the junction of both of these vessels, and have a tendency to point superiorly and lie against the medulla. The aneurysm usually has a close relationship with the vagal and hypoglossal nerves. SAH hemorrhage is the most common presentation, often accompanied by a palsy of the sixth or lower cranial nerves. Headache is usually localized to the neck and occipital region.

EPIDEMIOLOGY AND NATURAL HISTORY

The precise prevalence of intracranial aneurysms is not known and varies widely in the literature. It is accepted that about 3% to 5% of the population should harbor an intracranial aneurysm. The frequency of intracranial aneurysms in adult autopsy studies ranges from 1% to 6%.[25] According to angiographic series, the incidence of intracranial aneurysms varies from 0.65% to 7%.[9] Berry aneurysms are multiple in about 20% to 30% of cases. Intracranial aneurysms are also more prevalent in females,[2] and are lesions of adulthood with the peak prevalence in the fourth and sixth decades. Aneurysms in the pediatric population are rare, accounting for 2% to 4% of all aneurysms; they are often are found in males, and tend to be larger and of the dissecting variety.[26–28]

Several medical conditions are associated with the development of intracranial aneurysms, including systemic lupus erythematosus, Takayasu disease, giant cell arteritis, autosomal polycystic kidney disease, type IV Ehlers-Danlos syndrome, Marfan syndrome, fibromuscular dysplasia, type 1 neurofibromatosis, pseudoxanthoma elasticum, hereditary hemorrhagic telangiectasia, coarctation of the aorta, and α1-antitrypsin.[29–37]

Genetics also plays a role in the formation of intracranial aneurysms. If 2 first-degree relatives in the same family have an intracranial aneurysm with no heritable connective tissue disorder, immediate family members have up to a 17% incidence of harboring an unruptured aneurysm.[38] Furthermore, first-degree and second-degree relatives of a patient with aneurysmal SAH are at 4.1- to 6.6-fold increased risk for aneurysmal SAH.[39,40] Therefore, screening is suggested in patients who have 2 or more family members with intracranial aneurysms.

Other risk factors for the development of an intracranial aneurysm formation include cigarette smoking, cocaine use, and heavy consumption of alcohol.[41–44] Infections from bacterial or fungal colonization of vessel walls, head trauma, and intracranial neoplasms or neoplastic emboli are rare causes of intracranial aneurysms.

The predominant location for saccular intracranial aneurysms is the anterior circulation (90%), with most arising from the circle of Willis.[45] The anterior communicating complex (30%–35%) is the most common location, followed by the internal carotid artery (30%), including the carotid bifurcation, posterior communicating artery, and ophthalmic artery. The next most common location is the middle cerebral artery bifurcation (20%), followed by the basilar apex (5%), superior cerebellar artery (3%), inferior cerebellar artery (3%), and the vertebrobasilar junction (2%).[45]

The natural history of unruptured intracranial aneurysm is uncertain and is surrounded by controversy. The most known studies on the subject include a comprehensive cohort study (2000) with a patient follow-up of 18 years,[46] a large meta-analysis (1998) that included studies from 1955 to 1966,[47] a systematic review of literature from Japan (2005),[48] and the International Study of Unruptured Intracranial Aneurysms (ISUIA) (part 1, 1998 and part 2, 2003),[49,50] which compromise the majority of this discussion. Prior studies have extrapolated results from patients with small unruptured intracranial aneurysms (UIAs) diagnosed after SAH to infer that these aneurysms are at a considerable increased risk of rupture.[51] Other studies have used SAH incidence rates to infer prevalence of UIAs in the general population.[9] However, it is important to distinguish UIAs from ruptured intracranial aneurysms, as these separate entities are managed differently. Therefore, the goal in management of UIAs is to identify which

UIAs have the greatest risk of rupture and rerupture after treatment.

Results from the 1998 meta-analysis demonstrated an overall 2% prevalence of UIA in the population, with the vast majority of aneurysms being small (10 mm), having an estimated annual risk of rupture of approximately 0.7%. The male/female ratio was approximately 1:1.3 and incidence of an aneurysm increased with age, peaking in the 60- to 79-year-old age group. The main limitation of the study was that the meta-analysis included retrospective studies and was performed before the CT era.[47]

The cohort study published in 2000,[52] performed in Finland from 1956 to 1978, consisted of 142 patients with a mean follow-up of 18 years. Results from the study included an overall frequency of 1.0% UIA with no history of SAH and 1.3% UIA with history of SAH, 2.6% of aneurysms being symptomatic. Frequency of aneurysm by size was 1.1% (2–6 mm), 2.3% (7–9 mm), and 2.8% (10–26 mm). The mortality rate with rupture was 52%. Limitations of the study included lack of power of the test (N = 142), a homogeneous population, and 92% of the patients having a history of SAH.[52]

The 2005 meta-analysis of 13 Japanese studies (3801 patient-years) demonstrated rupture in 104 patients with the annual rupture rate of 2.7% (95% confidence interval [CI] 2.2%–3.3%). Large, posterior circulation, and symptomatic aneurysms were associated with significantly higher rates of rupture (relative risk 6.4, 2.3, and 2.1, respectively). The risk of rupture was significantly higher for the Japanese population when compared with results reported by investigators from international cohort studies. Limitations of the study included retrospective studies and a homogeneous population (single ethnic group).[48,53]

The ISUIA is the largest study evaluating the history of UIAs (N = 4060) at 53 international centers including Canada, Europe, and the United States. Data acquired from the ISUIA, a large, comprehensive multicenter study with retrospective and prospective cohorts, analyzed the natural history of UIA as well as the morbidity and mortality associated with rupture. In addition, subgroup analysis was performed according to aneurysmal size, aneurysmal location, and history of SAH from a separate aneurysm. The patients were divided into 2 groups. Group 1 included patients with unruptured intracranial aneurysm and no prior SAH, and group 2 consisted of patients with UIA and prior SAH. Overall, rupture rates with UIA smaller than 7 mm were statistically significantly higher (P<.01) in group 2 when compared with group 1. The site distribution of UIA in patients with no prior history of SAH was 16.9% for cavernous carotid artery, 24.8% for internal carotid artery, 10.0% for anterior cerebral artery and anterior communicating artery, 22.7% for middle cerebral artery, 13.9% for posterior communicating artery, 6.6% for vertebrobasilar or posterior cerebral artery, and 5.1% for basilar artery apex.

In the retrospective cohort, rupture rate was 0.1% per year for patients in group 1 who had UIAs smaller than 10 mm. The rupture rate for aneurysms larger than 10 mm was 1%, and 6% for aneurysms larger than 25 mm. Although aneurysm size was the best predictor, aneurysm location also predicted risk of rupture, with the posterior communicating artery and vertebrobasilar circulation aneurysms more likely to rupture. The rupture rates for the prospective cohorts were higher for aneurysms larger than 7 mm. Averages calculated for predetermined 3-mm successive size categories used in the retrospective cohort allowed the establishment of well-defined cutoff points to less than 7 mm, 7 to 12 mm, 13 to 24 mm, and greater than 25 mm, with each category having statistically significant rates of rupture that allowed for the establishment of prediction models. The 5-year cumulative rate for rupture in group 1 patients with aneurysms in the anterior circulation, excluding cavernous and posterior communicating arteries, was 0 for aneurysms smaller than 7 mm, 2.6 for aneurysms 7 to 12 mm, and 14.5 for aneurysms 13 to 24 mm in size, compared with 2.5, 14.5, and 18.4, respectively for aneurysms in the posterior circulation.

In the retrospective cohort, group 2 rupture rates were 11 times higher than rupture rates in group 1 for UIAs smaller than 10 mm of the same size. Therefore, size alone was not a clear predictor of future risk of rupture.[49] The only clear predictor of the future risk of rupture was aneurysmal location. In the prospective cohort, UIA rupture rates were statistically higher in group 2 with aneurysms smaller than 7 mm, which is of high relevance because a considerable portion of group 2 patients had UIAs smaller than 7 mm. Otherwise, the pattern and rupture rates for UIAs in the group 2 retrospective and prospective cohorts were almost the same.[50]

There is some controversy regarding the ISUIA results because there is an apparent discrepancy between the low rupture rates in the study and the number of SAHs observed in clinical practice. Critics state that the study suffers from selection and intervention bias because most aneurysms observed in practice are 6 mm to 7 mm, which falls within the benign natural history of the study, and the annual prevalence of UIA (2%) does not match the average rupture rates (0.7%) found in the study.

The incidence of aneurysmal SAH is approximately 10 in 100,000[8,54,55] with 21,000 to 33,000 new cases occurring in the United States each year.[56] Women have an increased risk when compared with men and African Americans (1.6×), and Hispanics (1.3×) have greater risks in comparison with Caucasians.[55] The mean age of presentation is 55 years.[57] SAH accounts for 4.4% of stroke mortality and 27.3% of all stroke-related years of potential life lost before age 65.[58] The in-hospital mortality rate is 26.3%[59] and the 30-day case-fatality rate is 38%.[59,60] Prospective studies, which include deaths occurring before hospital admission, have shown consistently higher mortality rates, ranging from 56% to 86%,[2,61,62] with 61% of deaths occurring within 48 hours and most deaths within 2 weeks.[63] Patients with posterior circulation aneurysms are 3 times more likely to die before reaching the hospital or within 48 hours when compared with those with anterior circulation SAH,[40,64] and 10% to 20% of SAH survivors remain dependent.[65,66]

Associated Complications of Aneurysmal SAH

Associated complications of aneurysmal SAH include rehemorrhage, hydrocephalus, and seizures. The peak rate of rebleeding occurs within the first 24 hours and is as high as 19%, 20% in the first 2 weeks, and 40% at 1 month,[66–68] with a mortality rate of up to 74%.[46,69,70] Approximately 20% of patients experience ventricular enlargement after aneurysmal SAH. Risk factors for hydrocephalus include subarachnoid and intraventricular hemorrhage; older age of the patient, and posterior circulation aneurysm.[71] Studies have demonstrated that seizures can occur in approximately 8% of patients, with 90% occurring in the first 24 hours after aneurysmal SAH.[72–74] Multisystemic medical complications are associated with high morbidity and mortality. Approximately 40% of patients have a life-threatening medical complication, and 23% of deaths can be attributed to a medical complication.[75] Hyperglycemia occurs in 30% of patients and is an independent predictor of poor outcome.[76,77] Hyponatremia occurs in 30% to 43% of patients, and has a strong association with vasospasm.[78–80] Morinaga and colleagues[81] demonstrated that as much as 84% of patients with hyponatremia had symptomatic vasospasm. Cardiopulmonary complications can occur in patients with aneurysmal SAH and may be related to sympathetic system activation. Serious cardiac arrhythmias occur in 1% to 4% and malignant arrhythmias in up to 4%.[75,82] Reversible cardiomyopathy (stunned myocardium) and left ventricular dysfunction has been reported in about 10% of cases.[83,84] The incidence of neurogenic pulmonary edema has been reported at 20% to 27%.[75,85,86] Of all medical complications, the leading cause of mortality and morbidity is vasospasm in patients with aneurysmal SAH. Prior studies have demonstrated that varying degrees of vasospasm occur in 70% of patients[87,88] and is symptomatic (clinical vasospasm) in 20% to 25% of patients.[89,90] Risk factors for vasospasm include amount of intracranial hemorrhage, age (<50 years), hyperglycemia, hyponatremia, hypertension, aneurysm size, and cocaine use.[91] Therefore, optimal medical management is of paramount importance and, as a result, hyperdynamic therapy (triple-H [permissive hypertension, hypervolemia, and hemodilution]) has become the first-line therapy for patients who have undergone treatment of ruptured aneurysmal SAH.

DIAGNOSTIC IMAGING

Current neuroimaging techniques for intracranial aneurysms include intra-arterial 3-dimensional (3D) digital subtraction angiography (DSA), intra-arterial DSA, multislice computed tomographic (MSCT) angiography, CT angiography with a dual-source CT scanner, MR angiography, and transcranial Doppler ultrasonography. Intra-arterial DSA is still the gold standard for evaluation of a patient with a suspected aneurysm, given its high spatial resolution; however, currently MSCTA has a similar specificity and sensitivity for detecting an intracranial aneurysm, except for aneurysm smaller than 3 mm. The spatial resolution for DSA is 0.2 mm, and about 0.15 mm for 3D-DSA.[92] Intra-arterial DSA is an invasive test with a 1% risk of transient neurologic complications and a 0.5% risk of permanent neurologic complications, whereas there is no risk of neurologic complications with MSCTA or MR angiography.[93,94]

To a large extent, sensitivity for detection of aneurysms depends on spatial resolution, which itself is dependent on the number of detector rows available on a helical CT scanner. The highest current spatial resolution of CT angiography is 0.4 to 0.7 mm on a 64-MSCT scanner.[92,95] When compared with DSA as the reference standard, CT angiography has an average reported specificity rate of 96% to 98% (90% to 94% for aneurysms smaller than 3 mm and up to 100% for aneurysms larger than 4 mm) and sensitivity rates of 96% to 98%.[96] With the advent of multidetector CT scanners with a very high number of detectors (eg, 256-slice and 320-detector row scanners), further improvements in spatial resolution and accuracy are expected.

The spatial resolution of MR angiography at 1.5 T is on the order of 1 mm.[97] With 3-T scanners, spatial resolution may reach 0.6 mm.[98–100] When compared with DSA, MR angiography reported specificity rates for detection of intracranial aneurysms ranging from 69% to 100%, with a sensitivity rate of 75% to 100%.[101–104]

TREATMENT
Conventional Coiling of a Simple Saccular Aneurysm

Technique
At the authors' institution, all intracranial aneurysm coiling procedures are performed under general anesthesia with neurologic monitoring. An arterial line is placed in the radial artery to closely monitor the patient's blood pressure. The anesthesiologist is aware of the need to avoid transient blood pressure spikes, especially when intubating or extubating the patient; this is particularly important in a patient who has a ruptured aneurysm. The procedure can sometimes take a few hours, therefore anesthesia is necessary to maintain immobility because 3D imaging and a fluoroscopic roadmap is very motion sensitive. A 6F sheath is inserted into the right common femoral artery. If balloon remodeling or additional microcatheters are needed, puncture of the left common femoral artery may be necessary. Just after the sheath is inserted in the groin, a baseline activated clotting time (ACT) is drawn. Sixty to 100 international units (IU) of heparin per kilogram are then given intravenously as a bolus. For patients with unruptured aneurysms the ACT is checked every 30 minutes throughout the procedure, and heparin is given intermittently to keep the ACT between 250 and 300 seconds.[105] For patients with a ruptured aneurysm, 3000 IU of heparin is given initially, and after placement of framing coils the patient is then given additional heparin to maintain an ACT range of 250 to 300. A syringe of protamine is prepared in advance and is readily available to be injected in case of aneurysm rupture. The usual dose is 10 mg of protamine per 1000 IU of heparin. After the procedure, the heparin is reversed, and hemostasis can be obtained with manual compression if the ACT is less than 200 seconds. Likewise, for patients with unruptured aneurysms who have been treated preoperatively with dual antiplatelet therapy, a 5-pack of unpooled platelets is kept in preparation in case of rupture.

Patients who have not suffered a recent SAH are preoperatively given 75 mg clopidogrel and 81 mg aspirin orally, starting 7 days before the procedure, to prevent thromboembolic complications. If emergent platelet inhibition is needed, the patient is loaded with 600 mg clopidogrel and 325 mg aspirin. Full platelet inhibition occurs 2 hours afterward. If the procedure needs to be performed urgently, the patient may be given a glycoprotein IIa/IIIb inhibitor. A platelet inhibition assay is drawn for clopidogrel and aspirin before treatment, because approximately 25% of patients will have clopidogrel or aspirin resistance.[106,107]

A complete cerebral angiogram is performed before treatment with a 4F or 5F catheter, including injections of the bilateral common carotid, internal carotid, and vertebral arteries. Additional 3D rotational images are obtained to more accurately define the neck, dome, and size of the aneurysm. Once the diagnostic portion of the procedure is performed the catheter is exchanged for a 6F guide catheter, which is positioned as close as possible to the aneurysm. It is necessary for the guide catheter to have a stable position so as to be able to introduce a microcatheter safely into the aneurysm. For this reason, the guide catheter should be positioned as close to the aneurysm as possible. This positioning gives optimal stability of the guide catheter and allows the operator to monitor the guide position on the same roadmap as the microcatheter during advancement of the coil into the aneurysm. New guide catheters that are more flexible, such as the Neuron (Penumbra, Alameda, CA), Navien (eV3, Irvine, CA), or distal accesses catheters (DAC) (Stryker, Fremont, CA) can be introduced further into the intracranial circulation, and can be routinely placed in the cavernous internal carotid artery or the distal vertebral artery.[108–111] This placement allows more stability in advancing devices into the intracranial circulation. This increased stability has been a major innovation in the endovascular treatment of aneurysms over the last 3 years. If additional stability is needed to treat an aneurysm, a triple coaxial system consisting of a long sheath introduced into the origin of the great vessel followed by a guide catheter through this may offer enhanced stability in advancing devices through tortuous anatomy for the treatment of intracranial aneurysms. If an aneurysm cannot be treated from a femoral artery approach, a brachial, radial, direct carotid or vertebral artery puncture is another option.[112–114]

Microcatheter placement into the aneurysm All microcatheters have an outer hydrophilic coating; this reduces the friction between the catheter and inner wall of the blood vessel, thus facilitating distal catheterization of the intracranial circulation. The microcatheter is advanced over a microwire into the aneurysm under roadmap. The microcatheter is never advanced into the aneurysm without using a wire, because this may perforate the aneurysm. Once the microcatheter is positioned within the aneurysm, the slack within the system is carefully removed and the wire slowly withdrawn to prevent forward movement of the microcatheter tip. The best microcatheter position depends on the size and shape of the aneurysm; however, the best position is usually in the middle of the aneurysm or at the origin of the neck. This configuration usually allows the coil to form within the aneurysm with minimal resistance. Some operators in large aneurysms will wrap the microcatheter around the dome of the aneurysm and place the tip of the catheter at the neck. These surgeons claim that this allows for placement of more coil loops across the neck of the aneurysm, thus limiting the possibility of prolapse of additional coils into the parent vessel during filling of the aneurysm.

Coil selection The choice of the coil is based on the size and shape of the aneurysm as seen on the angiogram and 3D reconstruction. The purpose of the first coil (framing coil or complex shape coil) is to create a support basket for the subsequent introduction of additional coils, and to provide a bridge to prevent additional coils from migrating into the parent vessel. The first coil is sized to the largest dimension of the aneurysm sac. The first coil should be as large and long as possible to fully appose the aneurysm wall, and provide a sound basket and stability to prevent the coil from prolapsing into the parent vessel. This maneuver will also provide the maximum number of coil loops across the neck of the aneurysm, thus preventing herniation of additional coils placed into the aneurysm from compromising the parent vessel (**Fig. 1**).

If the aneurysm sac has a sausage-like appearance, the principle guiding the selection of the first coil is different. In such aneurysms, a helical coil is preferred to a complex-shaped coil, and the first coil is sized to the smallest sac diameter. The subsequent coils are similar in size and length, with the aneurysm coiled from the dome toward the neck.

Coil placement Through the microcatheter, the platinum portion of the coil is introduced into the aneurysm sac while still on the delivery wire. In the microcatheter, the coil assumes a straight configuration; however, as soon as the coil leaves the microcatheter it assumes the manufactured memory shape. The coil is radiopaque under fluoroscopy and is visualized under live roadmap as it is placed into the aneurysm sac with the neck in profile. There should be limited resistance when introducing the coil into the aneurysm sac. If there

is any resistance, the coil maybe oversized. It is important not to force the coil into the aneurysm sac, to prevent possible rupture. If the coil is correctly sized it will readily adapt to the shape of the aneurysm. If the coil is undersized, it will not be stable within the aneurysm sac and may herniate into the parent vessel. If the coil is oversized, it will not form with the aneurysm sac and will herniate into the parent vessel. Oversizing the coil may also cause excessive pressure on the wall of the aneurysm sac, possibly risking perforation.

Before detachment of the coil, an angiogram is performed to determine how the coil is confined within the aneurysm sac and to determine if there is compromise of the parent vessel. If there is movement of the coil during the angiogram, this may indicate that the coil is undersized and may migrate out of the aneurysm sac after detachment. If the coil appears properly sized and there is no compromise of the parent vessel, the coil is detached under fluoroscopy. The detachment wire is then slowly pulled back through the microcatheter to make sure the coil has detached from the wire and to ensure that the coil does not move.

Additional coils of various sizes and shapes are subsequently introduced into the aneurysm sac until the sac is densely packed and no longer filling with contrast or the microcatheter is pushed outside the sac. The first coils used for the treatment of intracranial aneurysms were made of platinum; however, there were aneurysm recurrences after treatment, so bioactive coils were introduced with the goal of inducing an exuberant healing response and improved filling volume of the coiled aneurysm. The first bioactive coil was the Matrix (Stryker, Fremont, CA), introduced in 2002. The FDA approved the Matrix coil based on equivalency with the conventional GDC coil. Four bioactive coils are now available for clinical use: Matrix, Hydrocoil (Microvention, Tustin, CA), Cerecyte (Codman Neurovascular, Raynham, MA), and Axium (Ev3, Irvine, CA). The newer coils are manufactured so that the aneurysm sac is filled in a Russian nesting doll manner from the periphery toward the center.[115] Filling coils are placed into the aneurysm sac after the placement of framing coils; once the aneurysm is nearly densely packed, the final coils usually placed into the aneurysm sac are finishing coils.[116] These coils are very short and soft. Once the aneurysm is densely packed the microcatheter is removed slowly from the aneurysm, and a posttreatment angiogram is performed to assess the degree of aneurysm occlusion, the parent vessel, and the patency of the distal vasculature.

The heparin is reversed after the procedure with protamine, and manual pressure or a closure

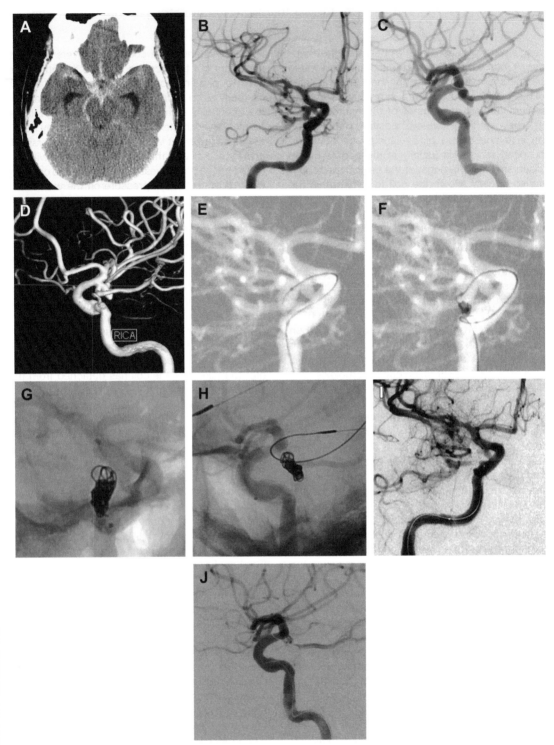

Fig. 1. A 73-year-old woman who presented with a Hunt and Hess grade 3 subarachnoid hemorrhage (SAH). (*A*) Axial computed tomography (CT) of the brain shows diffuse SAH, asymmetric in the region of the right posterior communicating artery. (*B, C*) Frontal oblique (*B*) and lateral (*C*) projections of a right internal carotid angiogram show a multilobulated aneurysm arising off the proximal right posterior communicating artery. (*D*) Three-dimensional (3D) right internal carotid angiogram shows the right posterior communicating artery aneurysm. (*E*) Saved roadmap; frontal oblique projection of a right internal carotid angiogram shows microcatheter within the aneurysm. (*F*) Saved roadmap shows placement of first coil within the aneurysm. (*G, H*) Unsubtracted frontal oblique projection and lateral (*H*) of a right internal carotid angiogram shows final coil mass within the aneurysm, with a patent right internal carotid artery and posterior communicating artery. (*I, J*) Final subtracted frontal oblique (*I*) and lateral (*J*) projections of a right internal carotid angiogram show no filling of the aneurysm.

device is used to obtain hemostasis at the femoral puncture site.[117] Pressure is usually held on the puncture site for 20 to 30 minutes after removal of the sheath if manual compression is used, and the leg immobilized for 6 hours to prevent groin complications. If a closure device is used, ambulation can occur as early as 2 hours after placement.[118,119] If there is compromise of the parent vessel, protrusion of coils, or thrombus formation during the coiling procedure, the heparin may be continued overnight with the sheath left in place. Antiplatelet therapy may also be given.

After endovascular treatment of nonruptured intracranial aneurysms, the patient is kept in the neurointensive care unit (NICU) for at least 24 hours for close monitoring of blood pressure, neurologic status, and puncture site. SAH patients are kept in the NICU for at least 14 days under close neuromonitoring and are prophylactically treated for vasospasm.

Results of endovascular treatment of ruptured aneurysms

Three prospective randomized trials have compared outcomes of endovascular coiling versus surgical clipping.

The first study was performed in Finland,[120] and randomized 109 patients with SAH who were suitable for either surgery or endovascular coiling. Angiographic outcome in the posterior circulation was significantly better for endovascular coiling, whereas angiographic outcome in the anterior circulation was significantly better for surgery. Angiographic outcomes in the internal carotid artery and middle cerebral artery were similar in both groups. Glasgow Outcome Scale scores were equivalent in both groups at 3 months. Mortality for technical reasons during surgery was twice that of the endovascular group (4% vs 2%). One patient in the endovascular group suffered rebleeding following incomplete coiling of the aneurysm.

The second study was the ISAT,[3,121,122] in which nearly 2000 patients with SAH from predominantly Europe were randomized to surgery or endovascular coiling based on judgment of the treating team. Outcomes analysis on the basis of death or dependence at 2 months and 1 year based on the Modified Rankin score (mRS) was the primary parameter of interest in the first 2002 publication. At 1 year postprocedure, 250 of 1063 (23.5%) of the endovascular patients were dead or dependent while 326 of 1055 (30.9%) of the surgical patients had died. This figure represents an absolute risk reduction of 7.4% for those patients' treated from an endovascular approach. Delayed rebleeding was more common in the endovascular group; however, several of the cases were due to incomplete treatments. Seizures were also less common in the endovascular group. In the most recent follow-up report there was an increased risk of recurrent bleeding from a coiled aneurysm in comparison with a clipped aneurysm, but the risk was small. The risk of death at 5 years was significantly lower in the coiled group than in the clipped group.[123] Scott and colleagues[124] showed improved cognitive outcomes with endovascular coiling of ruptured intracranial aneurysms from the ISAT trial.

A third study performed at the Barrow Institute examined the null hypothesis that no difference exists between microsurgical clipping and endovascular coil embolization for acutely ruptured cerebral aneurysms.[125] The investigators screened 725 patients with SAH, resulting in 500 eligible patients who were enrolled prospectively in the study. Patients were assigned in an alternating fashion to surgical aneurysm clipping or endovascular coil embolization. Two hundred thirty-eight patients were assigned to aneurysm clipping and 233 to coil embolization. The 2 groups were well matched. One year after treatment, 403 patients were available for evaluation and of these, 358 patients had actually undergone treatment. The remainder either died before treatment or had no identifiable source of SAH. A poor outcome (mRS >2) was observed in 33.7% of the patients assigned to aneurysm clipping and in 23.2% of the patients assigned to coil embolization (odds ratio 1.68, 95% CI 1.08–2.61; P = .02). No patient treated by coil embolization suffered a recurrent hemorrhage. The conclusion of the study 1 year after treatment favored coil embolization.

The CLARITY trial was a prospective, multicenter, consecutive series that compared patients treated with GDC or Matrix coils for ruptured aneurysms.[126,127] Five hundred seventeen patients harboring aneurysms were treated with GDC (276 patients) or Matrix coils (241 patients). Postoperative and midterm anatomic results were evaluated blindly using the Modified Montreal Scale (complete occlusion, neck remnant, and aneurysm remnant). At the midterm follow-up (mean 16.7 months in the GDC group and 15.4 months in the Matrix group), complete occlusion was reported in 95 of 276 aneurysms (34.4%) in the GDC group and 80 of 241 (33.2%) in the Matrix group; neck remnant in 127 of 276 (46.0%) in the GDC group and 118 of 241 (49.0%) in the Matrix group; and aneurysm remnant in 54 of 276 (19.6%) in the GDC group and 43 of 241 (17.8%) in the Matrix group. Aneurysm occlusion was improvement in 35 of 272 aneurysms (12.9%) in the GDC group and 27 of 239 (11.3%) in the Matrix group; stable situation in 98 of 272 (36.0%) in the GDC group and 97 of 239 (40.6%) in the Matrix group; and worsening in 139 of 272 (51.1%) in the GDC group and 115 of 239 (48.1%) in the Matrix group. A total of 32 out of 517 patients were retreated during the follow-up period: 9 of 276 (3.3%) in the GDC group and 23 of 241 (9.5%) in the Matrix group (P = .003). The study concluded that the midterm anatomic results and evolution of aneurysm occlusion were not different in patients with ruptured aneurysms treated with GDC or Matrix coils.

The CONSCIOUS-1 trial showed that aneurysm coiling was associated with less angiographic vasospasm and delayed ischemic neurologic deficit than was surgical clipping, whereas no effect on cerebral infarction or clinical outcome was observed in patients presenting with SAH.[128]

Results of endovascular treatment of unruptured aneurysms

The data from endovascular treatment versus surgical clipping for unruptured aneurysms does not show a clear benefit for one form of treatment over the other. A review of modern large clipping and coiling trials for unruptured aneurysms was published in 2005.[129] A majority of these trials were nonrandomized and retrospective. Adverse outcomes were estimated at 8.8% for endovascular coiling and 17.8% for clipping. In the International Study of Unruptured Intracranial Aneurysm (USUIA),[50] adverse outcomes were less common with endovascular treatment (9.3%) than with surgery (13.7%). However, the study was nonrandomized, and the endovascular treatment group included a higher number of elderly patients, larger aneurysms, and aneurysms within the posterior circulation. Surgical adverse outcomes in the USUIA study correlated with patient age greater than 50 years, aneurysm size greater than 12 mm, location in the posterior circulation, previous ischemic cerebrovascular disease, and symptoms of mass effect from the aneurysm. Endovascular outcomes were less influenced by these factors.

The Analysis of Treatment by Endovascular approach of Nonruptured Aneurysms (ATENA), published by Pierot and colleagues,[130] has been one of the most comprehensive studies on the treatment of unruptured aneurysms. The study included 649 patients harboring 739 aneurysms. Seven hundred twenty-seven aneurysms were treated using coils (98.4%). Coils alone were used in 396 aneurysms (54.4%), with balloon remodeling in 271 cases (37.3%), intracranial stents in 57 cases (7.8%), and the Trispan neck bridge in 3 cases (0.4%). Initial results indicated that postoperative occlusion was complete in 436 aneurysms (59.0%), with neck remnant in 160 aneurysms (21.7%) and aneurysm remnant in 143 aneurysms (19.3%). Additional trials on unruptured aneurysms are needed.

Results of endovascular treatment of ruptured and unruptured aneurysms

The Hydrocoil Endovascular Aneurysm Occlusion and Packing Study (HELPS) trial compared hydrogel-coated coils with bare platinum coils for the endovascular treatment of intracranial aneurysms.[131] This randomized controlled trial was performed in 24 centers in 7 countries. Patients with a previously untreated ruptured or unruptured cerebral aneurysm of 2 to 25 mm in maximum diameter were randomly allocated (1:1) to aneurysm coiling with either hydrogel-coated coils or standard bare platinum coils. Primary outcome was a composite of angiographic and clinical outcome at 18-month follow-up. Two hundred forty-nine patients were allocated to the hydrogel coil group and 250 to the control group. Seventy (28%) patients in the hydrogel group and 90 (36%) control patients had an adverse composite primary outcome, giving an absolute reduction in the proportion of adverse composite primary outcomes with hydrogel of 7.0% (95% CI 1.6–15.5) and odds ratio (OR) of 0.73 (95% CI 0.49–1.1, P = .13). In subgroup analysis of recently ruptured aneurysms, there were more adverse composite primary outcomes in the control group than in the hydrogel group (OR 2.08, 95% CI 1.24–3.46; P = .014). There were 8.6% fewer major angiographic recurrences in patients allocated to hydrogel coils (OR 0.7, 95% CI 0.4–1.0; P = .049). The study was inconclusive as to whether hydrogel coils reduce late aneurysm rupture or improve long-term clinical outcome, but their use does lower major recurrence.

The Cerecyte coil trial evaluated the procedural safety and clinical outcomes in patients with ruptured and UIA.[132] Five hundred patients with a ruptured or unruptured aneurysm were randomized to receive Cerecyte or bare platinum coils. Two hundred forty-nine patients were allocated to Cerecyte coils and 251 to bare platinum coils. There was a statistical excess of poor outcomes in the Cerecyte arm at discharge in the ruptured aneurysm groups and at 6-month follow-up in the unruptured group.

The Matrix and Platinum Science (MAPS) trial was recently presented in abstract form at several national meetings. Trial results demonstrated that overall, Matrix^2 detachable coils are as effective as GDC detachable coils with target aneurysm recurrence (TAR) rates of 13.3% versus 14.6%, respectively. In aneurysms with good occlusion immediately postprocedure, Matrix^2 detachable coils demonstrated a statistically significant, superior long-term TAR rate of 2.7% compared with the GDC detachable coils' rate of 9.6%.[133]

Coiling of Wide-Necked Aneurysms

Balloon remodeling technique

Side-wall wide-necked aneurysm The main feature that limits the endovascular treatment of aneurysms is the width of the neck. Other features that may limit treatment include the shape of the aneurysm. In 1992, Moret and colleagues[134,135] introduced the balloon remodeling technique for the treatment of wide-necked intracranial aneurysms. The technique involves placing a nondetachable balloon across the neck of the aneurysm during each coil placement. The coils remain molded around the balloon after deflation of the balloon, essentially "remodeling the arterial wall." The technique has been improved over the last 17 years with better coils and balloons. It is routinely used today to treat wide-necked aneurysms particularly in patients with SAH, thus eliminating stent placement and the use of antiplatelet agents. Most interventionists consider an aneurysm neck to be wide when the ratio between the maximum diameter of the aneurysm sac and the size of the neck is 1 or less.

To treat wide-necked side-wall aneurysms not at an arterial bifurcation, the authors routinely use the over-the-wire compliant HyperGlide balloon (Ev3, Irvine, CA). If distal catheterization of the neck of the aneurysm is difficult they have used the less compliant gateway balloon (Stryker, Fremont, CA) over a more torquable Synchro 14 wire (Boston Stryker, Fremont, CA) to perform balloon remodeling.

The authors prefer to perform the procedure using a 6F shuttle sheath (Cook, Bloomington, IN) or a 0.073 Navien guide catheter (eV3, Irvine, CA) with a dual Y-adapter, so that the microcatheter and balloon can be introduced separately. However, they have also performed the procedure by puncturing both groins and introducing 2 separate guide catheters. With this technique a 5F and 6F guide catheter are usually introduced into the target vessel.

Under roadmap, the balloon first is advanced across the neck of the aneurysm. The microcatheter is then advanced into the aneurysm. The balloon is inflated across the neck of the aneurysm, causing temporary occlusion of the neck and parent vessel. The first coil is positioned within the aneurysm sac. The balloon is deflated to test the stability of the coil within the aneurysm sac. If no movement of the coil is observed, the balloon is reinflated and the coil detached. The coil is not detached if coil movement (meaning that the coil is not well anchored in the sac) is detected after balloon deflation. An angiogram is then performed. This procedure is repeated multiple times until the aneurysm no longer fills with contrast or has a dense coil mass within the confines of its lumen (Fig. 2).

The balloon acts as a temporary wall across the neck of the aneurysm, allowing coils to be deflected off the balloon back into the aneurysm sac during placement. The choice of the first coil is the most crucial decision in being able to treat a wide-necked aneurysm. The coil diameter should be large enough to fully oppose the aneurysm wall and cross the neck well, thus providing friction between the coil and wall and limiting migration of the coil outside of the aneurysm. The coil diameter should be the largest that will form within the aneurysm sac. The coil length should also be the longest that will fit within the aneurysm sac. The large basket thus provided allows the coils to be strongly anchored within the aneurysm sac, and will also form a bridge across the neck to help prevent additional coils from migrating into the parent vessel. The balloon occlusion should not last more than 5 minutes. The size of the balloon depends on the volume of contrast and saline mixture introduced into the balloon; therefore, the balloon should only be inflated with the cadence syringe provided by the manufacture. Overinflation of the balloon may cause rupture of the parent vessel or aneurysm. The authors believe the balloon is best inflated with a 60:40 contrast/saline mixture, which provides good visibility of the balloon under roadmap and still leads to relative rapid deflation of the balloon. The balloon is tested on the table before introducing it into the patient. The balloon is also inflated in the lower cervical carotid or vertebral artery before introducing into the intracranial circulation, to determine if the balloon is working properly and to see if it can easily be seen under fluoroscopy. If the balloon will not deflate, the manufacturer recommends pulling negative pressure on the syringe connected to the Y-adapter. If all else fails, removing the wire from the balloon catheter will usually deflate the balloon; however, the entire system then has to be removed and prepped again before introducing it back into the body, because thrombus formation can occur within the balloon catheter, possibly making the balloon malfunction. Two other recently approved balloons that can be used for remodeling are the Ascent (Codman Neurovascular, Raynham, MA) and Scepter C Occlusion Balloon (Microvention-Terumo, Inc, Tustin, CA). The benefit of these two balloons is that they have a dual coaxial lumen, allowing for balloon inflation and coiling of the aneurysm with a single catheter. These balloons can

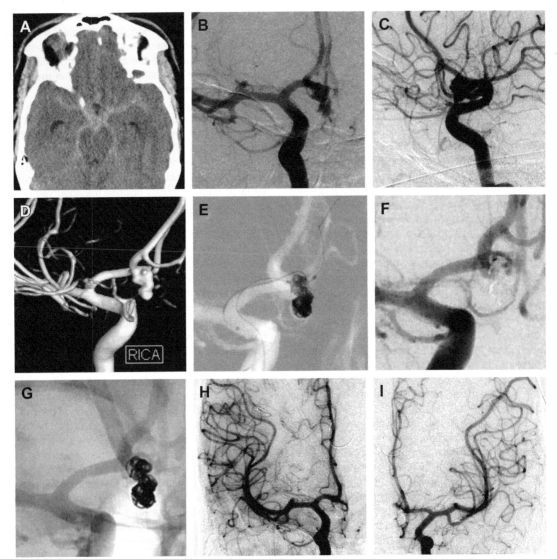

Fig. 2. A 54-year-old man who presented with a Hunt and Hess grade 4 SAH. (A) Axial CT of the brain shows diffuse SAH. (B, C) Anterior-posterior (AP) (B) and lateral (C) projections of a right internal carotid angiogram show an anterior communicating artery aneurysm pointing inferiorly. (D) 3D right internal carotid angiogram shows a multilobulated anterior communicating artery aneurysm with a wide neck. (E) Saved roadmap shows a balloon across the neck of the aneurysm with a microcatheter and coils within the anterior communicating artery aneurysm. (F, G) Oblique AP right internal carotid angiogram, subtracted (F) and unsubtracted (G), shows no filling of the aneurysm with the final coil mass within the aneurysm. (H) Final AP right internal carotid angiogram shows thrombosis of the aneurysm with a patent right anterior cerebral artery and anterior communicating artery. (I) Final AP left internal carotid angiogram shows no filling of the aneurysm with a patent left anterior cerebral artery and anterior communicating artery.

also be advanced over a torquable .014 inch microwire.

Bifurcation wide-necked aneurysm To treat a bifurcation aneurysm, the authors use a HyperForm balloon (Ev3), a very compliant low-pressure over-the-wire balloon that can conform to the vasculature being treated. Most interventionists believe this to be the balloon best suited for treating aneurysms located at arterial bifurcations or within small arteries. When the balloon is inflated, it may partially herniate into the aneurysm neck or the origin of the arterial branches emerging from the neck of the aneurysm. This configuration allows the parent vessel and arterial branches emerging from the neck of the aneurysm to remain patent with no compromise from the coils placed within the aneurysm sac.

Double-remodeling technique

Certain bifurcation aneurysms may not be able to be treated by a single-balloon remodeling technique. In these situations, another approach is to place two balloon catheters in a Y-configuration, one beside the other, both beginning proximally in the parent artery and ending distally within each of the branch vessels. The aneurysm is then coiled in a manner similar to that for the single-balloon remodeling technique. This technique allows the operator to treat certain aneurysms that would otherwise not be treatable by coil embolization.

A variation of the balloon remodeling technique is the conglomerate mass technique whereby multiple coils are placed into the aneurysm while the balloon is being inflated across the neck of the aneurysm for 5 to 10 minutes.[136] Another variant is the balloon-in-stent technique for constructive endovascular treatment of ultra–wide-necked circumferential aneurysms, as reported by Fiorella and colleagues.[137]

Results

In 2012, Pierot and colleagues[138] published a review and concluded that the remodeling technique provides equivalent safety and better anatomic results in comparison with standard coiling, and can be widely used in the management of both ruptured and unruptured aneurysms. Spiotta and colleagues[139] found no significant relationship between balloon inflation practices and ischemic events in a group of 147 patients undergoing balloon remodeling. Diabetic and older patients were more likely to have ischemic events develop. In 2008, Shapiro and colleagues[140] published a literature review with a meta-analysis of the safety and efficacy of adjunctive balloon remodeling during endovascular treatment of intracranial aneurysms. These investigators concluded that there was no higher incidence of thromboembolic events or iatrogenic rupture with the use of adjunctive balloon remodeling in comparison with unassisted coiling, and also commented that balloon remodeling appears to result in higher initial and follow-up aneurysm occlusion rates. Forty wide-necked aneurysms were successfully treated with the HyperForm balloon remodeling technique by Mu and colleagues[141] in 2008, with only 2 failed cases. Final results consisted of total occlusion in 34 cases (80.9%), subtotal occlusion in 4 (9.5%), and incomplete occlusion in 2 (4.8%). Of 22 patients treated in 2001 by Nelson and Levy,[142] aneurysm occlusion was found in 17 of 20 patients on follow-up angiography at a mean of 19 months, the other 2 patients having died before follow-up. Layton and colleagues[143] treated 73 of 221 aneurysms with balloon-assisted coiling over a 3-year period, and found no increased risk in thromboembolic complications in comparison with simple coiling techniques. In conclusion, there appears to be no increased risk of complications with the balloon remodeling technique. Aneurysm occlusion rates may be higher than with standard endovascular techniques, although there are few studies reporting the results of this form of treatment.

Stent-Assisted Coiling

Stent characteristics

Certain wide-necked and dysplastic aneurysms may not be treated with simple coiling or balloon remodeling; however, with the current availability of stents made to navigate the intracranial circulation, treatment from an endovascular approach is now possible. The disadvantages are that a permanent implant is placed into the artery, there is a lack of data on long-term patency, and the patient is subjected to the risk associated with the long-term use of antiplatelet medication. The stent acts as a scaffold that prevents the coils placed into the aneurysm sac from herniation into the parent vessel. The stent may also reduce the inflow into the aneurysm, promoting stasis and thrombosis of the aneurysm. In addition, the struts of the stent may provide a matrix for the growth of endothelial cells across the neck of the aneurysm.

A standard cerebral angiogram is obtained along with a 3D angiogram of the vessel in question. The dimension of the artery above and below the aneurysm is measured along with the size of the aneurysm and length of the neck. The targeted landing zone of the stent is determined. The self-expandable stent is sized to a nominal diameter 0.5 to 1.0 mm greater than the parent vessel at the targeted landing zone. The stent length should be centered on the aneurysm neck. The stent length is chosen to provide at least 5 mm of coverage proximal and distal to the aneurysm neck. If the parent vessel is tortuous, an attempt is made to place the distal and proximal aspect of the stent within a straight segment of the parent vessel.

Initially, balloon-expandable coronary stents were used; however, these were difficult to navigate into the intracranial circulation. Inflating the balloon also subjected the patient to possible rupture of the parent vessel, which is not possible with a self-expanding stent. Three self-expandable intracranial stents are currently available on the market: Neuroform (Stryker), Leo (Balt Extrusion, Montmorency, France), and Enterprise (Codman Neurovascular, Raynham, MA). The Neuroform and Enterprise are only available in the United States. The major differences between these stents are the delivery system and whether they are closed-cell or open-cell. The Neuroform is an open-cell stent, whereas the Enterprise and Leo are closed-cell stents.

The self-expandable stent that comes preloaded into the delivery microcatheter is the Neuroform. The advantage is that the microwire remains within the lumen of the stent after its deployment, which may allow easier delivery of overlapping stents and catheterization of the aneurysm. The disadvantage is that navigating this system through the intracranial circulation can be difficult, owing to the poor torquability of the microwire because it is in contact with the stent. The system is also less flexible because the stent is loaded into the microcatheter during navigation. To overcome these problems, many operators will navigate a standard microcatheter and microwire into the distal intracranial circulation past the neck of the aneurysm. The wire is then exchanged for a 300-cm exchange-length microwire. This step is crucial, as during the exchange the distal tip of the microwire may produce a perforation of the distal vessel. The delivery microcatheter carrying the stent is then brought up over the exchange-length microwire, and the stent deployed. This step in the procedure is also crucial in that the distal tip of the microwire should also be observed to prevent perforation. Because of these difficulties the manufacturer has changed the platform for the delivery method so that it is similar to the methods of deployment of the Leo and Enterprise stent **Fig. 3**.

The self-expandable stents that are loaded into the delivery catheter only when it has reached its proper position are the Leo and Enterprise stent. The advantage of this system is that the delivery microcatheter is placed past the aneurysm without the necessity for an exchange wire, and without the stent in place in the microcatheter. Theoretically this allows easier navigation through the vasculature because the operator can use the microwire of choice; moreover, the system is not rigid because the stent is absent from the microcatheter, and there is also no friction on the wire from it contacting the stent, thus make it more readily torquable. Because there is no need for an exchange-length wire, the risk of distal perforation is greatly reduced. The disadvantage of this system is that the microwire must be removed before stent deployment, thus possibly making placement of overlapping stents or catheterization of the aneurysm more difficult.

Technique of coiling with stent assistance

The aneurysm may be coiled by 3 different techniques using a stent assistant. With the first technique the microcatheter is placed into the aneurysm sac, then the stent is placed across the aneurysm neck; this is called the jailed microcatheter technique. The second technique consists of placing the stent across the neck of the aneurysm, then navigating a microcatheter through the struts of the stent into the aneurysm sac. In the final technique, the aneurysm is first coiled using the balloon remodeling technique, then the stent is placed across the neck of the aneurysm at the end of the procedure, with the idea that the stent struts will serve as a surface for endothelial cell growth across the neck of the aneurysm, thus preventing recanalization of the aneurysm. In a broad-necked dysplastic aneurysm or when the neck is not definable, the balloon may be inflated through the stent to define the parent vessel and prevent herniation of coils into the parent vessel.[137]

Antiplatelet treatment regimen for intracranial stenting

A stent is a metallic foreign body, thus introducing it into the cerebral vasculature will cause thrombus formation and platelet aggregation. To prevent this from occurring, it is important to administer antiplatelet agents before placement of an intracranial stent. This point has been eloquently elaborated in the coronary literature where a combination of aspirin and clopidogrel has been shown to prevent stent thrombosis and occlusion.[144] The optimal dose and treatment regimen, however, has not been determined. Given that the average life span of a platelet is 7 days, the authors administer aspirin (81 mg/d orally) and clopidogrel (75 mg/d orally) for 7 days before the procedure. If a stent needs to be placed on an emergent basis the authors will load the patient with clopidogrel (600 mg orally) and aspirin (325 mg orally), wait 2 hours, and then perform the procedure. If a stent needs to be placed during the course of an endovascular procedure and the patient has not been treated preoperatively with antiplatelet medications, the patient is loaded with the glycoprotein IIa/IIIb inhibitor abciximab at the cardiac dose of 0.25 mg/kg, then started on a 12-hour intravenous infusion at 0.125 µg/kg/min. The patient is also started on aspirin and clopidogrel. Most endovascular specialists avoid placement of a stent in patients with an acutely ruptured broad-necked aneurysm, because the patient will need to be placed on antiplatelet medications and will most likely need a ventriculostomy given the SAH. Also, if the patient develops vasospasm in the subacute period, intracranial balloon angioplasty can be more difficult with a stent placed in the intracranial circulation.

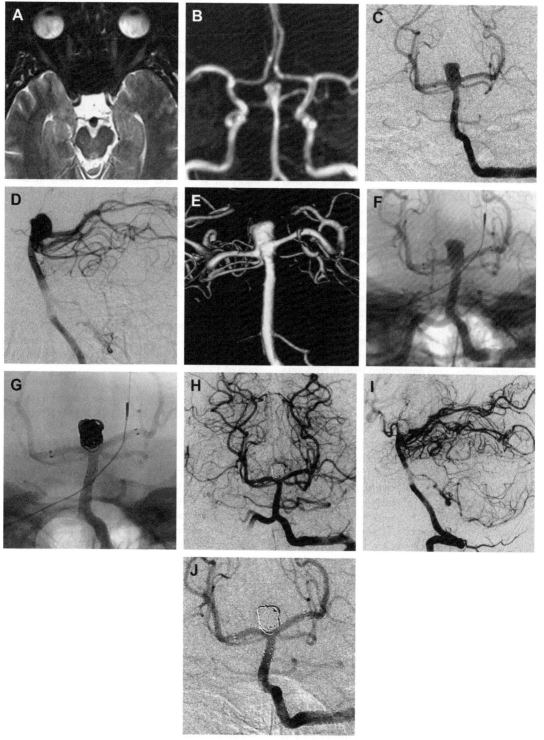

Fig. 3. A 45-year-old woman who presented with headaches and a family history of SAH. (*A*) Axial T2-weighted magnetic resonance (MR) image of the brain shows the top of the basilar artery aneurysm. (*B*) MR angiography better shows the wide-necked basilar artery aneurysm. (*C, D*) AP and lateral left vertebral artery angiogram shows the wide-necked basilar artery aneurysm. (*E*) 3D left vertebral artery angiogram better shows the basilar artery aneurysm. (*F*) Unsubtracted AP left vertebral artery angiogram shows 2 Neuroform stents in a Y-configuration, extending from the right and left P1 segment into the mid-basilar artery. (*G*) Unsubtracted AP left vertebral artery angiogram shows the final coil mass within the aneurysm with 2 Neuroform stents in a Y-configuration. (*H, I*) AP (*H*) and lateral (*I*) left vertebral angiogram shows no filling of the aneurysm with a patent basilar artery and both posterior cerebral arteries. (*J*) AP left vertebral angiogram at 6-month follow-up shows no recurrence of the aneurysm.

Results

Multiple articles have been published on the use of intracranial stents for the treatment of wide-necked intracranial aneurysms. Given the limitations of space, this article limits the discussion to those reports with a larger series of patients. Higashida and colleagues[145] initially reported the use of the Enterprise stent, all 5 cases of which were technically successful. The stent was well visualized, easily deployed, could be repositioned if needed, and was accurately placed without technical difficulties. In 2007, Weber and colleagues[146] described the use of the stent in 31 saccular wide-necked aneurysms. Follow-up angiography of 30 lesions after 6 months demonstrated 15 complete aneurysm occlusions, 8 aneurysm neck remnants, and 7 residual aneurysms. Two patients experienced possible device-related serious adverse events. The Enterprise stent multicenter registry was published in 2009, and included 141 patients with 142 aneurysms who underwent 143 attempted stent deployments.[147] The use of stent assistance with aneurysm coiling was associated with a 76% rate of at least 90% occlusion. The stent could not be navigated to the desired location in 3% of cases, and there was a 2% occurrence of inaccurate deployment. Procedure data demonstrated a 6% temporary morbidity, 2.8% permanent morbidity, and 2% mortality. A midterm follow-up report of 213 patients with 219 aneurysms treated with the Enterprise stent at a mean follow-up of 174.6 days demonstrated total occlusion of the aneurysm in 40% of the patients, with 88% having at least 90% aneurysm occlusion.[148] Three percent of patients demonstrated significant ($\geq$50%) in-stent stenosis or occlusion. Seven delayed thrombotic events occurred because of cessation of double antiplatelet therapy. Lv and colleagues,[149] in a report of 50 (31 saccular, 19 dissecting) complex intracranial aneurysms, reported a 2% complication rate (1 death). At mean 9.1-month follow-up, results were good in all dissecting cases and good in 30 saccular cases. There was 1 recurrence in each group.

In 2006, Kis and colleagues[150] described the successful deployment of the Leo stent in 24 of 25 aneurysms. There were 2 thromboembolic events related to the deployment of the Leo stent, 1 failure of stent deployment, difficulties in stent positioning in 3 cases, and 1 asymptomatic parent vessel occlusion after 7 months. Follow-up at an average of 5 months revealed aneurysm recurrence in 3 lesions, which were retreated.

The largest experience to date is with the Neuroform stent. The Neuroform was the first intracranial stent available for the treatment of wide-necked aneurysms. Gao and colleagues,[151] in a retrospective study of 232 patients with 239 wide-necked aneurysms, reported results of patients treated with Neuroform stent-assisted coil embolization. Stent placement was successful in 237 of 239 aneurysms. Favorable clinical outcome (mRS $\leq$2) was observed in 88.3% of the patients. Procedure complications included thromboembolism (n = 13), intraprocedural rupture (n = 8), coil protrusions (n = 5), new mass effect (n = 3), vessel injury (n = 3), and stent dislodgment (n = 2). Procedure-related morbidity and mortality were 4.2% and 1.3%. The overall recanalization rate was 14.5%. Delayed complications included in-stent stenosis (n = 2) and penetrating artery occlusion (n = 2) during the follow-up period.

Liang and colleagues[152] reported a series that included 110 wide-necked aneurysms. In all cases, the Neuroform system was delivered and deployed accurately. Procedure-related morbidity was 5.6% and procedural-related mortality 0.9%. Angiographic follow-up in 51 aneurysms at an average of 37 months showed an overall recanalization rate of 13.7%.

In 2005, Lylyk and colleagues[153] reported on 46 patients with 48 intracranial aneurysms treated using the Neuroform stent. There was a 92% technical success rate. Approximately 19% of the stents were placed in a suboptimal location. In 31% of the cases, the stent was difficult to place. Procedure-related morbidity and mortality were 8.6% and 2.1%, respectively. Since this report, there have been at least 2 newer generations of the device, allowing easier placement.

In 2007, Biondi and colleagues[154] reported on 42 patients with 46 wide-necked aneurysms. The balloon remodeling technique was performed in 77% of patients before stent placement. The stent was successfully deployed in 94% of the cases. Angiographic and clinical follow-up was available in 31 patients with 33 aneurysms. In the 30 aneurysms treated with stent-assisted coiling, there were 17 (57%) aneurysm occlusions, 7 (23%) neck remnants, and 6 (20%) residual aneurysms. In 3 recanalized aneurysms treated with stent alone, 2 (67%) neck remnants remained unchanged, and 1 (33%) neck remnant decreased in size.

Shapiro and colleagues[155] performed a comprehensive literature survey of stent-supported aneurysm coiling. Thirty-nine articles with 1517 patients met inclusion criteria. The overall procedure complication rate was 19%, with a periprocedural mortality of 2.1%. Approximately 45% of aneurysms were completely occluded at first treatment session, which increased to 61% on follow-up. An approximate 3.5% in-stent stenosis and 0.6% stent occlusion rate were observed at angiographic follow-up.

Fargen and colleagues[156] compiled data of patients treated with the Enterprise stent-assisted coiling of aneurysms at 9 high-volume centers. Two hundred twenty-nine patients with 229 aneurysms, 32 of which were ruptured, were included in the study. Fifty-nine percent of patients demonstrated 100% coil obliteration, and 81% had 90% or higher occlusion on the last follow-up angiogram. A total of 19 patients (8.3%) underwent retreatment of their aneurysms during the follow-up period. Angiographic in-stent stenosis was seen in 3.4% of patients, and thromboembolic events occurred in 4.4%. Overall, 91% of patients who underwent Enterprise-assisted coiling had an mRS of 2 or less at the last follow-up.

Trispan Device

Characteristics of the device
Another device used to treat wide-necked intracranial aneurysms is the Trispan device (Stryker). This device was never marketed in the United States but is widely available in Asia, Canada, and Europe. The Trispan device is composed of 3 loops of nitinol wire in the shape of a 3-leaf clover. The device is delivered through a microcatheter into the aneurysm and deployed. It is held in place by its detachable wire. Once the Trispan device is positioned to cover the neck of the aneurysm without compromise of the parent vessel, a microcatheter is placed through the device into the aneurysm, and the coils are delivered. After the aneurysm is adequately filled with coils, the Trispan device is detached. Since the introduction of dedicated intracranial stents for wide-necked aneurysms the use of this device has decreased, and the authors have no experience with its use.

Results
The largest experience using the Trispan for treating intracranial aneurysms has been in Montreal. In 2001, Raymond and colleagues[157] reported on 25 patients with 19 basilar bifurcation and 6 anterior circulation aneurysms. All aneurysms except 1 were wide-necked. The procedure was successful in all patients, with complete obliteration of the aneurysm in 3, residual necks in 13, and a minimal sac in 7. Follow-up angiogram in 16 patients revealed complete obliteration in 4 patients, a residual neck in 1, a persistent residual neck in 4, and recurrent aneurysm in 7. In 2008, DeKeukeleire and colleagues[158] reported on 14 patients in whom 16 Trispan devices were placed to assist coiling of wide-necked aneurysms in the anterior circulation. Trispan-assisted embolization was successful in 15 of 16 (93.8%) procedures, with complete occlusion in 2 of 16 (12.5%), near

complete occlusion in 10 of 16 (62.5%), and incomplete occlusion in 3 of 16 (18.75%).

Liquid Embolic Agents

Technique Onyx 500
Numerous publications throughout the late 1980s and early 1990s described various techniques using liquid embolic agents to treat intracranial aneurysms. There were problems with the control of these agents during delivery into the aneurysm and nontarget embolization of the material distally into the intracranial circulation. Onyx (Ev3) is a liquid embolic agent designed for endovascular use. It is an ethylene-vinyl-alcohol (EVOH) biocompatible copolymer used in conjunction with dimethyl sulfoxide (DMSO) as the solvent. Tantalum powder is added to the mixture to provide visualization under fluoroscopy. Onyx 500 used for aneurysm treatment contains 20% EVOH.

When the material comes in contact with an aqueous solution (ie, blood or water), it precipitates and forms a soft spongy polymer cast, with the outer layer solidifying first and the central portion remaining in a semiliquid state. As further material is injected, it fills the space within the aneurysm. The material does not fragment during injection, but remains in a cohesive semiliquid state, similar to lava from a volcano.

In treatment of intracranial aneurysms, the material is kept within the aneurysm sac by placement of a DMSO-compatible balloon (HyperGlide or HyperForm; Ev3) across the neck. The first step of the procedure consists of performing a seal test. During balloon inflation, contrast is injected through a DMSO-compatible microcatheter placed within the aneurysm sac to confirm any leakage of contrast into the parent vessel. If there is leakage of contrast into the parent vessel, patients are not treated with Onyx (Fig. 4).

Depending on the therapeutic strategy, coils or liquid embolic agents are delivered first to occlude the major part of the aneurysm sac. The dead space of the microcatheter is first filled with the solvent DMSO to prevent precipitation of the liquid embolic agent within the lumen of the microcatheter. The aneurysm is then obliterated slowly by injecting (0.1–0.2 mL/min) Onyx 500 with a cadence syringe. During each injection the balloon remains inflated across the neck of the aneurysm. The balloon is deflated after about 5 minutes, allowing the polymer to solidify. Angiography is performed to confirm the polymer's location relative to the aneurysm, and this process is continued until the aneurysm is occluded. After the last injection the material solidifies completely over a period of

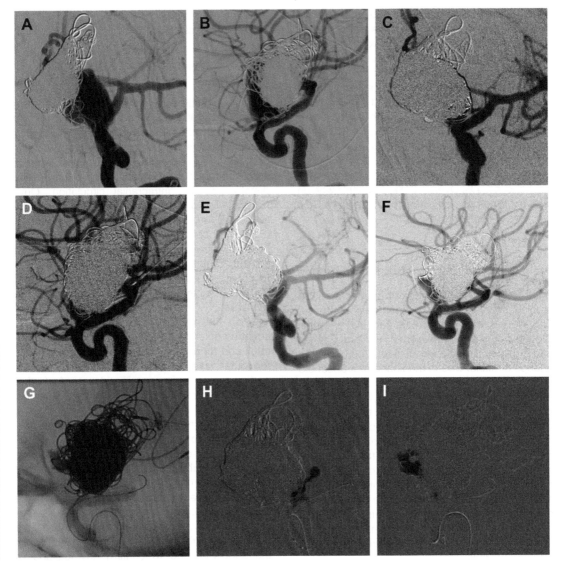

Fig. 4. A 45-year-old woman with a history of left retro-orbital headaches. (*A, B*) Oblique frontal (*A*) and lateral (*B*) left internal carotid angiogram shows recurrence of a large left supraclinoid aneurysm previously coiled. (*C, D*) After placement of additional coils within the aneurysm, repeat oblique frontal (*C*) and lateral (*D*) left internal carotid angiogram shows near complete thrombosis of the aneurysm with a large dense coil mass within the aneurysm. (*E, F*) Oblique frontal (*E*) and lateral (*F*) left internal carotid angiogram at 6-month follow-up shows an area of recurrence of the anterior and medial portion of the aneurysm. (*G*) Lateral spot fluoroscopic image shows a 5 × 15-mm Hyperglide balloon across the neck of the left supraclinoid aneurysm during the seal test. Oblique frontal (*H*) and (*I–K*) saved lateral roadmap images show filling of the area of aneurysm recurrence with Onyx HD 500. (*L, M*) Oblique frontal (*L*) and lateral (*M*) left internal carotid angiogram shows complete occlusion of the aneurysm. (*N, O*) Oblique frontal (*N*) and lateral (*O*) left internal carotid angiogram at 6-month follow-up shows continued occlusion of the aneurysm.

about 10 minutes, with diffusion of the solvent DMSO.

Results

Ev3 sponsored the Cerebral Aneurysm Multicenter European Onyx (CAMEO) trial in 20 centers.[159] CAMEO was a prospective, observational trial

that enrolled 119 consecutive patients with 123 aneurysms. Follow-up results were reported for 100 of these patients. CAMEO reported complete occlusion in 79% of aneurysms, subtotal occlusion in 13%, and incomplete occlusion in 8%. Delayed occlusion of the parent vessel occurred in 9 patients, 5 of whom were asymptomatic. In 2009,

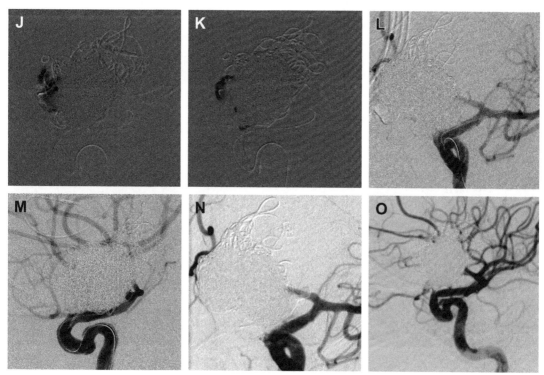

Fig. 4.

Piske and colleagues[160] treated 69 patients with 84 aneurysms, all of which had a wide neck. Fifty aneurysms were small (<12 mm), 30 were large (12 to <25 mm), and 4 were giant. Angiographic follow-up was available for 65 of the 84 aneurysms at 6 months. Complete aneurysm occlusion was seen in 65.5% of aneurysms on immediate control, in 84.6% at 6 months. The rates of complete occlusion were 74% for small aneurysms and 80% for large aneurysms. Progression from incomplete to complete occlusion was seen in 68.2% of all aneurysms, with a higher percentage in small aneurysms (90.9%). Aneurysm recanalization was observed in 3 patients (4.6%), with retreatment in 2 patients (3.3%).

Cekirge and colleagues[161] presented the long-term clinical and angiographic follow-up results of 100 consecutive intracranial aneurysms treated with Onyx. Intracranial stenting was used adjunctively in 25 aneurysms, including 19 during initial treatment and 6 during retreatment. Of the 100 aneurysms, 35 were giant or large/wide-necked, and 65 were small. Follow-up angiography was performed in all 91 surviving patients (96 aneurysms) at 3 and/or 6 months. Overall, aneurysm recanalization was observed in 12 of 96 aneurysms on follow-up angiography (12.5%). All 12 were large or giant aneurysms, resulting in a 36% recanalization rate in the large and giant aneurysm

group. One aneurysm of 25 treated with the combination of a stent and Onyx showed recanalization.

Flow Diversion

Characteristics

A new generation of endovascular devices has appeared over the last 3 years, called flow diverters.[162] These devices have been developed to treat aneurysms from an endoluminal rather than an endosaccular approach. Such stent-like devices are designed to reconstruct the parent vessel and to divert flow away from the aneurysm lumen without the use of coils. The device promotes thrombus formation within the aneurysm by decreasing the hemodynamic effects within the aneurysm sac, promoting stasis. In addition, the device has a tighter scaffolding than a conventional intracranial stent, providing a means over which endothelial cells can grow to seal off the neck of the aneurysm. Kallmes and colleagues[163,164] have characterized the effects of the pipeline embolization device (PED) in an experimental rabbit aneurysm model. The PED (Ev3) is one of the first flow-diversion devices used in humans, and was approved by the FDA for the treatment of aneurysms on April 10, 2011 (**Fig. 5**). The PED is a cylindrical, stent-like construct composed of 48 braided

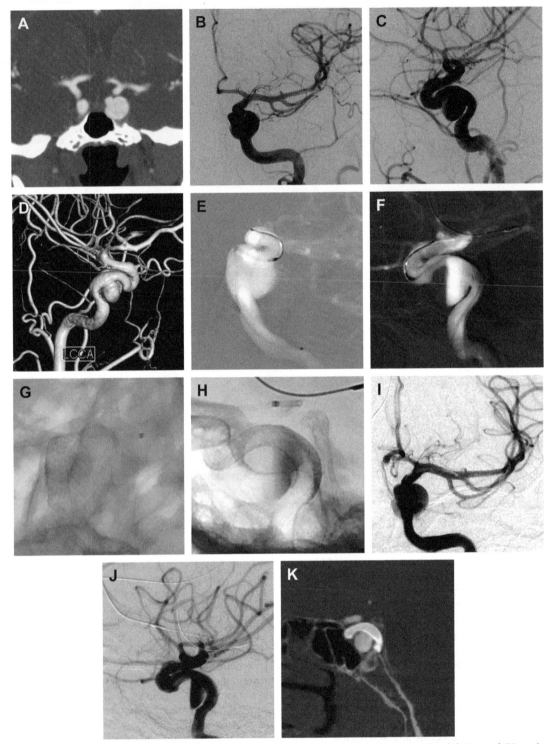

Fig. 5. A 66-year-old woman who presented with a headache and a right sixth nerve palsy. (*A*) Coronal CT angiogram shows a left cavernous carotid artery aneurysm. (*B, C*) AP (*B*) and lateral (*C*) left internal carotid artery angiogram shows a left cavernous carotid artery aneurysm. (*D*) 3D left internal carotid artery angiogram better defines the wide-necked left cavernous carotid artery aneurysm. (*E, F*) Saved oblique (*E*) and lateral (*F*) left internal carotid artery roadmap images show the pipeline stent within the microcatheter across the neck of the aneurysm. (*G, H*) Spot oblique (*G*) and lateral (*H*) fluoroscopic images show 2 pipeline stents across the neck of the aneurysm. (*I, J*) AP (*I*) and lateral (*J*) left internal carotid artery angiogram shows decrease in the inflow to the left cavernous carotid artery aneurysm. (*K*) Sagittal DynaCT image shows the pipeline stents across the neck of the cavernous carotid artery aneurysm.

strands of cobalt chromium and platinum. Its appearance is similar to that of the Wallstent; however, there is a more dense wire mesh. The Silk stent (Balt Extrusion, Montmorency, France) is a braided, self-expanding, high-metal surface area coverage construct that has CE Mark approval in Europe. Other devices are in development at the time of writing. The flow diverters are delivered and placed in a fashion similar as the current conventional intracranial stents already described.

Results

Lylyk and colleagues[165] recently reported their single-center results of 53 patients treated with the PED. No major procedure-related complications were reported in their series. On angiographic follow-up, there was a 93% and 95% rate of complete aneurysm occlusion observed at 6 and 12 months, respectively. Fiorella and colleagues[166] reported 2 cases of fusiform vertebral artery aneurysms treated successfully with the PED. Kadziolka and colleagues[167] reported on 6 patients with intracranial aneurysms treated with the Silk stent. The stent was deployed in all cases with no morbidity or mortality; however, the results were not commented on in the abstract. The Pipeline Embolization Device in the Intracranial Treatment of Aneurysms (PITA) was a multicenter, single-arm clinical trial of the PED conducted at 3 medical centers in Europe.[168] Subjects were included if they had a wide-necked intracranial aneurysm (neck of >4 mm or dome/neck ratio of <1.5) or intracranial aneurysm that had failed previous endovascular treatment attempts. Aneurysms were treated with the PED with or without adjunctive coil embolization. Thirty-one patients with 31 intracranial aneurysms were treated. Mean aneurysm size was 11.5 mm and mean neck size was 5.8 mm. PED placement was technically successful in 30 of 31 patients (96.8%). Two patients experienced a major periprocedural stroke. Follow-up angiography at 6 months demonstrated complete aneurysm occlusion in 28 (93.3%) of the 30 patients who underwent angiographic follow-up. Byrne and colleagues[169] reported the results of a multicenter prospective study using Silk that included 70 patients with 70 aneurysms. In 3 cases (4%) the stent could not be deployed. Fifty-seven aneurysms (81%) were treated with a single Silk and 10 (14%) with a combination of Silk and coils. At follow-up, complete occlusion was observed in 24 of 49 (49%), neck remnant in 13 of 49 (26%), and residual aneurysm filling in 12 of 49 (25%) aneurysms. Parent vessel occlusion was observed in 7 of 49 (14%) cases, and arterial narrowing in 3 of 49 (6%) of cases. The Pipeline for Uncoilable or Failed Aneurysms

(PUFS) study was able to show safety and efficacy of PED in large or giant wide-necked aneurysms.[170] A follow-up report of 12 wide-necked or otherwise untreatable aneurysms in 12 patients treated with the PED showed complete angiographic occlusion at 27 months.[171] In a prospective registry established at 3 Australian centers, a total of 57 aneurysms in 54 patients were treated with PED or PED and coils. Clinical follow-up was available in 57 aneurysms, with imaging follow-up at 6 months in 56. Permanent morbidity and mortality in the series was 0% at 6 months. Four transient ischemic attacks and 1 small retinal branch occlusion occurred, but no cerebral infarction was noted. The aneurysm occlusion rate at 1 month was 61.9%, and the overall occlusion rate at 6 months was 85.7%. In cases previously untreated, the 6-month occlusion was 92.5%. Three of 6 aneurysms with a previous stent in situ were occluded. Two patients (3.5%) had asymptomatic in-construct stenosis of greater than 50%. Acute aneurysm–provoked mass effect resolved or improved significantly in all cases.[172,173] The PUFS trial has been completed and presented in abstract form; however, there is no report in the literature. The Complete Occlusion of COilable Intracranial Aneurysms (COCOA) trial with the pipeline device is ongoing.

COMPLICATIONS OF ENDOVASCULAR COILING AND THEIR TREATMENT
Introduction

Every periprocedural or postprocedural complication needs to be examined thoroughly before corrective action is taken. For example, further manipulation of a single malpositioned loop of coil in a parent vessel may lead to aneurysm rupture and death or further thrombus formation and a cerebral infarction. If a single loop of coil is within the parent vessel and there is no thrombus formation on the coil or compromise of antegrade flow within the parent vessel, it may be prudent to just watch the situation by placing the patient on intravenous heparin overnight and antiplatelet medications, and avoid possible significant morbidity or mortality.

Alongside the risks, the advantages and disadvantages of endovascular coiling should be weighed against the risk of surgical treatment or a conservative approach before treatment, to determine the best option for the optimal clinical outcome. Patients should be given their full options along with extensive information before treatment. In the case of a ruptured aneurysm this information should be given to the patient's relatives whenever possible. The information provided must include the natural history of the disease, goals of treatment, and the potential risks involved.

Coil Malposition

Deposition of a coil outside the aneurysm sac can occur. Most commonly it is a single loop of coil protruding into the parent vessel, which seldom causes a thromboembolic complication. However, if thrombus forms around the loop of coil, a glycoprotein IIa/IIIb inhibitor can be given at the site of thrombus formation to dissolve the clot. The coil should then be removed with one of the retrieval devices. If this is not possible, the single loop of coil should be pushed against the vessel wall by placement of a self-expanding intracranial stent. Malposition of a coil is infrequent and is usually the result of a poor coil choice, poor catheter position, or poor technique. The authors commonly apply some minimal forward force on the microcatheter during coiling of the aneurysm in the late stages to prevent the microcatheter from being kicked out of the aneurysm and coil loop being deposited outside of the aneurysm sac.

Stretched Coil

Stretching of a coil is one of the biggest fears for the endovascular neurosurgeon; however, the incidence of this occurring has significantly decreased dramatically since the introduction of stretch-resistant coils. To avoid this from happening, retraction of the coil under fluoroscopy must be one-to-one with the delivery wire and hand movements at the groin. If the coil is not responding one-to-one under fluoroscopy with hand movements at the groin, or if difficulty is encountered in repositioning of the coil, it most likely has stretched. In this situation, the coil and microcatheter should be removed together as a unit from the patient. If this is not possible, the coil should be stretched as long as possible and positioned into the external carotid artery or descending thoracic aorta to prevent migration distally and to prevent a large coil mass from occluding the parent vessel. A majority of patients will tolerate stretching of a single loop of coil into the parent vessel, without a thromboembolic event or vessel occlusion. If this occurs, the patient should be kept anticoagulated overnight in the NICU and given an antiplatelet agent. A layer of endothelial cells will form over the stretched coil in about 8 to 10 weeks.

Broken Coil

A broken coil usually occurs when a stretched coil is pushed to mechanical failure. If a large portion of the coil is left in the parent vessel, thrombus formation with platelet aggregation may occur very rapidly. In these cases, it may be necessary to give a glycoprotein IIa/IIIb inhibitor at the site of thrombus formation and to make sure the patient is fully anticoagulated. An attempt at retrieving the coil with a dedicated device such as a loop snare, alligator clip, or the Merci device (Concentric Medical, Mountain View, CA) can then be made. If this cannot be performed and the coil is compromising antegrade flow within the parent vessel, the coil can be pushed against the vessel wall and trapped with a self-expanding stent.

Rupture of Aneurysm

Aneurysm rupture, the most dreaded complication, can occur spontaneously because of the fragile nature of the aneurysm. It may also occur iatrogenically from the cerebral angiogram or placement of a microcatheter or coil into the aneurysm.[174] When this occurs, there is a rapid severe transient elevation of intracranial pressure causing severe elevation of the blood pressure. If electroencephalograph monitoring is being performed, electrical activity will seize. The aneurysm needs to be secured quickly, because a ruptured aneurysm can easily cause death to the patient.[175,176] If the patient is anticoagulated, this must be immediately reversed with protamine (ie, 10 mg protamine per 1000 units heparin given), so that the ACT is less than 150 seconds. If the patient has been premedicated with aspirin or Plavix, an attempt at reversal of platelet inhibition should be made with the infusion of platelets. The authors have a prepared, nonpooled 5-pack of platelets ready in the operating room before coil placement in preparation for this event. The blood pressure should also be lowered immediately by pharmaceutical means in an attempt to prevent any further extravasation of blood into the subarachnoid space. If a balloon is present within the parent vessel, this should be carefully inflated and the aneurysm rapidly packed with additional coils. If the microcatheter is within the subarachnoid space this should not be removed, but coiling should be performed from the subarachnoid space into the aneurysm. After the aneurysm is secure, CT of the head should be immediately performed to assess for hydrocephalus and the need for placement of a ventriculostomy catheter. Vasospasm should be treated by intra-arterial injection of a pharmacologic agent (ie, verapamil, nicardipine, nimodipine) once the aneurysm is secure.

Rupture of Vessel

Perforation of a blood vessel by a microguide wire is rare. This rupture may be self-limiting and seal, or may lead to life-threatening hemorrhage. If life-threatening hemorrhage is identified, permanent occlusion of the vessel may be life-saving. A liquid embolic agent or coils can be used.[177] On rare occasions, rupture of a blood vessel after placement of a balloon-expandable stent can be managed conservatively with prolonged balloon inflation across the area of rupture.[178]

Procedural Thrombus Formation

A thromboembolic event is probably the most common complication related to endovascular management of an aneurysm. These events have decreased over the last few years, mainly attributable to better and more liberal use of antiplatelet agents. Patients are now routinely placed on clopidogrel and aspirin 7 days before treatment based on the coronary intervention literature, which has shown a significant decrease in the risk of thromboembolic events in patients treated with this regimen. Furthermore, to prevent thrombus formation during the procedure patients are fully anticoagulated so that the ACT range is between 250 and 300 seconds. Bivalirudin (Angiomax) is a direct thrombin inhibitor with a better anticoagulation profile and a shorter half-life than heparin; however, it does not have a reversal agent, which limits its use in the cerebral vascular circulation. If thrombus forms on coils placed at the neck of the aneurysm, most interventionists prefer local infusion of a glycoprotein IIa/IIIb receptor.[179] Abciximab (Reopro), which is mainly used in the authors' center, is administered intra-arterially through the microcatheter at a dose of 4 to 10 mg over 10 to 20 minutes.[180] Abciximab has also been shown to be effective in ruptured aneurysms, with no increased risk of bleeding complications. Three glycoprotein IIa/IIIb receptor inhibitors are available on the market, the most common being abciximab; however, eptifibatide (Integrilin) may be the preferred agent because of its shorter half-life and reversible binding to the glycoprotein IIa/IIIb receptor.

SUMMARY

Most intracranial aneurysms are asymptomatic and remain undetected until the time of rupture when they present with SAH. Patients in the ISUIA trial who had a UIA smaller than 10 mm had a low rate of rupture compared with historical controls. Diagnostic angiography is still the gold standard for the detection of intracranial aneurysms; however, CT angiography and MR angiography have shown significant improvement over the last 10 years with new and better scanners. A majority of intracranial aneurysms can now be treated from an endovascular approach with various coils,

balloons, and stents, with few complications, as discussed in this article. Microsurgery is still an important treatment option for patients with a wide-necked intracranial aneurysm.

REFERENCES

1. Le Roux PD, Winn HR, Newell DW. Management of cerebral aneurysms. Philadelphia: Saunders; 2004.
2. Wiebers DO, Whisnant JP, Huston J 3rd, et al. Unruptured intracranial aneurysms: natural history, clinical outcome, and risks of surgical and endovascular treatment. Lancet 2003;362:103–10.
3. Molyneux AJ, Kerr RS, Yu LM, et al. International Subarachnoid Aneurysm Trial (ISAT) of neurosurgical clipping versus endovascular coiling in 2143 patients with ruptured intracranial aneurysms: a randomised comparison of effects on survival, dependency, seizures, rebleeding, subgroups, and aneurysm occlusion. Lancet 2005;366:809–17.
4. Guglielmi G, Vinuela F, Dion J, et al. Electrothrombosis of saccular aneurysms via endovascular approach. Part 2: preliminary clinical experience. J Neurosurg 1991;75:8–14.
5. Guglielmi G, Vinuela F, Sepetka I, et al. Electrothrombosis of saccular aneurysms via endovascular approach. Part 1: electrochemical basis, technique, and experimental results. J Neurosurg 1991;75:1–7.
6. Raymond J, Roy D. Safety and efficacy of endovascular treatment of acutely ruptured aneurysms. Neurosurgery 1997;41:1235–45 [discussion: 1245–6].
7. Roy D, Milot G, Raymond J. Endovascular treatment of unruptured aneurysms. Stroke 2001;32: 1998–2004.
8. Menghini VV, Brown RD Jr, Sicks JD, et al. Incidence and prevalence of intracranial aneurysms and hemorrhage in Olmsted County, Minnesota, 1965 to 1995. Neurology 1998;51:405–11.
9. Winn HR, Jane JA Sr, Taylor J, et al. Prevalence of asymptomatic incidental aneurysms: review of 4568 arteriograms. J Neurosurg 2002;96:43–9.
10. Iwamoto H, Kiyohara Y, Fujishima M, et al. Prevalence of intracranial saccular aneurysms in a Japanese community based on a consecutive autopsy series during a 30-year observation period. The Hisayama study. Stroke 1999;30:1390–5.
11. Yamaura A, Ono J, Hirai S. Clinical picture of intracranial non-traumatic dissecting aneurysm. Neuropathology 2000;20:85–90.
12. Ostergaard JR. Headache as a warning symptom of impending aneurysmal subarachnoid haemorrhage. Cephalalgia 1991;11:53–5.
13. Raps EC, Rogers JD, Galetta SL, et al. The clinical spectrum of unruptured intracranial aneurysms. Arch Neurol 1993;50:265–8.

14. Yasargil MG, Gasser JC, Hodosh RM, et al. Carotid-ophthalmic aneurysms: direct microsurgical approach. Surg Neurol 1977;8:155–65.

15. Almeida GM, Shibata MK, Bianco E. Carotid-ophthalmic aneurysms. Surg Neurol 1976;5:41–5.

16. Day AL. Clinicoanatomic features of supraclinoid aneurysms. Clin Neurosurg 1990;36:256–74.

17. Heros RC, Nelson PB, Ojemann RG, et al. Large and giant paraclinoid aneurysms: surgical techniques, complications, and results. Neurosurgery 1983;12:153–63.

18. al-Rodhan NR, Piepgras DG, Sundt TM Jr. Transitional cavernous aneurysms of the internal carotid artery. Neurosurgery 1993;33:993–6 [discussion: 997–8].

19. Day AL. Aneurysms of the ophthalmic segment. A clinical and anatomical analysis. J Neurosurg 1990;72:677–91.

20. Alexander MP, Freedman M. Amnesia after anterior communicating artery aneurysm rupture. Neurology 1984;34:752–7.

21. McMahon AJ. Diabetes insipidus developing after subarachnoid haemorrhage from an anterior communicating artery aneurysm. Scott Med J 1988;33:208–9.

22. Heros RC. Middle cerebral artery aneurysm. In: Wilkins RH, Rengachary SS, editors. Neurosurgery, vol. 2. New York: McGraw Hill; 1985. p. 1376–83.

23. Longheed WM, Marshall BM. Management of aneurysm of the anterior circulation by intracranial procedures. In: Youmans JR, editor. Neurological surgery, vol. 2. Philadelphia: WB Saunders; 1973. p. 742–50.

24. Campos J, Fox AJ, Vinuela F, et al. Saccular aneurysms in basilar artery fenestration. AJNR Am J Neuroradiol 1987;8:233–6.

25. Nakagawa T, Hashi K. The incidence and treatment of asymptomatic, unruptured cerebral aneurysms. J Neurosurg 1994;80:217–23.

26. Krishna H, Wani AA, Behari S, et al. Intracranial aneurysms in patients 18 years of age or under, are they different from aneurysms in adult population? Acta Neurochir 2005;147:469–76 [discussion: 476].

27. Kanaan I, Lasjaunias P, Coates R. The spectrum of intracranial aneurysms in pediatrics. Minim Invasive Neurosurg 1995;38:1–9.

28. Steinherz P, Meyers P, Wollner N, et al. Reinduction therapy for advanced or refractory acute lymphoblastic leukemia of childhood. Cancer 1989;63:1472–6.

29. Masuzawa T, Kurokawa T, Oguro K, et al. Pulseless disease associated with multiple intracranial aneurysms. Neuroradiology 1986;28:17–22.

30. Milgram JW, Stecher K Jr. Idiopathic arteritis with multiple intracranial aneurysms. Angiology 1974;25:89–119.

31. Mimori A, Suzuki T, Hashimoto M, et al. Subarachnoid hemorrhage and systemic lupus erythematosus. Lupus 2000;9:521–6.

32. Schievink WI. Genetics of intracranial aneurysms. Neurosurgery 1997;40:651–62 [discussion: 662–3].

33. Krog M, Almgren B, Eriksson I, et al. Vascular complications in the Ehlers-Danlos syndrome. Acta Chir Scand 1983;149:279–82.

34. Schievink WI, Link MJ, Piepgras DG, et al. Intracranial aneurysm surgery in Ehlers-Danlos syndrome Type IV. Neurosurgery 2002;51:607–11 [discussion: 611–3].

35. Schievink WI, Parisi JE, Piepgras DG, et al. Intracranial aneurysms in Marfan's syndrome: an autopsy study. Neurosurgery 1997;41:866–70 [discussion: 871].

36. Schievink WI, Puumala MR, Meyer FB, et al. Giant intracranial aneurysm and fibromuscular dysplasia in an adolescent with alpha 1-antitrypsin deficiency. J Neurosurg 1996;85:503–6.

37. Schievink WI, Katzmann JA, Piepgras DG, et al. Alpha-1-antitrypsin phenotypes among patients with intracranial aneurysms. J Neurosurg 1996;84:781–4.

38. Ronkainen A, Miettinen H, Karkola K, et al. Risk of harboring an unruptured intracranial aneurysm. Stroke 1998;29:359–62.

39. Bromberg JE, Rinkel GJ, Algra A, et al. Subarachnoid haemorrhage in first and second degree relatives of patients with subarachnoid haemorrhage. BMJ 1995;311:288–9.

40. Schievink WI, Schaid DJ, Michels VV, et al. Familial aneurysmal subarachnoid hemorrhage: a community-based study. J Neurosurg 1995;83:426–9.

41. Shinton R, Beevers G. Meta-analysis of relation between cigarette smoking and stroke. BMJ 1989;298:789–94.

42. Qureshi AI, Suarez JI, Parekh PD, et al. Risk factors for multiple intracranial aneurysms. Neurosurgery 1998;43:22–6 [discussion: 26–7].

43. Juvela S, Hillbom M, Numminen H, et al. Cigarette smoking and alcohol consumption as risk factors for aneurysmal subarachnoid hemorrhage. Stroke 1993;24:639–46.

44. Lichtenfeld PJ, Rubin DB, Feldman RS. Subarachnoid hemorrhage precipitated by cocaine snorting. Arch Neurol 1984;41:223–4.

45. Bonneville F, Sourour N, Biondi A. Intracranial aneurysms: an overview. Neuroimaging Clin N Am 2006;16:371–82, vii.

46. Juvela S. Rebleeding from ruptured intracranial aneurysms. Surg Neurol 1989;32:323–6.

47. Rinkel GJ, Djibuti M, Algra A, et al. Prevalence and risk of rupture of intracranial aneurysms: a systematic review. Stroke 1998;29:251–6.

48. Morita A, Fujiwara S, Hashi K, et al. Risk of rupture associated with intact cerebral aneurysms in the Japanese population: a systematic review of the literature from Japan. J Neurosurg 2005;102:601–6.

49. Unruptured intracranial aneurysms—risk of rupture and risks of surgical intervention. International Study of Unruptured Intracranial Aneurysms Investigators. N Engl J Med 1998;339:1725–33.

50. Wiebers DO. Unruptured intracranial aneurysms: natural history and clinical management. Update on the International Study of Unruptured Intracranial Aneurysms. Neuroimaging Clin N Am 2006; 16:383–90, vii.

51. Weir B. Unruptured intracranial aneurysms: a review. J Neurosurg 2002;96:3–42.

52. Juvela S, Porras M, Poussa K. Natural history of unruptured intracranial aneurysms: probability and risk factors for aneurysm rupture. Neurosurg Focus 2000;8. Preview 1.

53. Wiebers DO. The risk of rupture of unruptured cerebral aneurysms in the Japanese population: a systematic review of the literature from Japan by Morita, et al. J Neurosurg 2005;102:597 [discussion: 598].

54. Linn FH, Rinkel GJ, Algra A, et al. Incidence of subarachnoid hemorrhage: role of region, year, and rate of computed tomography: a meta-analysis. Stroke 1996;27:625–9.

55. Labovitz DL, Halim AX, Brent B, et al. Subarachnoid hemorrhage incidence among Whites, Blacks and Caribbean Hispanics: the Northern Manhattan Study. Neuroepidemiology 2006;26:147–50.

56. Roger VL, Go AS, Lloyd-Jones DM, et al. Heart disease and stroke statistics—2011 update: a report from the American Heart Association. Circulation 2011;123:e18–209.

57. Mayberg MR, Batjer HH, Dacey R, et al. Guidelines for the management of aneurysmal subarachnoid hemorrhage. A statement for healthcare professionals from a special writing group of the Stroke Council, American Heart Association. Stroke 1994; 25:2315–28.

58. Johnston SC, Selvin S, Gress DR. The burden, trends, and demographics of mortality from subarachnoid hemorrhage. Neurology 1998;50:1413–8.

59. Qureshi AI, Suri MF, Nasar A, et al. Trends in hospitalization and mortality for subarachnoid hemorrhage and unruptured aneurysms in the United States. Neurosurgery 2005;57:1–8 [discussion: 1–8].

60. Stegmayr B, Eriksson M, Asplund K. Declining mortality from subarachnoid hemorrhage: changes in incidence and case fatality from 1985 through 2000. Stroke 2004;35:2059–63.

61. Josephson SA, Dillon WP, Dowd CF, et al. Continuous bleeding from a basilar terminus aneurysm imaged with CT angiography and conventional angiography. Neurocrit Care 2004;1:103–6.

62. Ferrante L, Acqui M, Trillo G, et al. Aneurysms of the posterior cerebral artery: do they present specific characteristics? Acta Neurochir (Wien) 1996; 138:840–52.

63. Broderick JP, Brott TG, Duldner JE, et al. Initial and recurrent bleeding are the major causes of death following subarachnoid hemorrhage. Stroke 1994; 25:1342–7.

64. Schievink WI, Wijdicks EF, Parisi JE, et al. Sudden death from aneurysmal subarachnoid hemorrhage. Neurology 1995;45:871–4.

65. Hop JW, Rinkel GJ, Algra A, et al. Case-fatality rates and functional outcome after subarachnoid hemorrhage: a systematic review. Stroke 1997;28: 660–4.

66. Brilstra EH, Hop JW, Rinkel GJ. Quality of life after perimesencephalic haemorrhage. J Neurol Neurosurg Psychiatr 1997;63:382–4.

67. Inagawa T, Kamiya K, Ogasawara H, et al. Rebleeding of ruptured intracranial aneurysms in the acute stage. Surg Neurol 1987;28:93–9.

68. Fujii Y, Takeuchi S, Sasaki O, et al. Ultra-early rebleeding in spontaneous subarachnoid hemorrhage. J Neurosurg 1996;84:35–42.

69. Hijdra A, Vermeulen M, van Gijn J, et al. Rerupture of intracranial aneurysms: a clinicoanatomic study. J Neurosurg 1987;67:29–33.

70. Hijdra A, Braakman R, van Gijn J, et al. Aneurysmal subarachnoid hemorrhage. Complications and outcome in a hospital population. Stroke 1987;18: 1061–7.

71. Graff-Radford NR, Torner J, Adams HP Jr, et al. Factors associated with hydrocephalus after subarachnoid hemorrhage. A report of the Cooperative Aneurysm Study. Arch Neurol 1989;46:744–52.

72. Hasan D, Schonck RS, Avezaat CJ, et al. Epileptic seizures after subarachnoid hemorrhage. Ann Neurol 1993;33:286–91.

73. Baker CJ, Prestigiacomo CJ, Solomon RA. Short-term perioperative anticonvulsant prophylaxis for the surgical treatment of low-risk patients with intracranial aneurysms. Neurosurgery 1995;37:863–70 [discussion: 870–1].

74. Rhoney DH, Tipps LB, Murry KR, et al. Anticonvulsant prophylaxis and timing of seizures after aneurysmal subarachnoid hemorrhage. Neurology 2000; 55:258–65.

75. Solenski NJ, Haley EC Jr, Kassell NF, et al. Medical complications of aneurysmal subarachnoid hemorrhage: a report of the multicenter, cooperative aneurysm study. Participants of the Multicenter Cooperative Aneurysm Study. Crit Care Med 1995;23:1007–17.

76. Wartenberg KE, Schmidt JM, Claassen J, et al. Impact of medical complications on outcome after subarachnoid hemorrhage. Crit Care Med 2006;34: 617–23 [quiz: 624].

77. Frontera JA, Fernandez A, Claassen J, et al. Hyperglycemia after SAH: predictors, associated complications, and impact on outcome. Stroke 2006;37:199–203.

78. Hasan D, Wijdicks EF, Vermeulen M. Hyponatremia is associated with cerebral ischemia in patients with aneurysmal subarachnoid hemorrhage. Ann Neurol 1990;27:106–8.

79. Kurokawa Y, Uede T, Ishiguro M, et al. Pathogenesis of hyponatremia following subarachnoid hemorrhage due to ruptured cerebral aneurysm. Surg Neurol 1996;46:500–7 [discussion: 507–8].

80. Qureshi AI, Suri MF, Sung GY, et al. Prognostic significance of hypernatremia and hyponatremia among patients with aneurysmal subarachnoid hemorrhage. Neurosurgery 2002;50:749–55 [discussion: 755–6].

81. Morinaga K, Hayashi S, Matsumoto Y, et al. Hyponatremia and cerebral vasospasm in patients with aneurysmal subarachnoid hemorrhage. No To Shinkei 1992;44:629–32 [in Japanese].

82. Andreoli A, di Pasquale G, Pinelli G, et al. Subarachnoid hemorrhage: frequency and severity of cardiac arrhythmias. A survey of 70 cases studied in the acute phase. Stroke 1987;18:558–64.

83. Mayer SA, Lin J, Homma S, et al. Myocardial injury and left ventricular performance after subarachnoid hemorrhage. Stroke 1999;30:780–6.

84. Kono T, Morita H, Kuroiwa T, et al. Left ventricular wall motion abnormalities in patients with subarachnoid hemorrhage: neurogenic stunned myocardium. J Am Coll Cardiol 1994;24:636–40.

85. Friedman JA, Pichelmann MA, Piepgras DG, et al. Pulmonary complications of aneurysmal subarachnoid hemorrhage. Neurosurgery 2003;52:1025–31 [discussion: 1031–2].

86. Kahn JM, Caldwell EC, Deem S, et al. Acute lung injury in patients with subarachnoid hemorrhage: incidence, risk factors, and outcome. Crit Care Med 2006;34:196–202.

87. Kassell NF, Sasaki T, Colohan AR, et al. Cerebral vasospasm following aneurysmal subarachnoid hemorrhage. Stroke 1985;16:562–72.

88. Dorsch NW. A review of cerebral vasospasm in aneurysmal subarachnoid haemorrhage Part III: mechanisms of action of calcium antagonists. J Clin Neurosci 1994;1:151–60.

89. Murayama Y, Malisch T, Guglielmi G, et al. Incidence of cerebral vasospasm after endovascular treatment of acutely ruptured aneurysms: report on 69 cases. J Neurosurg 1997;87:830–5.

90. Charpentier C, Audibert G, Guillemin F, et al. Multivariate analysis of predictors of cerebral vasospasm occurrence after aneurysmal subarachnoid hemorrhage. Stroke 1999;30:1402–8.

91. Conway JE, Tamargo RJ. Cocaine use is an independent risk factor for cerebral vasospasm after aneurysmal subarachnoid hemorrhage. Stroke 2001;32:2338–43.

92. Kallmes DF, Layton K, Marx WF, et al. Death by nondiagnosis: why emergent CT angiography should not be done for patients with subarachnoid hemorrhage. AJNR Am J Neuroradiol 2007;28:1837–8.

93. Fifi JT, Meyers PM, Lavine SD, et al. Complications of modern diagnostic cerebral angiography in an academic medical center. J Vasc Interv Radiol 2009;20:442–7.

94. Willinsky RA, Taylor SM, TerBrugge K, et al. Neurologic complications of cerebral angiography: prospective analysis of 2,899 procedures and review of the literature. Radiology 2003;227:522–8.

95. Villablanca JP, Rodriguez FJ, Stockman T, et al. MDCT angiography for detection and quantification of small intracranial arteries: comparison with conventional catheter angiography. AJR Am J Roentgenol 2007;188:593–602.

96. McKinney AM, Palmer CS, Truwit CL, et al. Detection of aneurysms by 64-section multidetector CT angiography in patients acutely suspected of having an intracranial aneurysm and comparison with digital subtraction and 3D rotational angiography. AJNR Am J Neuroradiol 2008;29:594–602.

97. Schellinger PD, Richter G, Kohrmann M, et al. Noninvasive angiography (magnetic resonance and computed tomography) in the diagnosis of ischemic cerebrovascular disease. Techniques and clinical applications. Cerebrovasc Dis 2007;24(Suppl 1):16–23.

98. Bernstein MA, Huston J 3rd, Lin C, et al. High-resolution intracranial and cervical MRA at 3.0T: technical considerations and initial experience. Magn Reson Med 2001;46:955–62.

99. Kaufmann TJ, Huston J 3rd, Cloft HJ, et al. A prospective trial of 3T and 1.5T time-of-flight and contrast-enhanced MR angiography in the follow-up of coiled intracranial aneurysms. AJNR Am J Neuroradiol 2010;31:912–8.

100. Hacein-Bey L, Provenzale JM. Current imaging assessment and treatment of intracranial aneurysms. AJR Am J Roentgenol 2011;196:32–44.

101. Wardlaw JM, White PM. The detection and management of unruptured intracranial aneurysms. Brain 2000;123(Pt 2):205–21.

102. Mallouhi A, Felber S, Chemelli A, et al. Detection and characterization of intracranial aneurysms with MR angiography: comparison of volume-rendering and maximum-intensity-projection algorithms. AJR Am J Roentgenol 2003;180:55–64.

103. Metens T, Rio F, Baleriaux D, et al. Intracranial aneurysms: detection with gadolinium-enhanced dynamic three-dimensional MR angiography-initial results. Radiology 2000;216:39–46.

104. Kouskouras C, Charitanti A, Giavroglou C, et al. Intracranial aneurysms: evaluation using CTA and

MRA. Correlation with DSA and intraoperative findings. Neuroradiology 2004;46:842–50.

105. Cognard C, Weill A, Castaings L, et al. Intracranial berry aneurysms: angiographic and clinical results after endovascular treatment. Radiology 1998;206:499–510.

106. Wang TH, Bhatt DL, Topol EJ. Aspirin and clopidogrel resistance: an emerging clinical entity. Eur Heart J 2006;27:647–54.

107. Tantry US, Bliden KP, Gurbel PA. Resistance to antiplatelet drugs: current status and future research. Expert Opin Pharmacother 2005;6:2027–45.

108. Spiotta AM, Hussain MS, Sivapatham T, et al. The versatile distal access catheter: the Cleveland Clinic experience. Neurosurgery 2011;68:1677–86 [discussion: 1686].

109. Hauck EF, Tawk RG, Karter NS, et al. Use of the outreach distal access catheter as an intracranial platform facilitates coil embolization of select intracranial aneurysms: technical note. J Neurointerv Surg 2011;3:172–6.

110. Binning MJ, Yashar P, Orion D, et al. Use of the outreach distal access catheter for microcatheter stabilization during intracranial arteriovenous malformation embolization. AJNR Am J Neuroradiol 2011;33(9):E117–9.

111. Park MS, Stiefel MF, Fiorella D, et al. Intracranial placement of a new, compliant guide catheter: technical note. Neurosurgery 2008;63:E616–7 [discussion: E617].

112. Schonholz C, Nanda A, Rodriguez J, et al. Transradial approach to coil embolization of an intracranial aneurysm. J Endovasc Ther 2004;11:411–3.

113. Nii K, Kazekawa K, Onizuka M, et al. Direct carotid puncture for the endovascular treatment of anterior circulation aneurysms. AJNR Am J Neuroradiol 2006;27:1502–4.

114. Blanc R, Piotin M, Mounayer C, et al. Direct cervical arterial access for intracranial endovascular treatment. Neuroradiology 2006;48:925–9.

115. Piotin M, Iijima A, Wada H, et al. Increasing the packing of small aneurysms with complex-shaped coils: an in vitro study. AJNR Am J Neuroradiol 2003;24:1446–8.

116. Piotin M, Liebig T, Feste CD, et al. Increasing the packing of small aneurysms with soft coils: an in vitro study. Neuroradiology 2004;46:935–9.

117. Shoulders-Odom B. Management of patients after percutaneous coronary interventions. Crit Care Nurse 2008;28:26–41 [quiz: 42].

118. Khaghany K, Al-Ali F, Spigelmoyer T, et al. Efficacy and safety of the Perclose Closer S device after neurointerventional procedures: prospective study and literature review. AJNR Am J Neuroradiol 2005;26:1420–4.

119. Assali AR, Sdringola S, Moustapha A, et al. Outcome of access site in patients treated with platelet glycoprotein IIb/IIIa inhibitors in the era of closure devices. Catheter Cardiovasc Interv 2003;58:1–5.

120. Vanninen R, Koivisto T, Saari T, et al. Ruptured intracranial aneurysms: acute endovascular treatment with electrolytically detachable coils—a prospective randomized study. Radiology 1999;211:325–36.

121. Molyneux A, Kerr R, Stratton I, et al. International Subarachnoid Aneurysm Trial (ISAT) of neurosurgical clipping versus endovascular coiling in 2143 patients with ruptured intracranial aneurysms: a randomised trial. Lancet 2002;360:1267–74.

122. Molyneux AJ, Kerr R, Langham J, et al. Applicability of coiling for subarachnoid haemorrhage. Lancet 2005;366:1924.

123. Molyneux AJ, Kerr RS, Birks J, et al. Risk of recurrent subarachnoid haemorrhage, death, or dependence and standardised mortality ratios after clipping or coiling of an intracranial aneurysm in the International Subarachnoid Aneurysm Trial (ISAT): long-term follow-up. Lancet Neurol 2009;8:427–33.

124. Scott RB, Eccles F, Molyneux AJ, et al. Improved cognitive outcomes with endovascular coiling of ruptured intracranial aneurysms: neuropsychological outcomes from the International Subarachnoid Aneurysm Trial (ISAT). Stroke 2010;41:1743–7.

125. McDougall CG, Spetzler RF, Zabramski JM, et al. The Barrow ruptured aneurysm trial. J Neurosurg 2012;116:135–44.

126. Pierot L, Cognard C, Ricolfi F, et al. Mid-term anatomic results after endovascular treatment of ruptured intracranial aneurysms with Guglielmi detachable coils and matrix coils: analysis of the CLARITY series. AJNR Am J Neuroradiol 2012;33(3):469–73.

127. Pierot L, Cognard C, Ricolfi F, et al. Immediate anatomic results after the endovascular treatment of ruptured intracranial aneurysms: analysis in the CLARITY series. AJNR Am J Neuroradiol 2010;31:907–11.

128. Dumont AS, Crowley RW, Monteith SJ, et al. Endovascular treatment or neurosurgical clipping of ruptured intracranial aneurysms: effect on angiographic vasospasm, delayed ischemic neurological deficit, cerebral infarction, and clinical outcome. Stroke 2010;41:2519–24.

129. Lee T, Baytion M, Sciacca R, et al. Aggregate analysis of the literature for unruptured intracranial aneurysm treatment. AJNR Am J Neuroradiol 2005;26:1902–8.

130. Pierot L, Spelle L, Vitry F. Immediate anatomic results after the endovascular treatment of unruptured intracranial aneurysms: analysis of the ATENA series. AJNR Am J Neuroradiol 2010;31:140–4.

131. White PM, Lewis SC, Gholkar A, et al. Hydrogel-coated coils versus bare platinum coils for the

endovascular treatment of intracranial aneurysms (HELPS): a randomised controlled trial. Lancet 2011;377:1655–62.

132. Coley S, Sneade M, Clarke A, et al. Cerecyte coil trial: procedural safety and clinical outcomes in patients with ruptured and unruptured intracranial aneurysms. AJNR Am J Neuroradiol 2012;33:474–80.

133. MAPS trial. In: Endovascular Today. July 2011.

134. Moret J, Cognard C, Weill A, et al. Reconstruction technic in the treatment of wide-neck intracranial aneurysms. Long-term angiographic and clinical results. Apropos of 56 cases. J Neuroradiol 1997; 24:30–44 [in French].

135. Aletich VA, Debrun GM, Misra M, et al. The remodeling technique of balloon-assisted Guglielmi detachable coil placement in wide-necked aneurysms: experience at the University of Illinois at Chicago. J Neurosurg 2000;93:388–96.

136. Fiorella D, Woo HH. Balloon assisted treatment of intracranial aneurysms: the conglomerate coil mass technique. J Neurointerv Surg 2009;1:121–31.

137. Fiorella D, Albuquerque FC, Masaryk TJ, et al. Balloon-in-stent technique for the constructive endovascular treatment of "ultra-wide necked" circumferential aneurysms. Neurosurgery 2005; 57:1218–27 [discussion: 1227].

138. Pierot L, Cognard C, Spelle L, et al. Safety and efficacy of balloon remodeling technique during endovascular treatment of intracranial aneurysms: critical review of the literature. AJNR Am J Neuroradiol 2012;33:12–5.

139. Spiotta AM, Bhalla T, Hussain MS, et al. An analysis of inflation times during balloon-assisted aneurysm coil embolization and ischemic complications. Stroke 2011;42:1051–5.

140. Shapiro M, Babb J, Becske T, et al. Safety and efficacy of adjunctive balloon remodeling during endovascular treatment of intracranial aneurysms: a literature review. AJNR Am J Neuroradiol 2008;29: 1777–81.

141. Mu SQ, Yang XJ, Li YX, et al. Endovascular treatment of wide-necked intracranial aneurysms using of "remodeling technique" with the HyperForm balloon. Chin Med J (Engl) 2008;121:725–9.

142. Nelson PK, Levy DI. Balloon-assisted coil embolization of wide-necked aneurysms of the internal carotid artery: medium-term angiographic and clinical follow-up in 22 patients. AJNR Am J Neuroradiol 2001;22:19–26.

143. Layton KF, Cloft HJ, Gray LA, et al. Balloon-assisted coiling of intracranial aneurysms: evaluation of local thrombus formation and symptomatic thromboembolic complications. AJNR Am J Neuroradiol 2007;28:1172–5.

144. Leon MB, Baim DS, Popma JJ, et al. A clinical trial comparing three antithrombotic-drug regimens after coronary-artery stenting. Stent Anticoagulation Restenosis Study Investigators. N Engl J Med 1998;339:1665–71.

145. Higashida RT, Halbach VV, Dowd CF, et al. Initial clinical experience with a new self-expanding nitinol stent for the treatment of intracranial cerebral aneurysms: the Cordis Enterprise stent. AJNR Am J Neuroradiol 2005;26:1751–6.

146. Weber W, Bendszus M, Kis B, et al. A new self-expanding nitinol stent (Enterprise) for the treatment of wide-necked intracranial aneurysms: initial clinical and angiographic results in 31 aneurysms. Neuroradiology 2007;49:555–61.

147. Mocco J, Snyder KV, Albuquerque FC, et al. Treatment of intracranial aneurysms with the Enterprise stent: a multicenter registry. J Neurosurg 2009; 110:35–9.

148. Mocco J, Fargen KM, Albuquerque FC, et al. Delayed thrombosis or stenosis following enterprise-assisted stent-coiling: is it safe? Midterm results of the interstate collaboration of enterprise stent coiling. Neurosurgery 2011;69:908–13 [discussion: 913–4].

149. Lv X, Li Y, Xinjian Y, et al. Results of endovascular treatment for intracranial wide-necked saccular and dissecting aneurysms using the Enterprise stent: a single center experience. Eur J Radiol 2012;81(6):1179–83.

150. Kis B, Weber W, Berlit P, et al. Elective treatment of saccular and broad-necked intracranial aneurysms using a closed-cell nitinol stent (Leo). Neurosurgery 2006;58:443–50 [discussion: 450].

151. Gao X, Liang G, Li Z, et al. Complications and adverse events associated with Neuroform stent-assisted coiling of wide-neck intracranial aneurysms. Neurol Res 2011;33:841–52.

152. Liang G, Gao X, Li Z, et al. Neuroform stent-assisted coiling of intracranial aneurysms: a 5 year single-center experience and follow-up. Neurol Res 2010; 32:721–7.

153. Lylyk P, Ferrario A, Pasbon B, et al. Buenos Aires experience with the Neuroform self-expanding stent for the treatment of intracranial aneurysms. J Neurosurg 2005;102:235–41.

154. Biondi A, Janardhan V, Katz JM, et al. Neuroform stent-assisted coil embolization of wide-neck intracranial aneurysms: strategies in stent deployment and midterm follow-up. Neurosurgery 2007;61: 460–8 [discussion: 468–9].

155. Shapiro M, Becske T, Sahlein D, et al. Stent-supported aneurysm coiling: a literature survey of treatment and follow-up. AJNR Am J Neuroradiol 2012;33:159–63.

156. Fargen KM, Hoh BL, Welch B, et al. Long-term results of enterprise stent-assisted coiling of cerebral aneurysms. Neurosurgery 2012;71(2):239–44.

157. Raymond J, Guilbert F, Roy D. Neck-bridge device for endovascular treatment of wide-neck bifurcation

aneurysms: initial experience. Radiology 2001;221:318–26.

158. De Keukeleire K, Vanlangenhove P, Defreyne L. Evaluation of a neck-bridge device to assist endovascular treatment of wide-neck aneurysms of the anterior circulation. AJNR Am J Neuroradiol 2008;29:73–8.

159. Molyneux AJ, Cekirge S, Saatci I, et al. Cerebral Aneurysm Multicenter European Onyx (CAMEO) trial: results of a prospective observational study in 20 European centers. AJNR Am J Neuroradiol 2004;25:39–51.

160. Piske RL, Kanashiro LH, Paschoal E, et al. Evaluation of Onyx HD-500 embolic system in the treatment of 84 wide-neck intracranial aneurysms. Neurosurgery 2009;64:E865–75 [discussion: E875].

161. Cekirge HS, Saatci I, Ozturk MH, et al. Late angiographic and clinical follow-up results of 100 consecutive aneurysms treated with Onyx reconstruction: largest single-center experience. Neuroradiology 2006;48:113–26.

162. Fiorella D, Kelly ME, Albuquerque FC, et al. Curative reconstruction of a giant midbasilar trunk aneurysm with the pipeline embolization device. Neurosurgery 2009;64:212–7 [discussion: 217].

163. Kallmes DF, Ding YH, Dai D, et al. A new endoluminal, flow-disrupting device for treatment of saccular aneurysms. Stroke 2007;38:2346–52.

164. Kallmes DF, Ding YH, Dai D, et al. A second-generation, endoluminal, flow-disrupting device for treatment of saccular aneurysms. AJNR Am J Neuroradiol 2009;30:1153–8.

165. Lylyk P, Miranda C, Ceratto R, et al. Curative endovascular reconstruction of cerebral aneurysms with the pipeline embolization device: the Buenos Aires experience. Neurosurgery 2009;64:632–42 [discussion: 642–3], [quiz: N6].

166. Fiorella D, Woo HH, Albuquerque FC, et al. Definitive reconstruction of circumferential, fusiform intracranial aneurysms with the pipeline embolization device. Neurosurgery 2008;62:1115–20 [discussion: 1120–1].

167. Kadziolka K, Estrade L, Leautaud A, et al. Flow diverter treatment for tiny, uncoilable, ruptured intracranial aneurysms: silk stent experience. Neuroradiology 2009;51(Suppl 1):S38.

168. Nelson PK, Lylyk P, Szikora I, et al. The pipeline embolization device for the intracranial treatment of aneurysms trial. AJNR Am J Neuroradiol 2011;32:34–40.

169. Byrne JV, Beltechi R, Yarnold JA, et al. Early experience in the treatment of intra-cranial aneurysms by endovascular flow diversion: a multicentre prospective study. PLoS One 2010;5. pii:e12492.

170. Summary of safety and effectiveness data PED, Food and Drug Administration, Advisory Committee. 2011. Available at: http://www.fda.gov/downloads/AdvisoryCommittees/CommitteesMeetingMaterials/NeurologicalDevicesPanel/UCM247165.pdf. Accessed April 12, 2012.

171. Deutschmann HA, Wehrschuetz M, Augustin M, et al. Long-term follow-up after treatment of intracranial aneurysms with the Pipeline embolization device: results from a single center. AJNR Am J Neuroradiol 2012;33:481–6.

172. McAuliffe W, Wycoco V, Rice H, et al. Immediate and midterm results following treatment of unruptured intracranial aneurysms with the pipeline embolization device. AJNR Am J Neuroradiol 2012;33:164–70.

173. McAuliffe W, Wenderoth JD. Immediate and midterm results following treatment of recently ruptured intracranial aneurysms with the Pipeline embolization device. AJNR Am J Neuroradiol 2012;33:487–93.

174. Doerfler A, Wanke I, Egelhof T, et al. Aneurysmal rupture during embolization with Guglielmi detachable coils: causes, management, and outcome. AJNR Am J Neuroradiol 2001;22:1825–32.

175. Hirai T, Suginohara K, Uemura S, et al. Management of aneurysm perforation during Guglielmi electrodetachable coil placement. AJNR Am J Neuroradiol 2002;23:738–9.

176. Ricolfi F, Le Guerinel C, Blustajn J, et al. Rupture during treatment of recently ruptured aneurysms with Guglielmi electrodetachable coils. AJNR Am J Neuroradiol 1998;19:1653–8.

177. Halbach VV, Higashida RT, Dowd CF, et al. Management of vascular perforations that occur during neurointerventional procedures. AJNR Am J Neuroradiol 1991;12:319–27.

178. Wada H, Piotin M, Boissonnet H, et al. Carotid rupture during stent-assisted aneurysm treatment. AJNR Am J Neuroradiol 2004;25:827–9.

179. Mounayer C, Piotin M, Baldi S, et al. Intraarterial administration of Abciximab for thromboembolic events occurring during aneurysm coil placement. AJNR Am J Neuroradiol 2003;24:2039–43.

180. Kwon OK, Lee KJ, Han MH, et al. Intraarterially administered abciximab as an adjuvant thrombolytic therapy: report of three cases. AJNR Am J Neuroradiol 2002;23:447–51.

Endovascular Treatment of Cerebral Vasospasm
Vasodilators and Angioplasty

Aditya S. Pandey, MD[a], Augusto E. Elias, DDS, MD[b],
Neeraj Chaudhary, MD, MRCS, FRCR[a],
Byron G. Thompson, MD[a], Joseph J. Gemmete, MD, FSIR[c],*

KEYWORDS

• Vasospasm • Balloon angioplasty • Triple-H therapy • SAH • Mechanical and chemical angioplasty

KEY POINTS

• Calcium channel blockers, magnesium, 3-hydroxy-3-methylglutaryl coenzyme A (HMG CoA) reductase inhibitors (statins), fasudil, thrombolytics, endothelial receptor antagonists, and tirilazad have all been used in attempts to prevent and treat vasospasm.

• Hypervolemia, hypertension, and hemodilution therapy (triple-H) has long been a mainstay of medical therapy in patients with aneurysmal SAH.

• Endovascular treatment with intra-arterial infusion of a vasodilator or balloon angioplasty is indicated in patients with symptomatic vasospasm refractory to medical therapy to prevent neurologic deficits referable to the vascular territory of the angiographic vasospasm.

• Papaverine, verapamil, nimodipine, and nicardipine have been used as intra-arterial vasodilators to treat patients with symptomatic vasospasm refractory to medical therapy.

• Two different balloon technologies have been used for treatment of vasospasm: coronary balloons and more compliant intracranial balloons.

INTRODUCTION

Cerebral vasospasm following aneurysmal subarachnoid hemorrhage (SAH) is a delayed, reversible narrowing of the intracranial vasculature that occurs most commonly 4 to 14 days after aneurysmal SAH and can lead to permanent ischemic injury (Fig. 1). Although it has been the focus of much research and clinical effort, vasospasm remains difficult to treat and is responsible for significant morbidity and mortality in patients with ruptured cerebral aneurysms. Angiographic spasm occurs in up to 70% of patients following SAH, and approximately half become symptomatic. In the past, mortality rates from vasospasm have been reported to range from 30% to 70%, with 10% to 20% of patients experiencing severe neurologic deficits.[1,2]

With advancements in diagnostic and interventional technology, estimates of patients who are disabled by vasospasm, or die because of it, range from 5% to 9%, with vasospasm accounting for 12% to 17% of all fatalities or cases of disability after SAH.[3,4] We have an incomplete understanding of the pathophysiology of vasospasm, and it is difficult to predict which patients will develop vasospasm after SAH. The Hunt and Hess grade, Fisher score, hypertension, smoking, cocaine

[a] Division of Interventional Neuroradiology, Departments of Neurosurgery and Radiology, University of Michigan Hospitals, 1500 East Medical Center Drive, Ann Arbor, MI 48109-5030, USA; [b] Division of Interventional Neuroradiology, Department of Radiology, University of Michigan Hospitals, 1500 East Medical Center Drive, Ann Arbor, MI 48109-5030, USA; [c] Division of Interventional Neuroradiology and Cranial Base Surgery, Departments of Radiology, Neurosurgery, and Otolaryngology, University of Michigan Hospitals, UH B1 D328, 1500 East Medical Center Drive, Ann Arbor, MI 48109-5030, USA
* Corresponding author.
E-mail address: gemmete@med.umich.edu

Neuroimag Clin N Am 23 (2013) 593–604
http://dx.doi.org/10.1016/j.nic.2013.03.008
1052-5149/13/$ – see front matter © 2013 Elsevier Inc. All rights reserved.

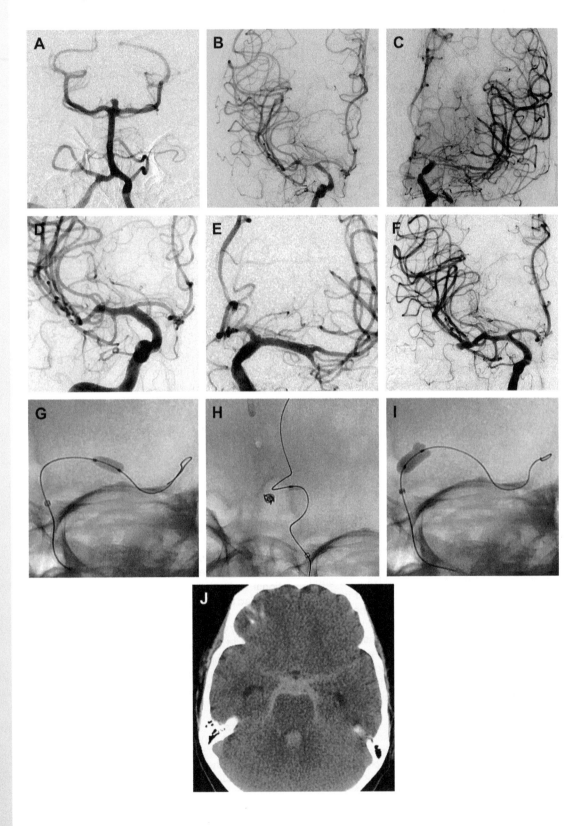

use, age range of 40 to 59 years, and early rise in the middle cerebral artery blood flow on transcranial Doppler have been shown to be independent risk factors for vasospasm.[4] Cerebral salt wasting has also been associated with vasospasm. This article discusses the multiple medical and endovascular therapies that are used to prevent or treat vasospasm.

VASOSPASM PROPHYLAXIS AND MEDICAL TREATMENT

Prophylactic treatment for cerebral vasospasm following aneurysmal SAH is controversial and varies among institutions. Calcium channel blockers, magnesium, 3-hydroxy-3-methylglutaryl coenzyme A (HMG CoA) reductase inhibitors (statins), fasudil, thrombolytics, endothelial receptor antagonists, and tirilazad have all been used in attempts to prevent and treat vasospasm. In addition, triple-H (hypervolemia, hypertension, and hemodilution) therapy has been a mainstay of vasospasm treatment for years. At our institution, we start all patients with SAH with triple H as soon as the aneurysm has been secured, as long as there are no medical contraindications, such as congestive heart failure or severe pulmonary disease. We use prophylactic nimodipine and magnesium sulfate and are considering using statins as new data emerge.

Calcium Channel Antagonists

Calcium channel antagonists have been shown to decrease the overall incidence of cerebral infarction after SAH by 34% and the incidence of poor outcomes by 40%.[5] The physiologic reasoning behind the use of calcium channel blockers is that the central event in vascular smooth muscle contraction is the influx of calcium into cells, which has been shown to occur after SAH.[6] This, in turn, leads to several downstream events, including free radical formation, production of vasoconstricting prostaglandins, and activation of the myosin light chain kinase that causes smooth muscle contraction. The most common calcium channel blocker used after SAH is nimodipine, which has a certain degree of specificity for the cerebral vessels. Multiple trials have shown its efficacy in improving outcomes, although it may not improve angiographic outcome.[5,7–12]

Two randomized controlled trials (RCTS) using nicardipine for treatment of and prevention of cerebral vasospasm have been performed. The largest RCT treated 449 patients with intravenous (IV) nicardipine (0.15 mg/kg/h) and 457 patient with placebo.[13] Patients treated with nicardipine had significantly reduced vasospasm compared with placebo ($P<.001$). Clinical outcomes were similar between the 2 groups at 3 months. Another small study that randomized 16 patients to receive nicardipine prolonged-release implants placed into the basal cisterns at the time of surgical clip placement demonstrated significantly reduced angiographic vasospasm incidence ($P<.05$) and improved modified Rankin Scale scores at 1 year.[14]

Magnesium

Obstetricians have used magnesium to treat eclampsia, as magnesium is thought to alter calcium physiology and thus alter vascular tone in the uterine circulation. Magnesium competes with calcium-binding sites, thus preventing muscular contraction and allowing vascular muscle relaxation. Level 1 evidence now exists for the usage of magnesium sulfate in the prevention of cerebral vasospasm. Westermaier and colleagues[15] have shown that magnesium sulfate significantly reduces cerebral ischemic events after SAH.[16–19]

Statins

Five RCTS have used statins for the prevention and treatment of cerebral vasospam following SAH.[20–24] Three of the trials have shown a benefit for statins in reducing vasospasm, delayed ischemic neurologic deficits (DINDs), and

---

Fig. 1. (*A*) Anterior posterior (AP) left vertebral angiogram shows a basilar tip aneurysm. (*B*) AP right internal carotid angiogram 10 days after hemorrhage demonstrates diffuse vasospasm involving the internal carotid artery, anterior cerebral artery, and middle cerebral artery. (*C*) AP left internal carotid angiogram 10 days after hemorrhage demonstrates diffuse vasospasm involving the internal carotid artery, anterior cerebral artery, and middle cerebral artery. (*D*) AP right internal carotid angiogram after balloon angioplasty and infusion of IA nicardipine shows angiographic resolution of the vasospasm. (*E*) AP left internal carotid angiogram after balloon angioplasty and infusion of IA nicardipine shows angiographic resolution of the vasospasm. (*F*) AP right internal carotid angiogram same patient shows an additional middle cerebral artery aneurysm. (*G*) Spot AP fluoroscopic image shows a hyperform balloon in the left middle cerebral artery. (*H*) Spot AP fluoroscopic images shows a gateway balloon in the left A1 segment. (*I*) Spot AP fluoroscopic images shows a hyperform balloon in the distal internal carotid artery, note a small portion of the balloon has herniated into the left A1 segment. (*J*) Axial CT of the head demonstrates diffuse high attenuation material within the subarachnoid space consistent with hemorrhage.

mortality.[20–22] However, 2 of the more recent trials have shown no significant difference in reducing vasospasm and clinical outcome.[23,24]

Fasudil

Fasudil acts as a calcium channel blocker via the Rho-kinase signaling pathway inhibition. It antagonizes the vasoconstrictive effects of endothelin by dilating cerebral arteries in an animal vasospasm model.[25] Fasudil has been studied in 2 RCTs.[25,26] Shibuya and colleagues[26] showed significant reductions in angiographic and symptomatic vasospasm, hypodensities on computed tomography (CT) scan, and poor outcome with use of the drug. In another study, Zhao and colleagues[25] compared IV fasudil to IV nimodipine and found no significant differences in vasospasm incidence or clinical outcome.

Thrombolytics

Two RCTs have been performed using thrombolytic therapy for the prevention or treatment of cerebral vasospasm.[27,28] Findlay[27] in an RCT of 100 patients who received either a 1-time intracisternal bolus of 10 mg of tissue plasminogen activator (t-PA) or placebo at the time of surgical clip placement found a significant reduction in severe vasospasm without improvement in outcome. Hamada and colleagues,[28] in another randomized controlled trial (RCT) of 110 patients who received either intrathecal urokinase (60,000 International units (IU) over 20 minutes) or no thrombolytic therapy following aneurysm coiling, showed a significant reduction in symptomatic vasospasm with improved outcome.

Endothelin receptor antagonists

A subclass of drugs has been developed to inhibit the binding of endothelin I, a potent vasoconstrictive peptide, to its target receptors of vascular smooth muscle cells. Two drugs in this class, clazosentan and TAK-044, have been studied in RCTs for the treatment and prevention of cerebral vasospasm following aneurysmal SAH.[29–31] Shaw and colleagues,[29] in study of 402 patients who were randomized to IV TAK-044 or placebo, found a decreased incidence of delayed cerebral infarction without improvement in the Glasgow Outcome Scale. Furthermore, Vajkoczy and colleagues,[30] in a small RCT comparing patients receiving IV clazosentan to placebo, found a significant reduction in cerebral vasospasm incidence and severity. Fifty percent of the crossover placebo patients had reversal of vasospasm following the initiation of clazosentan. The Clazosentan to Overcome Neurologic Ischemia and Infarction Occurring After Subarachnoid Hemorrhage (CONSCIOUS-I) trial randomized 413 patients to either dose-escalated clazosentan or placebo. Significant dose-dependent reductions in moderate and severe vasospasm were noted with increased pulmonary complications, hypotension, and anemia.[31]

TRIPLE-H THERAPY

Hypervolemia, hypertension, and hemodilution therapy (triple-H) has long been a mainstay of medical therapy in patients with aneurysmal SAH. The rationale behind triple-H therapy is that maintenance of high circulating blood volume, increased perfusion pressures, and decreased blood viscosity will enhance cerebral blood flow in the setting of vasoconstriction. Although in healthy adults, changes in cardiac output do not change the local cerebral flow, they do affect cerebral blood flow in patients suffering from cerebral vasospasm. Our goal is to maintain euvolemia as defined by the central venous/wedge pressure that allows for the highest cardiac output.

The vast majority of our patients with SAH receive central lines so that central venous pressures can be closely monitored to achieve optimized volume expansion without causing pulmonary edema. We prefer central venous pressures in the range of 8 to 12 mm Hg, but these are highly individualized and must be closely monitored in relation to the clinical findings in each patient. Patients with cardiopulmonary disease may need to be evaluated with a Swan Ganz catheter, as the ideal venous pressure in these patients needs to be related to the ideal cardiac output.[32] One series of 184 patients reported a 13% risk of device-related sepsis in patients with pulmonary artery catheters, as well as a 2.0% risk of congestive heart failure, 1.3% risk of subclavian vein thrombosis, and 1.0% risk of pneumothorax.[32] Most patients with SAH require invasive blood pressure monitoring. In the post-clipping or post-coiling vasospasm period, we often allow patients to autoregulate with systolic blood pressure in the range of 200 mm Hg. The role of red blood cell transfusion is not well studied, but transfusion could certainly increase the oxygen carrying capacity. Three RCTs have evaluated the efficacy of triple-H therapy.[33–35]

ENDOVASCULAR THERAPY

Endovascular treatment with intra-arterial (IA) infusion of a vasodilator or balloon angioplasty is indicated in patients with symptomatic vasospasm refractory to medical therapy to prevent neurologic deficits referable to the vascular territory of the angiographic vasospasm. Any patient who is a candidate for cerebral angioplasty in the context of cerebral vasospasm must be evaluated with a CT scan of the head to rule out hemorrhage and the presence of hypodensity in the vascular territory to undergo angioplasty. A vessel diameter reduction between 25% and 50% from the initial angiographic diameter is usually treated with IA infusion of vasodilators. Vessel diameter reductions greater than 50% from the initial angiographic diameter are treated with a combination of mechanical and chemical angioplasty. The timing of endovascular intervention for vasospasm is critical, and a 2-hour window from the time of symptoms may exist for restoration of blood flow to ultimately improve the patient's outcome.[36]

INTRA-ARTERIAL VASODILATORS
Papaverine

The most studied IA pharmacologic agent to date is papaverine. It is an opium alkaloid that is thought to alter adenosine $3',5'$–cyclic monophosphate levels in smooth muscles (Table 1).[37] The half-life is approximately 2 hours. In a review of IA agents for treatment of cerebral vasospasm, Hoh and Ogilvy[38] reported that papaverine produced clinical improvement in only 43% of the treated patients. The effectiveness of treatment was short given its half-life; therefore, multiple treatments were required, which led to a variable and increased risk of complications. Platz and colleagues[39] more recently reported a case of spontaneous hemorrhage following IA use of papaverine. They hypothesized that local increased levels of infused papaverine possibly led to a blood–brain barrier (BBB) breakdown with subsequent intracranial hemorrhage. Furthermore, there has been a recent report from Pennings and colleagues.[40]

They observed an abnormal response to topical application of papaverine on the cerebral cortical microvasculature during aneurysm surgery. They noted rebound vasoconstriction in 2 of 14 cases. In the cases in which there was some increase in vessel diameter compared with baseline, it did not reach statistical significance. There is wide variation in the IA use of papaverine in terms of dosage and duration of infusion.[40] Firlik and colleagues[41] demonstrated no correlation with the clinical response and angiographic picture in cases of vasospasm from aneurysmal SAH treated with IA papaverine. In their cohort of 15 patients, they had 23 IA treatments with papaverine, leading to partial angiographic reversal in 18 of the 23 IA treatments. However, major clinical improvement was seen in only 6 treatments and minor improvement or none in 17.

Papaverine hydrochloride is supplied as a 3% concentration, 30 mg/mL, in an acidic mixture of pH 3.3. Papaverine may form crystal precipitates, with crystal size up to 100 μm, when mixed with human serum at 3.0% or 0.3% concentrations. A precipitate has also been seen when 3% papaverine solution was mixed with heparinized saline in concentrations of 2000 to 10,000 units of heparin per liter. The typical papaverine concentration infused is 0.3%, produced by diluting 300 mg of papaverine in 100 mL of normal saline. The entire dose (300 mg) is given in a vascular territory over 20 to 30 minutes. If more than 1 vascular territory is involved, additional infusions of 300 mg can be given. The catheter for infusion in the anterior circulation should be placed past the ophthalmic artery to prevent possible precipitate being introduced into the retina. In the posterior circulation, the catheter should be positioned past the origin of the anterior inferior cerebellar artery to prevent

Table 1
Intra-arterial agents for the treatment of vasospasm

Agent	Typical Intra-arterial Dose	Half-Life, Hours	Side Effects
Papaverine	300 mg per vascular territory at 0.3% concentration over 20 min.	2	Cortical necrosis, permanent neurologic deficits, raised intracranial pressure, systemic hypotension
Verapamil	1–2-mg bolus over 2 min with maximum of 10 mg per vascular territory.	7	Increased intracranial pressure
Nimodipine	1–3 mg at 25% dilution over 10–30 min in each vascular territory; maximum dose 5 mg.	9	Increased intracranial pressure
Nicardipine	0.2–0.5 mg/mL in ml aliquots; maximum dose of 20 mg per vascular territory.	16	Increased intracranial pressure

respiratory arrest and the potential of cardiac dysfunction because of transient depression of the medullary respiratory and cardiovascular nuclei. Papaverine can cause systemic hypotension and elevation of intracranial pressure during infusion; therefore, these parameters should be monitored closely.

Side effects from IA infusion of papaverine also included transient neurologic deficits, such as mydriasis, transient hemiparesis, and respiratory depression. Given the short half-life, the transient effect on the local cerebral vasculature, and significant side effects, we no longer use papaverine for chemical angioplasty at our institution.

CALCIUM CHANNEL ANTAGONISTS

With the complications associated with papaverine, use of calcium channel antagonists (verapamil, nimodipine, nicardipine) for the treatment of cerebral vasospasm has become more typical. These agents are still not approved by the Food and Drug Administration in the United States for IA use in the cerebral vasculature.

Verapamil

Verapamil is a phenylalkylamine calcium channel blocker that inhibits voltage-gated calcium channels in the arterial wall smooth muscle cells, resulting in vasodilatation. The half-life is approximately 7 hours. Feng and colleagues[42] reported on the IA use of verapamil in 29 patients who underwent 34 procedures; 52% were treated with verapamil alone, which resulted in 44% experiencing increased vessel diameters and 33% exhibiting neurologic improvements without complications or intracranial pressure (ICP) issues. The vasodilation effects of verapamil are still transient and poorly sustained, and no studies thus far have demonstrated significant patient outcome benefit.

Verapamil is usually infused in a 1-mg to 2-mg bolus over 2 minutes, with a total maximal dose of 10 mg administered into each vascular territory. In their small cohort of 10 patients, Keuskamp and colleagues[43] have demonstrated the efficacy of using high doses of verapamil (total 41 ± 29 mg per procedure) without significant alteration of ICP, cerebral perfusion pressure, or other side effects. In their series, the neurologic deficits that prompted endovascular treatment of vasospasm improved in 8 of 12 procedures. In a recent report of a case series of again 12 patients, Albanese and colleagues[44] documented the use of ultra high doses of verapamil for treatment of vasospasm. They used an average dose of 164.6 mg (range 70 mg to 720 mg) of verapamil per vessel for infusion through an indwelling microcatheter. They

demonstrated improvement in 9 of 12 patients. Only 1 patient had the infusion stopped because of ICP increasing beyond 20 cm H_2O.

Major complications of intravenous verapamil are hypotension and bradycardia; however, no significant changes in blood pressure or heart rate have been reported with IA infusion. No prolonged or dramatic increase in ICP has been reported, as mentioned previously. IA verapamil administration appears to be safe with few systemic effects in the limited number of patients studied.

Nimodipine

Nimodipine is a dihydropyridine agent that has a mechanism of action similar to that of verapamil, but it has a slightly longer half-life of 9 hours. The systemic application of nimodipine has been proven to be an effective agent on clinical outcome after SAH in several clinical trials.[45] Hänggi and colleagues[46] recently analyzed the effect of IA nimodipine in the treatment of severe cerebral vasospasm due to aneurysmal SAH. In their small cohort of 26 patients, 8 (30.8%) had treatment failure with no angiographic response to IA nimodipine. Seven of the 18 patients who had angiographic response went on to develop additional cerebral infarctions related to the vasospasm. Although the results do not suggest nimodipine to have sustained benefit in improving patient outcome, they do demonstrate a trend toward improved cerebral perfusion parameters that were sustained for a period of 24 hours. The investigators conclude that the vasodilatory effect of IA nimodipine in the treatment of vasospasm is still transient albeit better than that of papaverine. In terms of patient numbers, Hänggi and colleagues[46] demonstrated that of the 11 patients who were clinically assessable, 7 had no change in neurologic status post-application of IA nimodipine, and only 2 had neurologic improvement, whereas 2 had worsening in their Glasgow Coma Scale (GCS) score. These results are in contrast to the 76% clinical improvement shown in another cohort of patients with aneurysmal SAH and vasospasm treated with IA nimodipine by Biondi and colleagues.[47]

Nimodipine is administered by diluting 1 to 3 mg with 15 to 45 mL of normal saline to obtain a dilution of 25%. This is then infused at a slow continuous infusion over 10 to 30 minutes (approximately 0.1 mg/min). The total dose reported in the literature has not been greater than 5 mg per procedure.[48] In their recent report of 19 patients treated with IA nimodipine, Kim and colleagues[48] demonstrated improvements in flow in 42 of

53 procedures and an improvement in clinical outcome after 23. They used nimodipine in a 10% concentration infused slowly at 0.1 mg nimodipine per minute. The main systemic complications of nimodipine include hypotension, rash, diarrhea, and bradycardia. No significant changes in heart rate, blood pressure, or ICP have been reported in the literature from IA administration.

Nicardipine

Nicardipine is also a dihydropyridine agent that has an even longer half-life of almost 16 hours. It has a more selective effect on vascular smooth muscle than cardiac muscle. Several studies have demonstrated that continuous IV nicardipine infusion significantly decreases the incidence of symptomatic, angiographic, and transcranial Doppler vasospasm, but the efficacy is limited by prolonged hypotension, pulmonary edema, and renal dysfunction. Badjatia and colleagues[49] previously demonstrated that the use of IA nicardipine induces more sustained reversal of vasospasm than does papaverine. They demonstrated a 42.1% neurologic improvement in patients following treatment with IA nicardipine. Although this is encouraging, the investigators also highlight the incidence of increased ICP following treatment in 6 patients. Tejada and colleagues[50] more recently showed that a higher-dose regimen of IA nicardipine is more efficacious. They used a total dose of 10 to 40 mg in each patient. GCS and Glasgow Outcome Scale (GOS) scores in 10 of 11 patients who were treated with the high-dose regimen improved. The investigators also demonstrated a low complication rate and a sustained clinical outcome benefit with a GOS score of 1 or 2 in 9 of 10 patients with at least 2-month follow-up.

Nicardipine is usually administered intraarterially by diluting with normal saline to a concentration of 0.2 mg/mL and infusing in 1-mL aliquots to a maximum dose between 2.5 and 20.0 mg per vessel.[50] At our institution we recently adopted a more aggressive approach, and use a 1-mg/mL dosage concentration infusing in 3-mL aliquots with a maximum dosage of 20 mg per vessel. Prolonged hypotension, pulmonary edema, and renal dysfunction have been reported following the IV administration of nicardipine; however, these findings have not been reported with IA administration.[50] The main adverse effect reported in the literature is an increase in ICP, which usually can be controlled with ventricular drainage. Tejada and colleagues demonstrated the safe use of a high dose of IA nicardipine in their series of 11 patients with vasospasm.[50] However, ICP monitoring was possible in only 2 of the 11 patients who did not demonstrate any change during IA infusion of nicardipine.

Other Agents

There are other pharmaceutical agents with various other mechanisms of vasodilatation, namely magnesium sulfate, HMG CoA reductase inhibitors, nitric oxide donors, and endothelin-1 antagonists. The neuroprotective and vasoprotective properties of magnesium sulfate have been well documented in the literature. Shah and colleagues[51] recently evaluated a cohort of patients in whom magnesium sulfate was used in conjunction with nicardipine for IA treatment of aneurysmal SAH-related vasospasm. They observed that this agent was well tolerated by the patients, with no adverse effects on ICP. They did not observe any statistically significant difference in clinical outcome improvement in comparison with other studies with cohorts treated only with nicardipine.

TRANSLUMINAL BALLOON ANGIOPLASTY

The mechanism of cerebral blood vessel narrowing in aneurysmal SAH is not clearly understood. Inflammatory changes mediating smooth muscle contraction, changes in the linkage of the protein matrix, and collagen deposition in the vessel wall have all been implicated as a possible cause of blood vessel narrowing in SAH related to aneurysm rupture (**Table 2**).

Mechanical dilation of intracranial vessels was performed first in 1984 by Zubkov and colleagues.[52] They reported their results in selected patients with large-vessel spasm. Balloons for intracranial angioplasty have developed considerably since then. The most significant limitation of these angioplasty balloons remains the inability to treat spasm affecting the distal cerebral vasculature. The current thinking is that transluminal balloon angioplasty (TBA) acts by stretching the vessel wall, leading to morphologic and functional changes in the smooth muscle fibers, resulting in impairment of contractility. At a cellular level it has been shown that there is fragmentation of the collagen matrix and flattening of the endothelial cells, resulting in permanent restoration of vessel diameter. This has been demonstrated to be durable in both canine and primate models.

Eskridge and colleagues[53] reported 50 patients with 170 treated arterial segments. They demonstrated sustained neurologic improvement in only 61% of patients within 72 hours following angioplasty. Rosenwasser and colleagues[36] sought to identify an optimal time frame for treatment of vasospasm from aneurysmal SAH. They demonstrated that 61% of patients treated within 2 hours had

Table 2
Balloons used for transluminal balloon angioplasty

Balloon Catheters	Technique	Dimensions	Manufacturer	Qualities
Hyperform	Over-the-wire balloon catheter with single lumen (0.010 expedion wire)	Balloon diameter: 4 mm, 7 mm Balloon length: 7 mm	ev3, Irvine, CA	Readily conformable
Hyperglide	Over-the-wire balloon catheter with single lumen (0.010 expedion wire)	Balloon diameter: 4 mm, 5 mm Balloon lengths (by diameter): 4/10, 4/15, 4/20, 4/30, 5/15, 5/20	ev3	Compliant balloon, rigid in longer length
Gateway	Over-the-wire balloon catheter with separate lumen for inflation, tracks over a 0.014 wire	Balloon diameter: 1.5, 2.0, 2.25, 3.0, 3.5, 4 mm Balloon lengths (by diameter): 1.5/9, 2.0/9, and 15, 20 mm in the other dimensions	(Stryker Neurovascular, Fremont, CA)	Comparatively rigid but available in smaller diameters
Scepter C	Over-the-wire balloon catheter with separate lumen for inflation, tracks over a 0.014 wire	Balloon diameter: 4.0 mm Balloon Lengths (10, 15, 20 mm)	(Microvention, Inc, Tustin, CA)	Compliant balloon catheter
Scepter XC	Over-the-wire balloon catheter with separate lumen for inflation, tracks over a 0.014 wire	Balloon diameter: 4.0 mm Balloon Length: 11 mm	Microvention	X-tra compliant occlusion balloon
Ascent	Over-the-wire balloon catheter with separate lumen for inflation, tracks over a 0.014 wire	Balloon diameter: 4.0, 6.0 mm Balloon lengths (by diameter): 4.0/7, 10, 15 and 6.0/9	(Codman Neurovascular, Raynham, MA)	Compliant balloon catheter

angiographic improvement in 90% of cases and a sustained clinical improvement in 70% of cases; in contrast, the other 39% of cases treated more than 2 hours later achieved 88% angiographic improvement but sustained only a 40% clinical improvement.[6] In summary, TBA has shown benefit in restoring antegrade flow in the treated cerebral vascular territory and some improvement in patient outcomes. Although anecdotal reports suggest that TBA provides durable relief of vasospasm, no RCTs using therapeutic angioplasty alone have been published to date. The only RCT of TBA compared prophylactic TBA or no prophylactic treatment within 96 hours of aneurysm rupture.[54] Patients undergoing prophylactic TBA experienced a nonsignificant reduction in DIND incidence ($P = .30$). A significant decrease in therapeutic angioplasty ($P = .03$) was observed, however, for patients who had prophylactic TBA compared with controls. There is still a lack of level 1 evidence

supporting balloon angioplasty for treatment of cerebral vasospasm in the literature, however.

Typical locations of vessels amenable to TBA are vertebral, basilar, supraclinoid internal carotid artery (ICA), and M1 segments. Less common locations, because of their small diameter, are the posterior communicating, A1, M2, and P1 arteries. In general, TBA in vessels with a diameter smaller than 2 mm may have a higher risk of vessel rupture. Hence, the posterior inferior communicating artery (PICA), anterior inferior communicating artery (AICA), A2, M3, and P2 arterial branches are usually avoided altogether.

Two different balloon technologies have been used for treatment of vasospasm: coronary balloons and more compliant intracranial balloons. The coronary balloon catheter technology comprises a stiff balloon membrane composed of polyethylene or nylon and a double-lumen shaft, one lumen for balloon inflation and the other for passage of a range of 0.014-inch guidewires. The short Maverick coronary balloons (Boston Scientific, Natick, MA) allow greater maneuverability and cause less vessel straightening and distortion. These balloons typically have tight size-to–inflation pressure calibration. Typically, a 2-mm-diameter balloon is used for the middle cerebral artery and 1.5 mm for A1 or M2 branches. Similar technology developed for dedicated intracranial use is the Gateway system (Boston Scientific), which is available in balloon sizes ranging from 1.5-mm-diameter to 4.0-mm-diameter (outer diameter at nominal inflation) and 10.0, 15.0, and 20.0 mm in length. This system has been designed for angioplasty of intracranial stenoses.

The other more compliant balloon catheter systems use a softer semipermeable silicone/elastomer membrane loaded on a single-lumen, more flexible catheter shaft. These balloons are designed to navigate over a 0.010-inch X-Pedion (ev3, Irvine, CA) guidewire. There are 2 types of balloons: HyperForm (ev3) and HyperGlide (ev3). The HyperForm is a softer balloon (4/7 × 7 mm) than the HyperGlide, which has a longer length (4 × 10/15/20/30 mm). These balloons are both over-the-wire systems. The distal end of the catheter has a small valve at the tip, which is occluded when the 0.010-inch wire passes 10 cm past the tip of the catheter. This design allows for a smaller profile, a less dense catheter, excellent distal access, and excellent guide-catheter compatibility. In addition, by using a mechanical seal for the balloon inflation, air management can be confidently and efficiently controlled. Some operators use a 0.08-inch wire, such as the Mirage wire (ev3), claiming that it allows the balloon to decompress if overinflated, thus conferring a possible safety mechanism. The wire should not be allowed to track proximal to the balloon in vivo, as this causes blood to track into the balloon and thus makes deflation difficult or inadequate and can potentially lead to complications, such as vessel rupture from overinflation of the balloon. The balloon is calibrated to the volume injected and is inflated with a highly calibrated threaded 1-mL Cadence (ev3) syringe that enables adjustments in the 0.01-mL range. The operator has to be very careful when inflating these balloons, as their maximum diameter is large; hence, inflation should cease once the soft balloon starts to conform to the vessel lumen diameter. All of the balloons mentioned previously should be inflated with a 50/50 or 60/40 concentration of 300 mg/mL iodinated contrast and saline for optimal visualization and deflation. Higher concentrations can lead to incomplete deflation and thus vessel damage.

Newer balloons have come on the market over the past 6 months including the Scepter and Ascent, which are compliant and track over a 0.014 wire. These are easier to prep and use than the older balloons and seem to navigate better in the intracranial circulation, given that they are delivered over a 0.014 wire.

Transluminal balloon angioplasty itself has some potential significant risks. These include vessel rupture due to the balloon being larger than the vessel diameter. In cases of critical spasm, there may be a poor roadmap because of minimal antegrade flow with the arterial vessels. This can lead to malpositioning of the balloon, which, for example, can accidentally get lodged in the posterior communicating artery rather than the supraclinoid ICA or in a lenticulostriate vessel rather than the M1, thus resulting in rupture of that vessel. Arterial dissection can also occur from angioplasty. These balloons can be flow limiting or may cause thrombus or pseudoaneurysm formation. Furthermore, thrombus or platelet aggregates can form around the balloon or in the catheter lumen, because of the increased thrombogenic state in patients with SAH. To avoid this, patients undergoing TBA typically are heparinized to an activated clotting time of 250 seconds unless contraindicated. Finally, there is the potential risk of hemorrhage or reperfusion injury by restoration of blood flow in a vascular territory with prolonged ischemia.

CURRENT CONCEPTS IN COMBINATION (eV3) THERAPY

The discrepancy in the clinical correlation with large-vessel vasospasm suggests that microvascular vasospasm is more crucial to overcome to improve clinical outcome. However, flow-limiting large-vessel luminal narrowing due to spasm can compromise the concentration of IA vasodilators in the distal cerebral microvasculature. It thus makes intuitive sense to combine both TBA, to improve proximal flow and thus to be able to deliver therapeutic and effective concentration and volume of IA vasodilators to the smaller distal cerebral microvasculature. It is controversial which should be performed first—TBA or IA vasodilator infusion. One argument is that initial IA vasodilator infusion may increase the proximal diameter of a target vessel to successfully place a balloon catheter in it for TBA. The durability of chemical angioplasty is unknown; however, TBA is thought to be a more durable modality than chemical angioplasty. Larger multicenter prospective randomized trials are necessary to create level 1 evidence to assess the efficacy of combination therapy with the newly available technology with compliant balloons and longer-acting IA vasodilators.

FUTURE ENDOVASCULAR THERAPIES

Our understanding of the phenomenon of vasospasm due to aneurysmal SAH is still evolving. A better understanding of the pathophysiologic insult to the brain at ictus will enable us to understand the phenomenon of vasospasm better and will enable better design in the therapy to improve patient outcome. Novel methods of production of animal vasospasm models are needed to evaluate various IA or TBA therapies to ultimately improve patient outcome. Animal models will play a key role in evaluating different variables in the understanding of cerebral vasospasm.

SUMMARY

The jury is still out on which IA endovascular pharmaceutical agent exclusively or in conjunction with TBA is the optimal treatment of cerebral vasospasm. There is a trend toward some benefit provided by the longer-acting calcium channel blockers in combination with TBA. Newer agents on the horizon specifically targeting the vascular endothelium without a wide spectrum of side effects need to be tried and tested in larger prospective randomized patient cohorts. Improved animal models of vasospasm are being validated in studies. These models should form the cornerstone of optimizing treatment by helping to develop a better understanding of the phenomenon of cerebral vasospasm due to SAH from a ruptured aneurysm.

REFERENCES

1. Hop JW, Rinkel GJ, Algra A, et al. Case-fatality rates and functional outcome after subarachnoid hemorrhage: a systematic review. Stroke 1997;28: 660–4.
2. Komotar RJ, Zacharia BE, Valhora R, et al. Advances in vasospasm treatment and prevention. J Neurol Sci 2007;261:134–42.
3. Roos YB, de Haan RJ, Beenen LF, et al. Complications and outcome in patients with aneurysmal subarachnoid haemorrhage: a prospective hospital based cohort study in the Netherlands. J Neurol Neurosurg Psychiatry 2000;68:337–41.
4. Zwienenberg-Lee M, Hartman J, Rudisill N, et al. Endovascular management of cerebral vasospasm. Neurosurgery 2006;59:S139–47 [discussion: S3–13].
5. Pickard JD, Murray GD, Illingworth R, et al. Effect of oral nimodipine on cerebral infarction and

6. Rothoerl RD, Ringel F. Molecular mechanisms of cerebral vasospasm following aneurysmal SAH. Neurol Res 2007;29:636–42.
7. Allen GS, Ahn HS, Preziosi TJ, et al. Cerebral arterial spasm—a controlled trial of nimodipine in patients with subarachnoid hemorrhage. N Engl J Med 1983;308:619–24.
8. Neil-Dwyer G, Mee E, Dorrance D, et al. Early intervention with nimodipine in subarachnoid haemorrhage. Eur Heart J 1987;8(Suppl K):41–7.
9. Ohman J, Servo A, Heiskanen O. Long-term effects of nimodipine on cerebral infarcts and outcome after aneurysmal subarachnoid hemorrhage and surgery. J Neurosurg 1991;74:8–13.
10. Petruk KC, West M, Mohr G, et al. Nimodipine treatment in poor-grade aneurysm patients. Results of a multicenter double-blind placebo-controlled trial. J Neurosurg 1988;68:505–17.
11. Philippon J, Grob R, Dagreou F, et al. Prevention of vasospasm in subarachnoid haemorrhage. A controlled study with nimodipine. Acta Neurochir (Wien) 1986;82:110–4.
12. Rinkel GJ, Feigin VL, Algra A, et al. Calcium antagonists for aneurysmal subarachnoid haemorrhage. Cochrane Database Syst Rev 2005;(1):CD000277.
13. Haley EC Jr, Kassell NF, Torner JC. A randomized controlled trial of high-dose intravenous nicardipine in aneurysmal subarachnoid hemorrhage. A report of the Cooperative Aneurysm Study. J Neurosurg 1993;78:537–47.
14. Barth M, Capelle HH, Weidauer S, et al. Effect of nicardipine prolonged-release implants on cerebral vasospasm and clinical outcome after severe aneurysmal subarachnoid hemorrhage: a prospective, randomized, double-blind phase IIa study. Stroke 2007;38:330–6.
15. Westermaier T, Stetter C, Vince GH, et al. Prophylactic intravenous magnesium sulfate for treatment of aneurysmal subarachnoid hemorrhage: a randomized, placebo-controlled, clinical study. Crit Care Med 2010;38:1284–90.
16. Muroi C, Terzic A, Fortunati M, et al. Magnesium sulfate in the management of patients with aneurysmal subarachnoid hemorrhage: a randomized, placebo-controlled, dose-adapted trial. Surg Neurol 2008;69:33–9 [discussion: 9].
17. van den Bergh WM, Algra A, van Kooten F, et al. Magnesium sulfate in aneurysmal subarachnoid hemorrhage: a randomized controlled trial. Stroke 2005;36:1011–5.
18. Veyna RS, Seyfried D, Burke DG, et al. Magnesium sulfate therapy after aneurysmal subarachnoid hemorrhage. J Neurosurg 2002;96:510–4.
19. Wong GK, Chan MT, Boet R, et al. Intravenous magnesium sulfate after aneurysmal subarachnoid

outcome after subarachnoid haemorrhage: British aneurysm nimodipine trial. BMJ 1989;298:636–42.

hemorrhage: a prospective randomized pilot study. J Neurosurg Anesthesiol 2006;18:142–8.

20. Lynch JR, Wang H, McGirt MJ, et al. Simvastatin reduces vasospasm after aneurysmal subarachnoid hemorrhage: results of a pilot randomized clinical trial. Stroke 2005;36:2024–6.

21. McGirt MJ, Woodworth GF, Pradilla G, et al. Galbraith Award: simvastatin attenuates experimental cerebral vasospasm and ameliorates serum markers of neuronal and endothelial injury in patients after subarachnoid hemorrhage: a dose-response effect dependent on endothelial nitric oxide synthase. Clin Neurosurg 2005;52:371–8.

22. Tseng MY, Czosnyka M, Richards H, et al. Effects of acute treatment with pravastatin on cerebral vasospasm, autoregulation, and delayed ischemic deficits after aneurysmal subarachnoid hemorrhage: a phase II randomized placebo-controlled trial. Stroke 2005;36:1627–32.

23. Chou SH, Smith EE, Badjatia N, et al. A randomized, double-blind, placebo-controlled pilot study of simvastatin in aneurysmal subarachnoid hemorrhage. Stroke 2008;39:2891–3.

24. Vergouwen MD, Meijers JC, Geskus RB, et al. Biologic effects of simvastatin in patients with aneurysmal subarachnoid hemorrhage: a double-blind, placebo-controlled randomized trial. J Cereb Blood Flow Metab 2009;29:1444–53.

25. Zhao J, Zhou D, Guo J, et al. Effect of fasudil hydrochloride, a protein kinase inhibitor, on cerebral vasospasm and delayed cerebral ischemic symptoms after aneurysmal subarachnoid hemorrhage. Neurol Med Chir (Tokyo) 2006;46:421–8.

26. Shibuya M, Suzuki Y, Sugita K, et al. Effect of AT877 on cerebral vasospasm after aneurysmal subarachnoid hemorrhage. Results of a prospective placebo-controlled double-blind trial. J Neurosurg 1992;76:571–7.

27. Findlay JM. A randomized trial of intraoperative, intracisternal tissue plasminogen activator for the prevention of vasospasm. Neurosurgery 1995;37: 1026–7.

28. Hamada J, Kai Y, Morioka M, et al. Effect on cerebral vasospasm of coil embolization followed by microcatheter intrathecal urokinase infusion into the cisterna magna: a prospective randomized study. Stroke 2003;34:2549–54.

29. Shaw MD, Vermeulen M, Murray GD, et al. Efficacy and safety of the endothelin, receptor antagonist TAK-044 in treating subarachnoid hemorrhage: a report by the Steering Committee on behalf of the UK/Netherlands/Eire TAK-044 Subarachnoid Haemorrhage Study Group. J Neurosurg 2000;93:992–7.

30. Vajkoczy P, Meyer B, Weidauer S, et al. Clazosentan (AXV-034343), a selective endothelin A receptor antagonist, in the prevention of cerebral vasospasm following severe aneurysmal subarachnoid

hemorrhage: results of a randomized, double-blind, placebo-controlled, multicenter phase IIa study. J Neurosurg 2005;103:9–17.

31. Macdonald RL, Kassell NF, Mayer S, et al. Clazosentan to overcome neurological ischemia and infarction occurring after subarachnoid hemorrhage (CONSCIOUS-1): randomized, double-blind, placebo-controlled phase 2 dose-finding trial. Stroke 2008;39:3015–21.

32. Rosenwasser RH, Jallo JI, Getch CC, et al. Complications of Swan-Ganz catheterization for hemodynamic monitoring in patients with subarachnoid hemorrhage. Neurosurgery 1995;37:872–5 [discussion: 5–6].

33. Egge A, Waterloo K, Sjoholm H, et al. Prophylactic hyperdynamic postoperative fluid therapy after aneurysmal subarachnoid hemorrhage: a clinical, prospective, randomized, controlled study. Neurosurgery 2001;49:593–605 [discussion: 6].

34. Lennihan L, Mayer SA, Fink ME, et al. Effect of hypervolemic therapy on cerebral blood flow after subarachnoid hemorrhage: a randomized controlled trial. Stroke 2000;31:383–91.

35. Rosenwasser RH, Delgado TE, Buchheit WA, et al. Control of hypertension and prophylaxis against vasospasm in cases of subarachnoid hemorrhage: a preliminary report. Neurosurgery 1983;12:658–61.

36. Rosenwasser RH, Armonda RA, Thomas JE, et al. Therapeutic modalities for the management of cerebral vasospasm: timing of endovascular options. Neurosurgery 1999;44:975–9 [discussion: 979–80].

37. Macdonald RL, Weir BK, Young JD, et al. Cytoskeletal and extracellular matrix proteins in cerebral arteries following subarachnoid hemorrhage in monkeys. J Neurosurg 1992;76:81–90.

38. Hoh BL, Ogilvy CS. Endovascular treatment of cerebral vasospasm: transluminal balloon angioplasty, intra-arterial papaverine, and intra-arterial nicardipine. Neurosurg Clin N Am 2005;16:501–16, vi.

39. Platz J, Barath K, Keller E, et al. Disruption of the blood-brain barrier by intra-arterial administration of papaverine: a technical note. Neuroradiology 2008;50:1035–9.

40. Pennings FA, Albrecht KW, Muizelaar JP, et al. Abnormal responses of the human cerebral microcirculation to papaverin during aneurysm surgery. Stroke 2009;40:317–20.

41. Firlik KS, Kaufmann AM, Firlik AD, et al. Intra-arterial papaverine for the treatment of cerebral vasospasm following aneurysmal subarachnoid hemorrhage. Surg Neurol 1999;51:66–74.

42. Feng L, Fitzsimmons BF, Young WL, et al. Intraarterially administered verapamil as adjunct therapy for cerebral vasospasm: safety and 2-year experience. AJNR Am J Neuroradiol 2002;23:1284–90.

43. Keuskamp J, Murali R, Chao KH. High-dose intraarterial verapamil in the treatment of cerebral vasospasm

after aneurysmal subarachnoid hemorrhage. J Neurosurg 2008;108:458–63.

44. Albanese E, Russo A, Quiroga M, et al. Ultrahigh-dose intraarterial infusion of verapamil through an indwelling microcatheter for medically refractory severe vasospasm: initial experience. Clinical article. J Neurosurg 2010;113:913–22.

45. Barker FG 2nd, Ogilvy CS. Efficacy of prophylactic nimodipine for delayed ischemic deficit after subarachnoid hemorrhage: a metaanalysis. J Neurosurg 1996;84:405–14.

46. Hänggi D, Beseoglu K, Turowski B, et al. Feasibility and safety of intrathecal nimodipine on posthaemorrhagic cerebral vasospasm refractory to medical and endovascular therapy. Clin Neurol Neurosurg 2008;110:784–90.

47. Biondi A, Ricciardi GK, Puybasset L, et al. Intra-arterial nimodipine for the treatment of symptomatic cerebral vasospasm after aneurysmal subarachnoid hemorrhage: preliminary results. AJNR Am J Neuroradiol 2004;25:1067–76.

48. Kim JH, Park IS, Park KB, et al. Intraarterial nimodipine infusion to treat symptomatic cerebral vasospasm after aneurysmal subarachnoid hemorrhage. J Korean Neurosurg Soc 2009;46:239–44.

49. Badjatia N, Topcuoglu MA, Pryor JC, et al. Preliminary experience with intra-arterial nicardipine as a treatment for cerebral vasospasm. AJNR Am J Neuroradiol 2004;25:819–26.

50. Tejada JG, Taylor RA, Ugurel MS, et al. Safety and feasibility of intra-arterial nicardipine for the treatment of subarachnoid hemorrhage-associated vasospasm: initial clinical experience with high-dose infusions. AJNR Am J Neuroradiol 2007;28:844–8.

51. Shah QA, Memon MZ, Suri MF, et al. Super-selective intra-arterial magnesium sulfate in combination with nicardipine for the treatment of cerebral vasospasm in patients with subarachnoid hemorrhage. Neurocrit Care 2009;11:190–8.

52. Zubkov YN, Nikiforov BM, Shustin VA. Balloon catheter technique for dilatation of constricted cerebral arteries after aneurysmal SAH. Acta Neurochir (Wien) 1984;70:65–79.

53. Eskridge JM, McAuliffe W, Song JK, et al. Balloon angioplasty for the treatment of vasospasm: results of first 50 cases. Neurosurgery 1998;42:510–6 [discussion: 6–7].

54. Zwienenberg-Lee M, Hartman J, Rudisill N, et al. Effect of prophylactic transluminal balloon angioplasty on cerebral vasospasm and outcome in patients with Fisher grade III subarachnoid hemorrhage: results of a phase II multicenter, randomized, clinical trial. Stroke 2008;39:1759–65.

Endovascular Treatment of Cerebral Arteriovenous Malformations

Mohammad Yashar Sorena Kalani, MD, PhD[a],
Felipe C. Albuquerque, MD[a],*, David Fiorella, MD[b,†],
Cameron G. McDougall, MD[a]

KEYWORDS

• Arteriovenous malformation • Complications • Endovascular embolization • Management

KEY POINTS

• In the year after a symptomatic hemorrhage from a cerebral arteriovenous malformation (AVM), the rate of hemorrhage is believed to be higher, in the order of 6% to 18% per year, returning to the 2% to 4% baseline over time.
• After an AVM ruptures, the risk of death is 10% and the risk of major disability is 20% to 30%.
• The operative morbidity and mortality rates are 1% and 3% for Grade I/II and Grade III cerebral AVMs, respectively.
• The morbidity and mortality rates in the immediate postoperative period associated with treating Grade IV and V cerebral AVMs may be as high as 31% and 50%, respectively.
• Grade IV and V cerebral AVMs are treated only in patients with progressive neurologic deficits attributable to repeated hemorrhage or disabling symptoms, such as intractable seizures.
• Current data suggest that partial treatment of cerebral AVMs increases the risk of future hemorrhage.
• In select patients with Grade IV and V AVMs, partial treatment targeted to eliminate an identified bleeding source (ie, intranidal aneurysm) may be undertaken.
• Embolization can be used to reduce the size of the AVM nidus to a range that is amenable to radio-surgical ablation.
• A small cerebral AVM with a limited number of feeding pedicles can be cured completely using endovascular embolization with a permanent agent (eg, n-butyl cyanoacrylate [NBCA] or Onyx, not particles).
• NBCA and Onyx are the primary liquid embolic agents used for endovascular treatment of cerebral AVMs.
• Flow-related aneurysms proximal to the nidus (feeding vessel or circle of Willis) and nidal aneurysms should be addressed before embolization of the AVM.
• A staged embolization for large cerebral AVMs is usually necessary with no more than 30% of the nidus obliterated in 1 session to prevent normal perfusion pressure breakthrough.
• Heparin is used when the venous outflow appears to be sluggish on the postembolization angiogram or if an important component of the venous outflow has been compromised.

[a] Division of Neurological Surgery, Barrow Neurological Institute, St. Joseph's Hospital and Medical Center, 350 West Thomas Road, Phoenix, AZ 85013, USA; [b] Department of Neurological Surgery, Stony Brook University Medial Center, 101 Nicolls Road, Stony Brook, NY 11794, USA
[†] Deceased.
* Corresponding author.
E-mail address: neuropub@dignityhealth.org

Neuroimag Clin N Am 23 (2013) 605–624
http://dx.doi.org/10.1016/j.nic.2013.03.009

INTRODUCTION

Arteriovenous malformations (AVMs) are relatively uncommon, highly complex vascular lesions that tend to occur in younger patients (20–40 years old).[1] These lesions often become symptomatic with hemorrhage, seizures, headache, or focal neurologic deficits. Although treatment paradigms differ across institutions, the most compelling reason for the treatment of these lesions is to prevent hemorrhage. Existing data indicate that partial treatment of AVMs is not helpful and may increase the rate of future hemorrhage. The goal in treatment, therefore, is complete obliteration of the AVM. Given the complex morphology of AVMs and their frequent location in eloquent regions of the brain, no single treatment modality has proved to be effective. More so than for any other vascular lesion, a combined multidisciplinary approach is essential to formulate a safe and effective treatment strategy.

FORMULATING A TREATMENT STRATEGY

The most critical step in the successful management of any AVM is formulation of a treatment plan based on an understanding of the natural history of the lesion and of the morbidity and mortality rates associated with various treatments.

Natural History

AVMs are usually identified after a hemorrhage[2]; therefore, the natural history of AVMs is not well described and is predominantly composed of retrospective analyses of selected populations (eg, those not undergoing surgery, patients with symptoms other than hemorrhage at presentation) yielding biased and relatively variable estimates of the rate of hemorrhage and its associated consequences.[3] Given this bias, most series estimate that the annual risk of hemorrhage is 2% to 4% per year.[4,5] In the year after a symptomatic hemorrhage, the rate of hemorrhage is believed to be higher, in the order of 6% to 18% per year, returning to the 2% to 4% baseline over time.[2,5–7] AVM hemorrhages are not as severe as those associated with aneurysmal subarachnoid hemorrhage; after an AVM ruptures, the risk of death is 10% and the risk of major disability is 20% to 30%.[2]

Morbidity and Mortality Rates Associated with Treatment

The risk of surgical intervention is directly related to the angioarchitecture and to the location of a particular AVM. This relationship is best represented by the Spetzler-Martin grading system,[8] as modified by Spetzler and Ponce.[9] In prospective studies, the Spetzler-Martin grade has been show to correlate reliably with surgical outcome.[9–12]

Hamilton and Spetzler reported favorable operative morbidity and mortality rates of 1% and 3% for Grade I/II and Grade III AVMs, respectively.[10] Morbidity and mortality rates in the immediate postoperative period associated with treating Grade IV and V AVMs may be as high as 31% and 50%, respectively. The morbidity and mortality rates decrease to 22% and 17%, respectively, at the time of the follow-up examination. Heros and colleagues[11] reported a similar relationship between Spetzler-Martin grade and outcome. The aforementioned studies have provided the foundation for most management decisions related to treating AVMs.

Based on these studies, the risk of hemorrhage from Grade I and II AVMs outweighs the risk of surgical resection; therefore, these lesions are treated surgically, frequently without preoperative embolization, the risk of which can approach or even surpass the risk of surgery. Grade III AVMs represent a complex and at times challenging treatment conundrum. These lesions can be heterogeneous and associated with highly variable rates of morbidity and mortality. Lawton[13] stratified these lesions into 3 additional angioarchitectural subcategories with low (2.9%), intermediate (7.1%), and high (14.8) risk of postsurgical death or new deficit. The treatment paradigm for these lesions involves preoperative embolization or radiosurgery followed by surgical resection.

The surgical resection of Grade IV and V AVMs is usually associated with a higher risk of morbidity and mortality than predicted from the natural history of these lesions. Han and colleagues[14] analyzed outcomes in a series of 73 consecutive patients with Grade IV and V AVMs and recommended observation in most cases (55 of 73). The annual risk of hemorrhage in this group was 1% per year. Given the low rate of hemorrhage and the increased likelihood of hemorrhage from a partially treated lesion, the investigators recommend treatment of Grades IV and V AVMs only in patients with progressive neurologic deficits attributable to repeated hemorrhage or disabling symptoms, such as intractable seizures.

INDICATIONS FOR ENDOVASCULAR THERAPY FOR AVMS

The role of endovascular therapy in the management of cerebral AVMs depends on the overall treatment plan. The indications for embolization of AVMs from most to least common are as follows: (1) preoperative embolization as a precursor to complete curative surgical resection, (2) targeted therapy to obliterate a source of hemorrhage, (3) preradiosurgery as a precursor to radiation therapy, (4) curative embolization to attempt to cure small lesions, and (5) palliative embolization to relieve symptoms attributed to shunting.

Preoperative Embolization

The embolization of an AVM is usually performed before curative surgical resection (Fig. 1). The goal of embolization is to decrease the blood supply to the malformation, thereby decreasing the level of technical difficulty and associated morbidity of surgical resection. The endovascular interventionist must be aware of the surgical complication rate associated with the resection of the lesion being treated and must assure that the risks of the embolization do not exceed those of the surgical resection. For example, the risk of embolizing a Grade II AVM cannot exceed the risk of surgical treatment, given that these lesions can be safely resected with minimal complications. A successful embolization reduces the size of the AVM nidus, occludes deep feeding vessels that are difficult to access and control surgically, reduces intraoperative hemorrhage, and delineates surgical resection planes by leaving behind a cast of the lesion. Aided by the embolization, the goal of the vascular neurosurgeon is to achieve a complete, curative resection of the AVM.

Current data suggest that partial treatment of AVMs increases the risk of future hemorrhage. Han and colleagues[14] observed a hemorrhage rate of 10.4% in patients with Grade IV and V AVMs after partial treatment, compared with a 1% risk in patients with observation. Miyamota

and colleagues[15] found an annual risk of hemorrhage of 14.6% in patients who underwent palliative treatment of cerebral AVMs. Wikholm and colleagues[16] observed an increased rate of hemorrhage and death in patients undergoing partial treatment that resulted in less than 90% obliteration of the nidus.

The efficacy of embolization of AVMs using n-butyl cyanoacrylate (NBCA) has been demonstrated in several clinical studies. Jafar and colleagues[17] demonstrated that the operative morbidity for large AVMs embolized preoperatively decreased to a level similar to that of small AVMs. DeMerritt and colleagues[18] reported similar results with preoperative embolization of large AVMs improving postsurgical outcomes in comparison with a control group of smaller AVMs that were not embolized. More recently, Weber and colleagues[19] reported their experience with Onyx for preoperative embolization and noted a mean nidus reduction of 84% after embolization in 47 patients. In their series of 28 patients, Natarajan and colleagues[20] obliterated a mean of 74.1% of the preoperative volume.

Targeted Therapy

Partial obliteration of an AVM increases the likelihood of hemorrhage. However, in select patients with Grade IV and V AVMs, partial treatment targeted to eliminate an identified bleeding source may be undertaken. AVM-associated aneurysms are identified in 7% to 20% of cases[21–24] and represent a significant risk factor for intracranial hemorrhage.[25] These aneurysms may be flow related and are located on a feeding vessel or

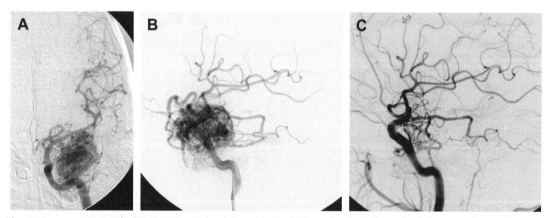

Fig. 1. Preoperative embolization. Posterior (A) and lateral (B) projections from the left internal carotid artery angiogram obtained from a 24-year-old man with a seizure disorder demonstrating a Grade III AVM involving the anterior left temporal lobe. (C) Angiogram shows that after 6 pedicle embolizations performed during a single session, the volume of the AVM is reduced substantially. (*From* Fiorella D, Albuquerque FC, Woo HH, et al. The role of neuroendovascular therapy for the treatment of brain arteriovenous malformations. Neurosurgery 2006;59(5 Suppl 3):S163–77; with permission.)

on vessels remote from the nidus.[26] In some cases, an intranidal aneurysm or intranidal pseudoaneurysm composed of an organized hematoma that communicates with the intravascular space formed after AVM hemorrhage may be present. Both intranidal and extranidal aneurysms are risk factors for intracranial hemorrhage in patients with AVMs. The increased risk of hemorrhage in the setting of an extranidal aneurysm may be attributed to aneurysm rupture rather than to hemorrhage from the AVM nidus.[21,26,27] When an unresectable AVM hemorrhages 1 or more times, endovascular exploration for a nidal aneurysm represents a reasonable strategy to embolize the aneurysm with a liquid embolic agent (nidal aneurysm) or coils (proximal flow-related aneurysm or remote aneurysm; Fig. 2).

Feeding vessel aneurysms can usually be identified by conventional angiography. Overlying vessels or other portions of the AVM nidus can obscure nidal aneurysms on conventional angiographic views. When aneurysms are difficult to visualize, superselective angiography, performed using high frame rates, can be used to identify and define the anatomy of lesions.

Preradiosurgery

A detailed discussion of the role of radiosurgery for the treatment of AVMs is beyond the scope of this article, and the reader is referred to excellent reviews on this topic.[28,29] The success of radiotherapy in treating AVMs is inversely proportional to the size of the nidus.[30,31] The goal of embolization is to reduce the size of the AVM nidus to a range that is amenable to radiosurgical ablation (Fig. 3), target nidal or feeding vessel aneurysms, and obliterate arteriovenous fistulae, which are usually refractory to treatment by radiosurgery. AVMs with nidal volume less than 10 mL (diameter <3 cm) can often be cured by radiosurgery, with rates of cure at 2 years estimated between 80% and 88%.[32,33] In preradiosurgical embolization, the use of a permanent embolizate, such as

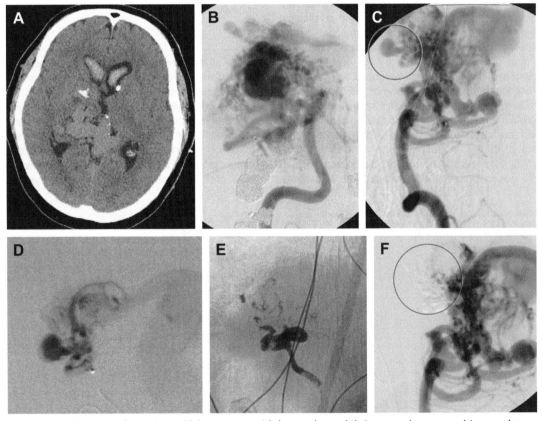

Fig. 2. Targeted therapy for an intranidal aneurysm with hemorrhage. (*A*) Computed tomographic scan shows a Grade V AVM in the right thalamic region with associated intraventricular hemorrhage. Posterior-anterior (*B*) and lateral (*C*) angiograms via the vertebral artery show an intranidal aneurysm projecting toward the ventricle (*circle*). (*D*) Superselective angiography shows the nidal aneurysm. (*E*) An unsubtracted fluoroscopic image shows the glue cast filling the nidal aneurysm. (*F*) Lateral vertebral artery angiogram shows no further filling of the aneurysm (*circle*). (*Courtesy of* Barrow Neurological Institute; with permission.)

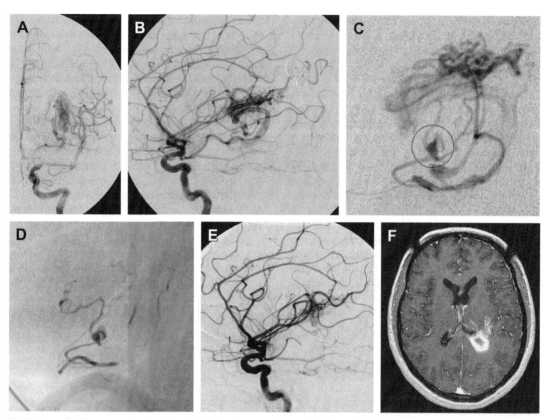

Fig. 3. Preradiotherapy embolization. (*A*) Posterior-anterior and (*B*) lateral left internal carotid artery angiograms show a deep frontoparietal AVM in a 38-year-old woman with intraventricular hemorrhage who presented with right hemiparesis. (*C*) Superselective angiogram shows a nidal aneurysm (*circle*). (*D*) Native fluoroscopic image shows the glue cast filling the nidal aneurysm. (*E*) Lateral angiogram shows no filling of the nidal aneurysm. (*F*) Soon thereafter the patient underwent Gamma Knife irradiation of her residual AVM. (*Courtesy of* Barrow Neurological Institute; with permission.)

NBCA (see later discussion), is essential to avoid recanalization of the portions of the embolized AVM not included in the radiation field.

The latency associated with radiosurgery to achieve a definitive effect on AVMs is 2 to 3 years. Of the available case series on combined endovascular/radiosurgical treatment of AVMs, most were conducted in the late 1980s and early 1990s, and many used particulate embolizates (eg, polyvinyl alcohol [PVA]).

The largest series, with 125 patients undergoing embolization (predominantly with NBCA) as a precursor to radiosurgery, achieved total occlusion in 11.2% of the AVMs after embolization alone; an additional 76% of lesions were reduced sufficiently to undergo radiotherapy.[34] A 65% rate of total occlusion was observed after radiotherapy in patients undergoing combined treatment. More recently, Henkes and colleagues[35] reported a series of 30 patients with high-grade AVMs undergoing combined embolization and radiotherapy. Their obliteration rate of 67% was less impressive.

Andrade-Souza and colleagues[36] reported nidus obliteration in 22 patients undergoing combined embolization and radiosurgery (47%) and in 33 patients (70%) undergoing radiosurgery alone. Their data suggest that preradiosurgery embolization may actually be detrimental to the effect of radiosurgery.

Several groups, however, have challenged this finding more recently. Back and colleagues[37] reported that their patients who underwent embolization followed by unstaged Gamma Knife surgery had a follow-up rate of 53.5% (15 of 28) and an obliteration rate of 60.0% (9 of 15). Patients who underwent embolization followed by staged Gamma Knife surgery had a follow-up rate of 85.7% (6 of 7) and an obliteration rate of 66.7% (4 of 6). Blackburn and colleagues[38] reported their experience with staged endovascular embolization followed by stereotactic radiosurgery for the treatment of large AVMs. Their AVM obliteration rate was 81% (13 of 16 cases). The newer data on combined endovascular/radiosurgical treatment of AVMs are more compelling and highlight this combined regimen as a viable option for the treatment of surgically challenging lesions.

Curative Therapy

Occasionally, a small AVM with a limited number of feeding pedicles can be cured completely using endovascular embolization with a permanent agent (eg, NBCA or Onyx, not particles, Fig. 4). Most studies on the isolated use of embolization for treating AVMs predate the advent of Onyx (ev3, Inc, Irvine, CA). With the widespread application of this agent, obliteration rates may be expected to increase. Vinuela and colleagues[39] reported a 9.7% cure rate for the embolization of small AVMs with few feeding pedicles. Gobin and colleagues[34] reported a cure rate of 11.2% (14 patients) in a series of 125 patients undergoing

preradiosurgical embolization. In this study, the chance of complete obliteration was inversely proportional to AVM volume and the number of feeding pedicles. Fournier and colleagues[40] reported a cure rate of 14% with embolization alone. Wikholm and colleagues[16] reported a complete obliteration rate of 13.3%, with success heavily dependent on the size of the AVM nidus: 71% for AVMs smaller than 4 mL and 15% for AVMs between 4 and 8 mL. Yu and colleagues[41] reported a 22% cure rate in 27 patients treated with cyanoacrylate embolization alone. These investigators found that the angiographic obliteration of the AVM was durable at 17 to 32 months with no recurrences or complications.

Katsaridis and colleagues[42] reviewed their experience with 101 patients treated with Onyx and identified total occlusion of AVMs in 28 of 101 (27.7%) and near total occlusion in 18 of 101

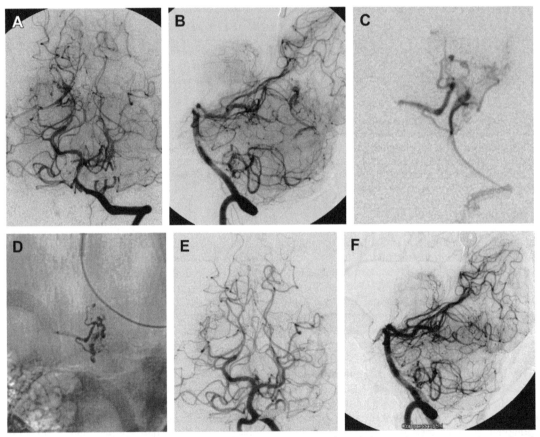

Fig. 4. Curative embolization. Towne (A) and (B) lateral projections from left vertebral artery angiography obtained from a 44-year-old woman who had undergone 2 previous unsuccessful attempts at AVM resection show a small diffuse AVM involving the right supracerebellar hemisphere. (C) Superselective angiography shows the small AVM fed from a single branch of the left superior cerebellar artery. (D) Native fluoroscopic image shows the glue cast filling the entire AVM. (E) Postembolization posterior-anterior angiography shows no evidence of residual AVM, which is confirmed on lateral angiography (F). ([A–E] From Fiorella D, Albuquerque FC, Woo HH, et al. The role of neuroendovascular therapy for the treatment of brain arteriovenous malformations. Neurosurgery 2006;59(5 Suppl 3):S163–77, with permission; [F] Courtesy of Barrow Neurological Institute; with permission.)

(17.8%). Their results are primary, as only 52 patients in their series had been treated completely; the remaining 49 required further embolization. They concluded that, with the introduction of Onyx, more AVMs would be amenable to complete curative embolization.

Similarly Maimon and colleagues[43] obtained complete obliteration by using embolization in 16 patients, resulting in a 55% cure rate in patients who concluded treatments (16 of 29). Abud and colleagues[44] used double arterial catheterization with simultaneous injection of Onyx in 17 patients and obtained curative embolization in 16 patients (94.1%). They advocated the use of this technique because it allows controlled hemodynamic filling of the AVM nidus.

Valavanis and Christoforidis[45] reported substantially higher cure rates (40%) in a consecutive series of 387 patients. These investigators identified the presence of direct, dominant feeding arteries, a monocompartmental nidus, and a dominant fistulous component of the nidus, without perinidal angiogenesis as the key characteristics predictive of endovascular cure. These investigators did not find size or number of feeding pedicles to be important determinants of the potential for endovascular obliteration. Others,[41] however, have clearly documented both size and feeding number of pedicles as important determinants of the likelihood for cure.

Palliative Therapy

Although the point is controversial, some investigators theorize that large AVMs cause progressive neurologic deficits, intellectual deterioration, or persistent headaches as a result of a vascular steal phenomenon, via shunting.[30,46] There is currently minimal evidence to support partial embolization in cases of suspected cerebrovascular steal.[47] Despite reports of increased likelihood of hemorrhage associated with partially treated AVMs, some investigators have advocated palliative, partial embolization to reduce the severity of arteriovenous shunting and to improve perfusion pressure in functional brain parenchyma.[14]

No large clinical series support this strategy, but several case reports have described success in small numbers of patients.[48,49] Fox and colleagues[50] reported that limb weakness improved in 3 patients after subtotal embolization of large AVMs located near the motor cortex. They attributed the improvement to a reduction in cerebrovascular steal. Rosenkranz and colleagues[51] reported 2 patients who underwent palliative embolization with resolution of the effects of shunting and intracranial hypertension secondary to inoperable AVMs. Simon and colleagues[52] report a single case of a patient whose symptoms of trigeminal neuralgia resolved after palliative embolization of a cerebellopontine angle AVM. The patient had a recurrence after 17 months and underwent another bout of palliative embolization. From a practical perspective, when such a strategy is undertaken, it is imperative to proceed cautiously and to avoid minimizing venous outflow.

EMBOLIZATES
Liquid Embolics

Liquid embolic agents are the most widely used and most effective for AVM embolization. The cyanoacrylate polymers (eg, NBCA) most commonly used of the liquid agents. The dimethyl sulfoxide (DMSO) solvent-based system ethylene-vinyl alcohol (EVOH) copolymer (Onyx) is a liquid nonadhesive embolic agent that became available in the United States in late 2005. In terms of its safety and efficacy, Onyx has recently been shown to be equivalent to NBCA as a preoperative embolic agent for reducing brain AVMs.[53] Ethanol (EtOH), an agent used effectively in treating peripheral AVMs, has been used successfully to treat cerebral AVMs.

Cyanoacrylate

Cyanoacrylates are liquid adhesive polymeric agents with several important advantages: (1) the potential for deep penetration into the AVM nidus; (2) permanent embolization with durable occlusion of the embolized vessel or pedicle; (3) the ability to be delivered through small, flexible, flow-directed catheters that can be manipulated safely and atraumatically into the most distal locations within the cerebrovasculature (Fig. 5); and (4) the ability to be delivered into the pedicle easily and quickly, with infusions usually requiring less than 1 minute. Several different cyanoacrylates have been used. The first agent available was iso-butyl-2-cyanoacrylate, but its use has now been discontinued after studies demonstrated that it possessed carcinogenic potential in animals.

NBCA is now the cyanoacrylate of choice for AVM embolization. Cyanoacrylates are introduced as liquid monomers that polymerize to form a stable solid when they contact a solution containing anions, such as the hydroxyl groups in blood. The rate of polymerization and the rate of injection determine how far the agent travels within the cerebral vasculature before solidifying. The NBCA itself is radiolucent and must be mixed with a radiopaque agent, typically ethiodized oil (eg, Lipiodol, Ethiodol). For most applications we use a

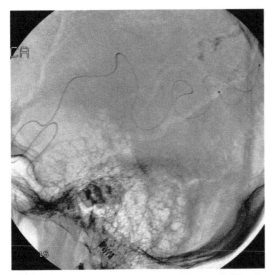

Fig. 5. Distal catheter position. Unsubtracted film obtained during the embolization of a left parietal lobe AVM providing an example of the extent to which the modern generation of flow-directed microcatheters (Elite 1.8-French; Boston Scientific, Natick, MA) can be efficiently and atraumatically manipulated into the most distal of locations within the cerebrovasculature. (*From* Fiorella D, Albuquerque FC, Woo HH, et al. The role of neuroendovascular therapy for the treatment of brain arteriovenous malformations. Neurosurgery 2006;59(5 Suppl 3):S163–77; with permission.)

1.5:1 to 3:1 (oil/NBCA) mixture. In addition to imparting radiopacity to the NBCA, the oil acts as a retardant, slowing the rate of polymerization and allowing the NBCA to travel further in the vessel before it solidifies.[54,55] Glacial acetic acid can also be added to the mixture in small quantities to retard the rate of further polymerization.[56]

After solidifying, the cyanoacrylates (if a sufficient volume has been injected) immediately occlude the embolized pedicle. The intense inflammatory reaction that follows leads to fibrous ingrowth, which, in turn, produces a durable occlusion.[16] Although recanalization can occur, it is rare after adequate embolization. Some disadvantages of the liquid adhesives include the high level of expertise required to control the injection safely to achieve adequate nidal penetration without allowing the agent to extend into the vein and the risk of NBCA adhering to the catheter, making it traumatic or impossible to withdraw the catheter.

EVOH Copolymer-DMSO Solvent

EVOH is a radiolucent polymeric agent that, in some respects, is similar to NBCA. This agent was first applied to the treatment of AVMs in the early 1990s[57] and has been commercially available in the United States as Onyx since late 2005. The most significant advantage of the EVOH copolymer is that it is nonadhesive, reducing the possibility of the catheter adhering to the injected polymer. The operator therefore has a greater degree of flexibility in terms of the volume and rate of the injection. Periodically, the operator may temporarily halt an EVOH-DMSO infusion to perform control angiography and to assess the status of the AVM nidus and draining veins before continuing the infusion.

Initial studies showed that the DMSO component of the mixture induced vasospasm and angionecrosis.[58,59] Jahan and colleagues[60] identified 1 complication (proximal reflux) related to distal vasospasm that developed during an injection. This same group also reported histopathologic evidence of angionecrosis in 2 AVM specimens resected 24 hours after embolization. Subsequent investigations indicated that the deleterious effects of DMSO could be eliminated by limiting its volume and rate of introduction.[61] Given the radiolucency of the EVOH-DMSO, tantalum powder must be mixed with the agent to provide radiopacity. Failure to mix the EVOH-DMSO-tantalum preparation constantly results in sedimentation of the tantalum from the mixture with subsequent variable opacification. The result is suboptimal visualization of the embolizate during its injection. Although long-term data are lacking, EVOH is, like NBCA, for all practical purposes, a permanent agent.[60,61]

EtOH

EtOH is a sclerosant, functioning to dehydrate and denude the endothelium, creating fractures within the vessel wall that extend to the level of the internal elastic lamina. These changes result in acute thrombosis of the vessel.[62] EtOH causes significant brain edema, necessitating treatment with high doses of steroids immediately before the procedure and for 2 weeks after. In some cases, brain edema and increases in intracranial pressure necessitate mannitol therapy.[63] In high doses, EtOH can induce pulmonary precapillary vasospasm, which can lead to cardiopulmonary collapse. This effect has been reported in humans after the embolization of peripheral AVMs with EtOH.

Based on the success associated with the use of EtOH in treating peripheral vascular malformations, Yakes and colleagues[62] advocated the use of undiluted absolute ethyl alcohol (98% dehydrated alcohol injection) for the embolization of AVMs involving the central nervous system. In their initial series of 17 patients, they obtained total occlusion in 7 patients with EtOH alone; 3 additional patients were cured after surgery and another 1 after radio-therapy.[62] Despite this impressive cure rate, there was a significant complication rate. Two patients with partially treated lesions died and 8 patients had treatment-related complications.

Others have reported intraprocedural complications associated with the use of EtOH. Unnikrishnan and colleagues[64] used EtOH to embolize a left parietooccipital AVM under general anesthesia. Despite general anesthesia, during injection of absolute EtOH into the AVM nidus, the patient developed hypertension and tachycardia coincident with a profound and sustained reduction of bispectral index values. This patient did not have a hemorrhage, but the hypertension and tachycardia are certainly worrisome byproducts of EtOH use. No other similar case series describing the application of EtOH have been reported to date. Given the risks associated with the use of EtOH, the high level of procedure-related complications, and the relatively widespread experience and comfort level with the cyanoacrylates, there has been a general reluctance among most endovascular interventionalists to use EtOH to embolize brain AVMs.

Particles

Many different particulate embolizates, including silk sutures, microfibrillar collagen material, PVA, and embolization microspheres, have been used to embolize AVMs.

PVA/Embospheres

Technically, embolization with particulate agents is fundamentally different from embolization with NBCA. To perform particulate embolization, a microcatheter with an internal diameter large enough to accept the particulate agent without clumping and clogging must be used. These catheters have a higher profile and are considerably less flexible than the smaller internal diameter flow-directed catheters. Given the structural limitations of these catheters, an over-the-wire technique must be used to negotiate the microcatheter into the region of the AVM nidus. These technical factors make superselective catheterization of pedicles feeding the nidus more labor intensive and more hazardous with a greater potential for vascular perforation.[65]

After a pedicle has been catheterized, the size of the particles chosen is based on the superselective angiogram. If superselective angiography shows large shunts, they must initially be occluded with coils to avoid direct arteriovenous shunting of the particles into the pulmonary circulation. Next, the particles must be injected through the catheter

gradually to occlude the vessels supplying the nidus with intermittent control angiography to assess flow. Unfortunately, the vessels coursing to the nidus are frequently of various calibers with differing degrees of shunting, making the selection of optimally sized particles challenging. Furthermore, multiple injections are typically required to occlude the pedicle over minutes rather than over seconds, as for NBCA.

In addition to the increased procedural time, there is the theoretic concern of temporarily pressurizing the nidus, as the higher flow, lower pressure, fistulous components become preferentially occluded. Theoretically, this situation increases the potential for intraprocedural hemorrhage. Particulate agents have also been reported to be more prone to recanalization than cyanoacrylates. Sorimachi and colleagues[66] reported a 43% rate of nidal recanalization after particulate embolization with PVA. Mathis and colleagues[67] reported a 12% recanalization rate for AVMs embolized with PVA in preparation for radiosurgery when portions of the AVM were not included in the radiation field.

Given the availability of more permanent embolizates, particulate agents are relatively contraindicated for the embolization of AVMs. Wallace and colleagues[68] reported a retrospective comparison of outcomes for 65 patients with AVMs embolized with either PVA or NBCA. The lowest complication rate was associated with NBCA embolization, which they attributed to a lower surgical complication rate. In a larger prospectively randomized trial comparing NBCA and PVA, the equivalency of the 2 agents was demonstrated with respect to the degree of nidal reduction, the number of vessels embolized, surgical resection times, transfusions, fluid replacement, and Glasgow Outcome Scale scores. A significant difference was identified only with respect to the rate of postsurgical hematoma, which was greater after PVA (8 of 45) than after NCBA (2 of 42).[65]

Coils

Coils, both detachable (eg, Guglielmi detachable coils) and injectable (Berenstein liquid coils), are useful for the occlusion of arteriovenous fistulae within the AVM nidus. The introduction of coils into the friable arterial feeders of an AVM, however, represents a risk of perforation. Detachable coils are most useful for the initial embolization of large fistulae. Depending on the size of the artery to be embolized, we usually select a complex three-dimensional geometry or a fibered 0.457 mm (0.018-in) detachable coil for the first coil. The coil is selected based on the size of the feeding artery as estimated on superselective angiography or guiding catheter angiography if the volume of shunting precludes complete opacification of the vessel after a microcatheter injection. We oversize the coil by 1 to 2 mm and choose the longest available coil that satisfies the diameter requirements. This coil can be manipulated within the feeding artery to achieve optimal positioning.

Visualization of the nondetached coil under fluoroscopy can provide some indication of its stability within the artery. After detachment of the first coil, a second soft coil of a diameter similar to the artery in the greatest length available is immediately introduced. After several coils have been introduced and a stable basket has been created, 1 or more liquid coils (0.254-mm [0.010-in] Berenstein liquid coils; Boston Scientific, Natick, MA) may be deployed. After the coil pack has adequately slowed the flow through the fistula, the pedicle may be occluded definitively with an injection of NBCA. Frequently, it is useful to induce hypotension (systolic blood pressure <90 mm Hg) for the NBCA injection to reduce the risk of NBCA passing through the fistula and into the venous system.

When detachable coils are used, the over-the-wire manipulation of a microcatheter with 2 distal markers into the pedicle is necessary, introducing the potential for vascular perforation. For this reason, it is useful to have an appropriate ethiodized oil/NBCA (2:1) mixture prepared for use before cannulization of the pedicle to be coiled.

If the coils are sized improperly, there is the potential for embolization through the fistula and into the venous system. If the arterial pedicle supplying the fistula is small enough, embolization with injectable or small 0.254 mm (0.010-in) pushable coils can be performed primarily. Liquid coils may be introduced through the smaller internal diameter, flexible, flow-directed microcatheters, eliminating the need for an exclusively over-the-wire catheterization.

PREOPERATIVE EMBOLIZATION TECHNIQUE
Goals of Embolization

Before initiation of the endovascular portion of AVM therapy, all members of the multidisciplinary team involved in the treatment of the lesion must understand the overall plan and goals of therapy, including the risks associated with microsurgical and endovascular treatment of the lesion. It is important to weigh these risks against those associated with each catheterization and each embolization. For example, if embolizing a Grade II AVM in a noneloquent region, it is critical that the risks of each embolization be minimized to avoid complicating an otherwise straightforward resection.

Imaging Assessment
Magnetic resonance imaging

The anatomic location of the lesion, including its size, location, proximity to venous structures and eloquence, is best defined on magnetic resonance (MR) imaging. MR imaging data provide important information about the status of the brain parenchyma surrounding the lesion, indicating regions of encephalomalacia or hemorrhage (recent or remote). The true size of the AVM nidus is sometimes better evaluated on conventional angiography, particularly if it has a diffuse component in which the small vessels are not well depicted on MR imaging.

Conventional angiography

AVMs are highly complex anatomic lesions; often with numerous tortuous arterial feeders winding around a nidus and rapidly flowing into 1 or more enlarged draining veins. In many cases, the specific arterial branches supplying the lesion can be difficult to identify without superselective angiography. However, the vascular distributions involved and the approximate number and size of the feeding arterial vessels can be ascertained. This information is usually sufficient to determine the number of staged embolizations needed.

When reviewing the angiographic images, the interventionalist should look for the presence of associated aneurysms. Flow-related aneurysms proximal to the nidus (feeding vessel or circle of Willis) and nidal aneurysms should be addressed before the AVM is embolized. The venous phase images represent a critical component of preembolization evaluation. During the venous phase, the operator should identify the number, size, and location of all draining veins before embolization. Not all draining veins are visualized with a single parent vessel injection because different parts of the nidus are opacified and are associated with patterns of contrast washout. The operator should be aware of the expected venous drainage pathways, including any venous stenoses that may be visualized from any given vascular injection. The inadvertent occlusion of venous efflux from the AVM nidus represents one of the most dangerous complications of embolization. Control angiography should be performed after each pedicle is embolized to reassess flow through the AVM and, in particular, to verify continued patency of venous efflux.

Staging

The number of embolizations that can be performed during a single session varies with the preference of the interventionist, the anatomy of the lesion, and the choice of the embolizate. One potential risk of over embolization of a large lesion is hemorrhage related to normal perfusion pressure breakthrough, the sequela of an abrupt reduction in arteriovenous shunting and sudden increase in the perfusion pressure of the adjacent normal brain parenchyma with impaired autoregulatory capacity (Fig. 6).[69]

In a patient with a large AVM scheduled for surgical resection the next day, we routinely perform between 5 and 7 NBCA embolizate infusions during a single session. Given the much larger volume of Onyx that can be injected from a single catheter position, the number of pedicles catheterized and the volume of embolizate injected are more variable and are assessed on a case-by-case basis. If a lesion is fed by multiple vascular distributions (eg, right internal carotid and vertebrobasilar arteries) and multiple sessions are to be performed, we prefer to embolize within only 1 vascular distribution during any given session. In general, we prefer multiple sessions to embolize AVMs larger than 3 cm (Fig. 7).

Technique

At Barrow Neurological Institute, all AVMs are embolized with the patient under general anesthesia and neuroelectrophysiologic monitoring (both somatosensory evoked potentials and electroencephalography). Although there is extensive debate about the benefit of awake continuous monitoring and Amytal testing, we prefer complete paralysis, tight control of the patient's blood pressure, and eradication of all motion during embolizate infusion. Before Onyx was introduced in 2005, all our embolization procedures were performed with NBCA. The following describes our technique using both agents. Regardless of the agent, we use the common femoral artery to obtain access and insert a 6-French sheath. Patients with unruptured AVMs are heparinized with a targeted activated coagulation time of 200 to 250 seconds throughout the procedure. For patients with ruptured AVMs, the decision to administer an anticoagulant is assessed on a case-by-case basis.

Using a 90-cm, 6-French guiding catheter (Envoy guiding catheter; Cordis Endovascular, Miami Lakes, FL), we gain access to the cervical segment of the artery targeted for embolization and identify the pedicles targeted for embolization. Depending on the choice of the embolizate, we prefer to use different catheters. If NBCA is to be used, we prefer the Elite microcatheter (Boston Scientific, Natick, MA) over a 0.20-mm (0.008-in) Mirage (ev3, Irvine, CA) microwire. If Onyx is to be used, we use either a Marathon (ev3) or Echelon microcatheter (ev3).

The Elite microcatheters are navigated primarily using a flow-directed technique. The microwire is usually maintained within the confines of the catheter to add support to the proximal aspect of the catheter as it is passed distally. Occasionally, the wire can be used to manipulate the catheter beyond small nontargeted branch vessels that repeatedly engage the tip of the flow-directed catheter or to engage a tortuous targeted branch that cannot be selected with the microcatheter alone. The Marathon and Echelon microcatheters are applied primarily using an over-the-wire technique. Typically, a 0.355-mm (0.014-in) microwire is used with the Echelon catheters and 0.254 mm (0.010-in) Expedion (ev3, Irvine, CA) or 0.203-mm (0.008-in) Mirage microwires are used with the Marathon catheter. Occasionally, the Marathon catheter can be navigated using a flow-directed technique. However, this is only feasible and safe in large, relatively straight vascular segments that can usually be captured easily with an over-the-wire technique.

After the microcatheter has been successfully manipulated into a perinidal position, contrast is gently injected on a blank roadmap. If the fluoroscopic images demonstrate catheterization of a potential pedicle for embolization, a superselective digital subtraction angiography run is performed. A higher frame rate (5–6 French) is sometimes helpful, particularly if the pedicle courses into a region with brisk arteriovenous shunting. The microcatheter run is then reviewed.

In reviewing the superselective runs, 4 factors need to be considered: (1) identification of normal parenchymal branches that may arise from the pedicle subject to embolization; (2) anatomy of the catheterized pedicle proximal to the catheter tip and AVM nidus, specifically identification of eloquent branches arising from the targeted pedicle that could be compromised by reflux of embolizate; (3) rate of transit of contrast through the nidus; and (4) anatomy of early draining veins.

The most important observation is the identification of parenchymal branches arising from the pedicle to be embolized. Arterial feeders range from vessels that course directly into the nidus to en passage vessels that course beside the nidus primarily to supply normal brain but that simultaneously give rise to multiple small side branches that extend into the nidus. We usually do not embolize pedicles that give rise to parenchymal branches.

If a branch supplies the nidus over a long segment of its course and then continues to normal parenchyma, the vessel can be occluded distally with coils to protect the normal parenchymal branches and then occluded proximally

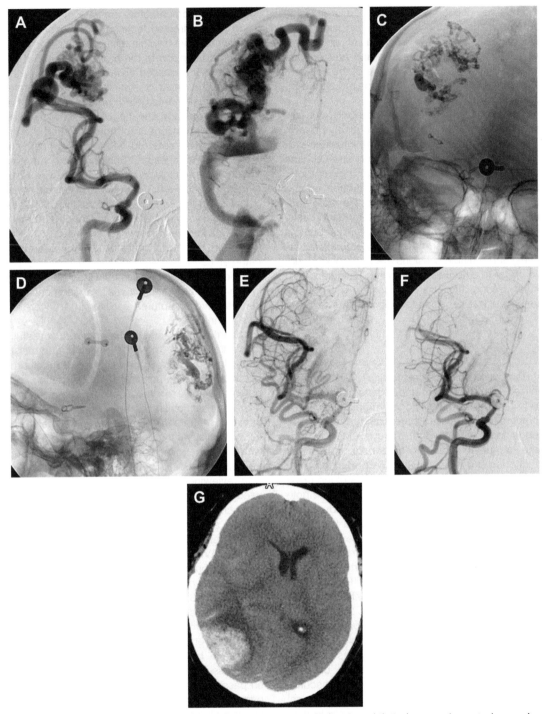

Fig. 6. Images demonstrating hemorrhage after aggressive embolization. (*A*) Early posterior-anterior angiography shows a large frontoparietal AVM. (*B*) Late phase posterior-anterior angiography shows the venous drainage pattern of the AVM. (*C*) Posterior-anterior fluoroscopic image after a single session of embolization shows the nidal glue cast, which is confirmed on (*D*) lateral fluoroscopy. (*E*) Early posterior-anterior angiography shows no filling of the AVM after preoperative embolization. (*F*) Later phase angiography confirms the obliteration of the AVM. The patient emerged from general anesthesia neurologically intact. She experienced a progressive headache and left hemiparesis 48 hours after the embolization on the morning of her surgical resection. (*G*) Computed tomographic scan, performed emergently, shows a left parietal hematoma. (*From* Fiorella D, Albuquerque FC, Woo HH, et al. The role of neuroendovascular therapy for the treatment of brain arteriovenous malformations. Neurosurgery 2006;59(5 Suppl 3):S163–77; with permission.)

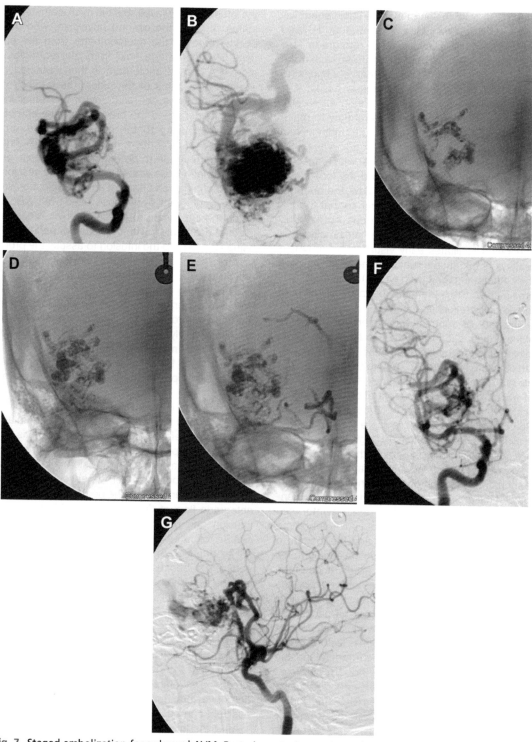

Fig. 7. Staged embolization for enlarged AVM. Posterior-anterior angiography in the early (A) and late (B) arterial phase show a large right frontal AVM. (C–E) Staged embolization over 3 days demonstrates a progressively enlarging glue cast within the AVM. After the third stage of embolization, posterior-anterior (F) and lateral (G) angiography show a substantial reduction in the AVM nidus. ([A, C–G] *From* Fiorella D, Albuquerque FC, Woo HH, et al. The role of neuroendovascular therapy for the treatment of brain arteriovenous malformations. Neurosurgery 2006;59(5 Suppl 3):S163–77, with permission; [B] *Courtesy of* Barrow Neurological Institute; with permission.)

with NBCA, with the hope that the liquid agent will penetrate the AVM nidus. This strategy is used only when there is evidence of retrograde flow (as indicated by washout of contrast) within the distal aspect of the branch that continues to normal brain parenchyma. In these cases, it is reasonable to assume that the branch will receive adequate leptomeningeal collateral flow to maintain the viability of functional surrounding brain tissue.

The position of the microcatheter with respect to the orientation of the pedicle and the location of the nidus is critical. In at least 1 view, the operator should orient the image intensifier so that the microcatheter is elongated and does not overlap either the nidus or draining vein proximally. This orientation facilitates early visualization of NBCA or Onyx reflux, thus minimizing the risks of gluing the catheter in place (with NBCA) or of occluding proximal eloquent branches because of reflux of the embolizate (either agent).

The rate of contrast transit through the AVM nidus provides data that can be helpful in determining the optimal composition of the NBCA/ethiodized oil mixture as well as the initial rate of the NBCA injection. When Onyx is used, the rate of transit defines the concentration of the agent used. We typically use Onyx-18 (6%) for most infusions, but Onyx-34 (8%), a more viscous mix, is available for embolization of high-flow pedicles that lead to fistulous portions of the AVM.

Next, the later phase images are evaluated to demonstrate the location and timing of the appearance of the draining vein. The vein should be identified in both planes so that the operator can immediately recognize when the liquid embolizate has passed through the nidus and has begun to approach the vein. After selecting the angiographic frame showing the pedicle and appearance of the draining vein, we display this frame as a reference image on an in-room monitor so that it can be visualized during injection of the glue as necessary. Two experienced physicians working in concert optimally perform NBCA infusions. Before gluing begins, both physicians need to understand the anatomy of the cast that they hope to achieve. Before preparing the NBCA, the neuroanesthesiologist should be informed of the NBCA infusion so that paralytics can be readministered to ensure prolonged apnea (90 seconds) and to obtain adequate control of the patient's blood pressure (systolic blood pressure <90 mm Hg).

After the microcatheter has been purged with a solution of 5% dextrose in water, the NBCA is injected with the patient apneic under blank fluoroscopic roadmap control. When the desired NBCA cast has been achieved, the physician performing the infusion gently aspirates the microcatheter and states "pull" to the second physician, who then briskly removes the microcatheter from the patient. The last image hold from the roadmap is stored. A control angiogram is then obtained to evaluate the status of the nidus, the patency of the draining veins, the anatomy of the remaining arterial feeders, and the presence of any complications (eg, injury to the parent vessel, thromboembolic complication, extravasation). A final evaluation is made to determine if any additional pedicles need to be embolized during the session.

The technique and pace of an Onyx injection are markedly different from those used with NBCA. Given the chemical properties of Onyx, it can be injected deliberately with the luxury of periodically being able to stop the infusion to assess the progress of the cast, the patency of the nidus and draining veins, and the status of any important vessels exiting the pedicle more proximally. The injection is performed under blank fluoroscopic roadmap control after the dead space of the catheter has slowly been purged with the solvent DMSO (0.25 mL/90 s). The initial infusion is continued until the agent is noted to reflux around the catheter tip into the proximal aspect of the pedicle.

When reflux is observed, the infusion is halted for 30 seconds to several minutes. Then the blank roadmap is refreshed, and the injection is resumed. This progression continues throughout the course of a typically long, slow infusion that is paused periodically after the observation of reflux and is resumed with the goal of reestablishing antegrade flow of Onyx into the AVM nidus. The infusion can be continued until no more reflux can be tolerated because of the risk of occluding an eloquent proximal branch of the targeted pedicle or because the agent has progressed into the vein and has potentially begun to interrupt the outflow of the nidus. The intermittent pauses between infusions allow the proximal Onyx material to precipitate around the catheter, thereby increasing the odds that antegrade flow of Onyx will be reestablished when the injection is resumed (ie, the plug-and-push technique). Using this technique, large-volume injections of Onyx, in the order of several milliliters from a single catheter position, can be injected into the AVM nidus.

After the injection is completed, the syringe is aspirated gently and slowly; gentle traction is applied to remove the microcatheter. Depending on the tortuosity of the targeted pedicle, the length of the injection, and the amount of refluxed Onyx surrounding the microcatheter, variable degrees of resistance can be experienced during catheter removal. The Onyx cast can demonstrate significant deflection while traction is being applied to the microcatheter. In such cases, slow constant traction, with an incremental increase over several minutes, should be maintained on the catheter. Again, patience is critical, because it is not unusual to maintain tension on the catheter for more than 5 to 10 minutes before freeing it from the Onyx cast. If the catheter cannot be retracted without placing undue stress on the cast or cerebrovasculature, the microcatheter can be left in place and cut off at the groin sheath.

POSTOPERATIVE CARE

For AVMs, we usually plan for a single session of embolization followed by surgical resection the next day. Large lesions are occasionally staged for embolization over multiple sessions.

In most cases, heparinization is reversed at the conclusion of the procedure. In adult patients, the arterial sheath is often left in situ in anticipation of performing intraoperative angiography after resection. When the venous outflow appears sluggish on the postembolization angiogram or if an important component of the venous outflow has been compromised (eg, a large AVM nidus with associated venous varices that is nearly totally obliterated), we put the patient on a heparin drip to prevent catastrophic thrombosis.

Normal pressure breakthrough is a theoretic possibility after embolization or resection of AVMs,[69] especially when a large arteriovenous shunt or a large volume of the nidus has been occluded. Consequently, we attempt to maintain a low systolic blood pressure (100–120 mm Hg), using a nicardipine or nitroprusside drip after the procedure. The level is determined empirically by the amount of shunting that has been reduced, the patient's baseline blood pressure, and the presence of any additional vascular lesions (eg, flow-related stenoses, carotid atheromatous stenoses). In cases of large AVMs that have been aggressively embolized in a single session, we pursue an even more aggressive hypotensive strategy, maintaining a systolic blood pressure of less than 90 mm Hg. Traditionally, we maintained the patient under continuous general anesthesia (usually using an agent such as propofol) and supplemented this regimen with antihypertensive medication to carry out the hypotensive strategy after the procedure.

With the introduction of dextromedetomidine (Precedex; Hospira, Lake Forest, IL), we are able to achieve continuous conscious sedation and hypotension in a controlled manner. Precedex offers the benefit of immediate extubation after the procedure and neurologic examination while the patient is on the drip medication. We maintain aggressive blood pressure control until the surgical resection on the next day. When patients are maintained under general anesthesia, a computed tomography scan of the head is obtained immediately after completion of the embolization and 4 hours later to monitor for possible hemorrhage.

Any increases in blood pressure that occur during the postembolization period represent a potential harbinger of intracranial hemorrhage and require immediate evaluation by computed tomography. We have found these strategies to be effective when inadvertent venous occlusion occurs early in the embolization of a large lesion (Fig. 8). If surgical resection cannot be performed on the same day after completion of the embolization, we embolize accessible arterial feeders during a single session and maintain the patient in this aggressive hypotensive state until the time of resection the next day.

COMPLICATIONS

Our experience with the embolization of AVMs at the Barrow Neurological Institute mirrors reports in the literature. Between 1995 and 2004, 508 vessels were embolized over 203 sessions in 153 patients with 17 unexpected neurologic deficits immediately after embolization (5 cases of visual field cuts, 7 cases of hemiparesis, 3 cases of aphasia, 1 case of diminished hearing, and 1 case of facial weakness). We identified 6 postembolization hemorrhages and 11 ischemia-related events. Six cases of intraprocedural thromboembolic events required intra-arterial thrombolytic treatment,[70] yielding an overall rate of neurologic morbidity per patient of 11.8% (8.6% permanent) and a 0.7% death rate.[70,71] Taylor and colleagues,[72] using PVA particles, NBCA, detachable coils, and/or the liquid polymer Onyx, reported a 2% death rate and a 9% rate of permanent neurologic deficits in 201 patients undergoing 339 embolization procedures during an 11-year period at their institution. Vinuela and colleagues[73] reported a morbidity rate of 13% and a single death in a series of 101 patients. Debrun and colleagues[74] reported a 5.6% rate of neurologic morbidity and 2 deaths (3.7%) in 54 patients undergoing NBCA embolization. Gobin and colleagues[34] reported permanent complications of 12.8% (minor deficits in 5.6%, moderate deficits in 4.8%, major deficits in 2.4%) and 2 deaths (1.6% mortality rate) in a series of 125 patients.

In an initial study comparing NBCA with PVA, 4 of the 22 patients who underwent particle embolization had ischemic neurologic complications (1 of which was major), whereas 4 of 23 patients who

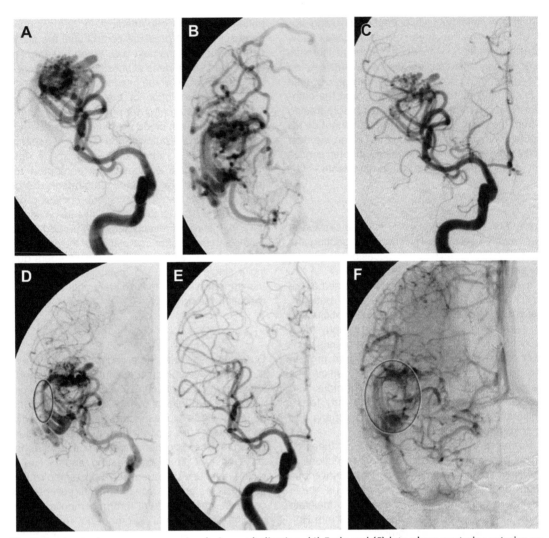

Fig. 8. Inadvertent venous compromise during embolization. (*A*) Early and (*B*) late phase posterior-anterior angiographs show a Grade III AVM of the right frontal lobe in a 57-year-old woman presenting with headaches. (*C*) Posterior-anterior angiography after 1 glue embolization shows substantial reduction in the nidus volume. (*D*) Later phase angiography in a posterior-anterior projection shows a substantial amount of glue within the large draining venous complex (*ellipse*). After 4 more pedicle embolizations, early posterior-anterior angiography (*E*) shows near-complete obliteration of the AVM. (*F*) On venous phase angiography, the large venous draining component (*circle*) remains patent. ([*A, B, D–F*] *From* Fiorella D, Albuquerque FC, Woo HH, et al. The role of neuroendovascular therapy for the treatment of brain arteriovenous malformations. Neurosurgery 2006; 59(5 Suppl 3):S163–77, with permission; [*C*] *Courtesy of* Barrow Neurological Institute; with permission.)

underwent acrylic embolization experienced minor neurologic deficits.[68] In a subsequent trial, an overall death rate of 3.9% was reported for 101 patients who underwent either NBCA or PVA embolization. Using Onyx, Jahan and colleagues[60] reported 4 adverse events (with a single permanent morbidity, 4%) and no deaths in a series of 23 patients. Hartmann and colleagues[75] reported a 14% rate of new deficits, a 2% rate of permanent disability, and a 1% death rate in 233 patients undergoing 545 sessions of embolization. In a compilation of all data from 1969 to 1993, a 10% rate of temporary morbidity, 8% rate of permanent morbidity, and 1% rate of death in 1246 patients with brain AVMs undergoing embolization were reported.[76] Although Onyx has superior handling properties that allow more aggressive embolization of AVMs, it is still too early to predict its affect on the complication rate associated with embolization (**Fig. 9**).

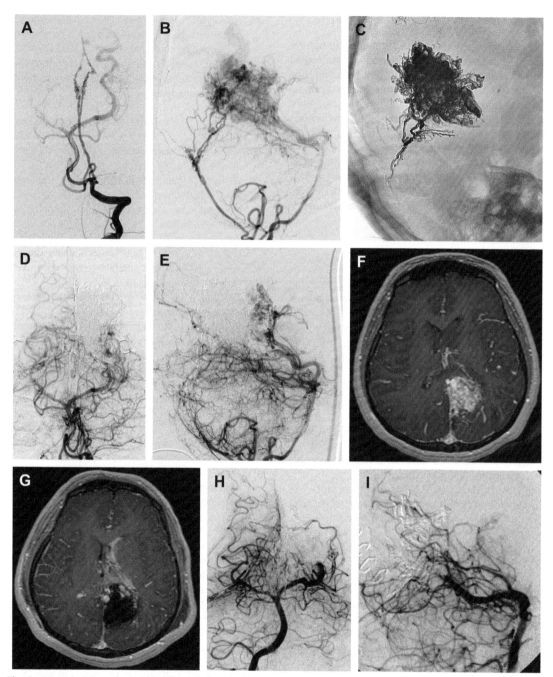

Fig. 9. Extensive Onyx (ev3, Inc, Irvine, CA) embolization of a large parietoccipital AVM in a 19-year-old girl with intraventricular and intracerebral hemorrhage. (*A*) Posterior-anterior angiography from the left vertebral artery shows the AVM. A large branch of the posterior meningeal artery is noted to fill the AVM and confirmed on (*B*) lateral angiography. (*C*) After the only posterior meningeal feeder is embolized, a dramatic amount of Onyx is visible within the AVM nidus. At the conclusion of embolization, (*D*) posterior-anterior and (*E*) lateral angiograms confirmed more than 90% obliteration of the AVM. (*F*) Preembolization magnetic resonance image with contrast demonstrates the large parietoccipital AVM. (*G*) After embolization there is a dramatic reduction in contrast enhancement reflecting the large amount of Onyx within the nidus. (*H*) Posterior-anterior and (*I*) lateral angiograms after surgical resection confirm complete removal of the AVM. (*Courtesy of* Barrow Neurological Institute; with permission.)

SUMMARY

A multidisciplinary team well versed in the natural history and complication management strategies for AVMs should perform treatment planning. Endovascular embolization continues to be a critical component of the multidisciplinary management of cerebral AVMs. With the advent of new embolizates and improved technical prowess of interventionalists, the next decade is sure to see a growing role for endovascular embolization as a stand-alone cure and in improving treatment outcomes for combined endovascular and open surgical approaches to formidable Grade IV and V AVMs.

REFERENCES

1. Berman MF, Sciacca RR, Pile-Spellman J, et al. The epidemiology of brain arteriovenous malformations. Neurosurgery 2000;47:389–96.
2. Itoyama Y, Uemura S, Ushio Y, et al. Natural course of unoperated intracranial arteriovenous malformations: study of 50 cases. J Neurosurg 1989;71:805–9.
3. Al-Shahi R, Warlow CP. Quality of evidence for management of arteriovenous malformations of the brain. Lancet 2002;360:1022–3.
4. Crawford PM, West CR, Chadwick DW, et al. Arteriovenous malformations of the brain: natural history in unoperated patients. J Neurol Neurosurg Psychiatry 1986;49:1–10.
5. Mast H, Young WL, Koennecke HC, et al. Risk of spontaneous haemorrhage after diagnosis of cerebral arteriovenous malformation. Lancet 1997;350:1065–8.
6. Graf CJ, Perret GE, Torner JC. Bleeding from cerebral arteriovenous malformations as part of their natural history. J Neurosurg 1983;58:331–7.
7. Jane JA, Kassell NF, Torner JC, et al. The natural history of aneurysms and arteriovenous malformations. J Neurosurg 1985;62:321–3.
8. Spetzler RF, Martin NA. A proposed grading system for arteriovenous malformations. J Neurosurg 1986;65:476–83.
9. Spetzler RF, Ponce FA. A 3-tier classification of cerebral arteriovenous malformations. J Neurosurg 2011;114:842–9.
10. Hamilton MG, Spetzler RF. The prospective application of a grading system for arteriovenous malformations. Neurosurgery 1994;34:2–6.
11. Heros RC, Korosue K, Diebold PM. Surgical excision of cerebral arteriovenous malformations: late results. Neurosurgery 1990;26:570–7.
12. Martin NA, King WA, Wilson CB, et al. Management of dural arteriovenous malformations of the anterior cranial fossa. J Neurosurg 1990;72:692–7.
13. Lawton MT. Spetzler-Martin Grade III arteriovenous malformations: surgical results and a modification of the grading scale. Neurosurgery 2003;52:740–8.
14. Han PP, Ponce FA, Spetzler RF. Intention-to-treat analysis of Spetzler-Martin grades IV and V arteriovenous malformations: natural history and treatment paradigm. J Neurosurg 2003;98:3–7.
15. Miyamoto S, Hashimoto N, Nagata I, et al. Post-treatment sequelae of palliatively treated cerebral arteriovenous malformations. Neurosurgery 2000;46:589–94.
16. Wikholm G, Lundqvist C, Svendsen P. The Goteborg cohort of embolized cerebral arteriovenous malformations: a 6-year follow-up. Neurosurgery 2001;49:799–805.
17. Jafar JJ, Davis AJ, Berenstein A, et al. The effect of embolization with N-butyl cyanoacrylate prior to surgical resection of cerebral arteriovenous malformations. J Neurosurg 1993;78:60–9.
18. DeMeritt JS, Pile-Spellman J, Mast H, et al. Outcome analysis of preoperative embolization with N-butyl cyanoacrylate in cerebral arteriovenous malformations. AJNR Am J Neuroradiol 1995;16:1801–7.
19. Weber W, Kis B, Siekmann R, et al. Preoperative embolization of intracranial arteriovenous malformations with Onyx. Neurosurgery 2007;61:244–52.
20. Natarajan SK, Ghodke B, Britz GW, et al. Multimodality treatment of brain arteriovenous malformations with microsurgery after embolization with onyx: single-center experience and technical nuances. Neurosurgery 2008;62:1213–25.
21. Kim EJ, Halim AX, Dowd CF, et al. The relationship of coexisting extranidal aneurysms to intracranial hemorrhage in patients harboring brain arteriovenous malformations. Neurosurgery 2004;54:1349–57.
22. Lasjaunias P, Piske R, terBrugge K, et al. Cerebral arteriovenous malformations (C. AVM) and associated arterial aneurysms (AA). Analysis of 101 C. AVM cases, with 37 AA in 23 patients. Acta Neurochir (Wien) 1988;91:29–36.
23. Marks MP, Lane B, Steinberg GK, et al. Hemorrhage in intracerebral arteriovenous malformations: angiographic determinants. Radiology 1990;176:807–13.
24. Redekop G, terBrugge K, Montanera W, et al. Arterial aneurysms associated with cerebral arteriovenous malformations: classification, incidence, and risk of hemorrhage. J Neurosurg 1998;89:539–46.
25. Brown RD Jr, Wiebers DO, Forbes GS. Unruptured intracranial aneurysms and arteriovenous malformations: frequency of intracranial hemorrhage and relationship of lesions. J Neurosurg 1990;73:859–63.
26. Mpotsaris A, Loehr C, Harati A, et al. Interdisciplinary clinical management of high grade arteriovenous malformations and ruptured flow-related

aneurysms in the posterior fossa. Interv Neuroradiol 2010;16:400–8.

27. da Costa L, Thines L, Dehdashti AR, et al. Management and clinical outcome of posterior fossa arteriovenous malformations: report on a single-centre 15-year experience. J Neurol Neurosurg Psychiatry 2009;80:376–9.

28. Foy AB, Wetjen N, Pollock BE. Stereotactic radiosurgery for pediatric arteriovenous malformations. Neurosurg Clin North Am 2010;21:457–61.

29. Starke RM, Komotar RJ, Hwang BY, et al. A comprehensive review of radiosurgery for cerebral arteriovenous malformations: outcomes, predictive factors, and grading scales. Stereotact Funct Neurosurg 2008;86:191–9.

30. Batjer HH, Devous MD Sr, Seibert GB, et al. Intracranial arteriovenous malformation: relationships between clinical and radiographic factors and ipsilateral steal severity. Neurosurgery 1988;23: 322–8.

31. Kwon Y, Jeon SR, Kim JH, et al. Analysis of the causes of treatment failure in gamma knife radiosurgery for intracranial arteriovenous malformations. J Neurosurg 2000;93(Suppl 3):104–6.

32. Lunsford LD, Kondziolka D, Flickinger JC, et al. Stereotactic radiosurgery for arteriovenous malformations of the brain. J Neurosurg 1991;75:512–24.

33. Steiner L, Lindquist C, Adler JR, et al. Clinical outcome of radiosurgery for cerebral arteriovenous malformations. J Neurosurg 1992;77:1–8.

34. Gobin YP, Laurent A, Merienne L, et al. Treatment of brain arteriovenous malformations by embolization and radiosurgery. J Neurosurg 1996;85:19–28.

35. Henkes H, Nahser HC, Berg-Dammer E, et al. Endovascular therapy of brain AVMs prior to radiosurgery. Neurol Res 1998;20:479–92.

36. Andrade-Souza YM, Ramani M, Scora D, et al. Embolization before radiosurgery reduces the obliteration rate of arteriovenous malformations. Neurosurgery 2007;60:443–51.

37. Back AG, Vollmer D, Zeck O, et al. Retrospective analysis of unstaged and staged Gamma Knife surgery with and without preceding embolization for the treatment of arteriovenous malformations. J Neurosurg 2008;109(Suppl):57–64.

38. Blackburn SL, Ashley WW, Rich KM, et al. Combined endovascular embolization and stereotactic radiosurgery in the treatment of large arteriovenous malformations. J Neurosurg 2011;114(6):1758–67.

39. Vinuela F, Duckwiler G, Guglielmi G. Contribution of interventional neuroradiology in the therapeutic management of brain arteriovenous malformations. J Stroke Cerebrovasc Dis 1997;6:268–71.

40. Fournier D, TerBrugge KG, Willinsky R, et al. Endovascular treatment of intracerebral arteriovenous malformations: experience in 49 cases. J Neurosurg 1991;75:228–33.

41. Yu SC, Chan MS, Lam JM, et al. Complete obliteration of intracranial arteriovenous malformation with endovascular cyanoacrylate embolization: initial success and rate of permanent cure. AJNR Am J Neuroradiol 2004;25:1139–43.

42. Katsaridis V, Papagiannaki C, Aimar E. Curative embolization of cerebral arteriovenous malformations (AVMs) with Onyx in 101 patients. Neuroradiology 2008;50:589–97.

43. Maimon S, Strauss I, Frolov V, et al. Brain arteriovenous malformation treatment using a combination of Onyx and a new detachable tip microcatheter, SONIC: short-term results. AJNR Am J Neuroradiol 2010;31:947–54.

44. Abud DG, Riva R, Nakiri GS, et al. Treatment of brain arteriovenous malformations by double arterial catheterization with simultaneous injection of Onyx: retrospective series of 17 patients. AJNR Am J Neuroradiol 2011;32:152–8.

45. Valavanis A, Christoforidis G. Endovascular management of cerebral arteriovenous malformations. Neurointerventionist 1999;1:34–40.

46. Marks MP, Lane B, Steinberg G, et al. Vascular characteristics of intracerebral arteriovenous malformations in patients with clinical steal. AJNR Am J Neuroradiol 1991;12:489–96.

47. Mast H, Mohr JP, Osipov A, et al. 'Steal' is an unestablished mechanism for the clinical presentation of cerebral arteriovenous malformations. Stroke 1995;26:1215–20.

48. Kusske JA, Kelly WA. Embolization and reduction of the "steal" syndrome in cerebral arteriovenous malformations. J Neurosurg 1974;40:313–21.

49. Luessenhop AJ, Mujica PH. Embolization of segments of the circle of Willis and adjacent branches for management of certain inoperable cerebral arteriovenous malformations. J Neurosurg 1981; 54:573–82.

50. Fox AJ, Girvin JP, Vinuela F, et al. Rolandic arteriovenous malformations: improvement in limb function by IBC embolization. AJNR Am J Neuroradiol 1985;6:575–82.

51. Rosenkranz M, Regelsberger J, Zeumer H, et al. Management of cerebral arteriovenous malformations associated with symptomatic congestive intracranial hypertension. Eur Neurol 2008;59:62–6.

52. Simon SD, Yao TL, Rosenbaum BP, et al. Resolution of trigeminal neuralgia after palliative embolization of a cerebellopontine angle arteriovenous malformation. Cent Eur Neurosurg 2009;70:161–3.

53. Loh Y, Duckwiler GR. A prospective, multicenter, randomized trial of the Onyx liquid embolic system and N-butyl cyanoacrylate embolization of cerebral arteriovenous malformations. Clinical article. J Neurosurg 2010;113:733–41.

54. Brothers MF, Kaufmann JC, Fox AJ, et al. n-Butyl 2-cyanoacrylate–substitute for IBCA in

interventional neuroradiology: histopathologic and polymerization time studies. AJNR Am J Neuroradiol 1989;10:777–86.

55. Spiegel SM, Vinuela F, Goldwasser JM, et al. Adjusting the polymerization time of isobutyl-2 cyanoacrylate. AJNR Am J Neuroradiol 1986;7:109–12.

56. Gounis MJ, Lieber BB, Wakhloo AK, et al. Effect of glacial acetic acid and ethiodized oil concentration on embolization with N-butyl 2-cyanoacrylate: an in vivo investigation. AJNR Am J Neuroradiol 2002;23:938–44.

57. Taki W, Yonekawa Y, Iwata H, et al. A new liquid material for embolization of arteriovenous malformations. AJNR Am J Neuroradiol 1990;11:163–8.

58. Chaloupka JC, Vinuela F, Vinters HV, et al. Technical feasibility and histopathologic studies of ethylene vinyl copolymer (EVAL) using a swine endovascular embolization model. AJNR Am J Neuroradiol 1994;15:1107–15.

59. Sampei K, Hashimoto N, Kazekawa K, et al. Histological changes in brain tissue and vasculature after intracarotid infusion of organic solvents in rats. Neuroradiology 1996;38:291–4.

60. Jahan R, Murayama Y, Gobin YP, et al. Embolization of arteriovenous malformations with Onyx: clinicopathological experience in 23 patients. Neurosurgery 2001;48:984–95.

61. Murayama Y, Vinuela F, Ulhoa A, et al. Nonadhesive liquid embolic agent for cerebral arteriovenous malformations: preliminary histopathological studies in swine rete mirabile. Neurosurgery 1998;43:1164–75.

62. Yakes WF, Rossi P, Odink H. How I do it. Arteriovenous malformation management. Cardiovasc Intervent Radiol 1996;19:65–71.

63. Yakes WF, Krauth L, Ecklund J, et al. Ethanol endovascular management of brain arteriovenous malformations: initial results. Neurosurgery 1997;40:1145–52.

64. Unnikrishnan KP, Sinha PK, Sriganesh K, et al. Case report: alterations in bispectral index following absolute alcohol embolization in a patient with intracranial arteriovenous malformation. Can J Anaesth 2007;54:908–11.

65. n-BCA Trail Investigators. N-Butyl cyanoacrylate embolization of cerebral arteriovenous malformations: results of a prospective, randomized, multicenter trial. AJNR Am J Neuroradiol 2002;23:748–55.

66. Sorimachi T, Koike T, Takeuchi S, et al. Embolization of cerebral arteriovenous malformations achieved with polyvinyl alcohol particles: angiographic reappearance and complications. AJNR Am J Neuroradiol 1999;20:1323–8.

67. Mathis JA, Barr JD, Horton JA, et al. The efficacy of particulate embolization combined with stereotactic radiosurgery for treatment of large arteriovenous malformations of the brain. AJNR Am J Neuroradiol 1995;16:299–306.

68. Wallace RC, Flom RA, Khayata MH, et al. The safety and effectiveness of brain arteriovenous malformation embolization using acrylic and particles: the experiences of a single institution. Neurosurgery 1995;37:606–15.

69. Spetzler RF, Wilson CB, Weinstein P, et al. Normal perfusion pressure breakthrough theory. Clin Neurosurg 1978;25:651–72.

70. Kim LJ, Albuquerque FC, Spetzler RF, et al. Postembolization neurological deficits in cerebral arteriovenous malformations: stratification by arteriovenous malformation grade. Neurosurgery 2006;59:53–9.

71. Fiorella D, Albuquerque FC, Woo HH, et al. The role of neuroendovascular therapy for the treatment of brain arteriovenous malformations. Neurosurgery 2006;59:S163–77.

72. Taylor CL, Dutton K, Rappard G, et al. Complications of preoperative embolization of cerebral arteriovenous malformations. J Neurosurg 2004;100:810–2.

73. Vinuela F, Dion JE, Duckwiler G, et al. Combined endovascular embolization and surgery in the management of cerebral arteriovenous malformations: experience with 101 cases. J Neurosurg 1991;75:856–64.

74. Debrun GM, Aletich V, Ausman JI, et al. Embolization of the nidus of brain arteriovenous malformations with n-butyl cyanoacrylate. Neurosurgery 1997;40:112–20.

75. Hartmann A, Pile-Spellman J, Stapf C, et al. Risk of endovascular treatment of brain arteriovenous malformations. Stroke 2002;33:1816–20.

76. Frizzel RT, Fisher WS III. Cure, morbidity, and mortality associated with embolization of brain arteriovenous malformations: a review of 1246 patients in 32 series over a 35-year period. Neurosurgery 1995;37:1031–9.

Endovascular Treatment of Cerebral Dural and Pial Arteriovenous Fistulas

Pascal Jabbour, MD*, Stavropoula Tjoumakaris, MD,
Nohra Chalouhi, MD, Ciro Randazzo, MD,
Luis Fernando Gonzalez, MD, Aaron Dumont, MD,
Robert Rosenwasser, MD

KEYWORDS

• Dural • Pial • Fistula • Endovascular • Arteriovenous • Embolization

KEY POINTS

• Dural arteriovenous fistulas (DAVFs) are arteriovenous shunts from a dural arterial supply to a dural venous channel, typically supplied by pachymeningeal arteries and located near a major venous sinus.
• DVAFs with retrograde venous drainage can result in hemorrhage or cause decreased regional cerebral blood flow in cortical regions involved.
• DAVFs can be treated with surgery, endovascular embolization (transarterial or transvenous approach), and radiosurgery.
• Elimination of the retrograde cortical venous drainage is the goal of any type of treatment for DAVFs.
• Pial Arteriovenous fistulas (PAVFs) are direct fistulas from an intracranial arterial feeder into a single venous channel and typically have high risk of intracranial hemorrhage and death if left untreated.
• PAVFs can be treated with surgery or endovascular embolization. Radiosurgery is not used because of the latent effect and difficulties in targeting the fistula.

DURAL ARTERIOVENOUS FISTULAS

Dural arteriovenous fistulas (DAVFs) are arteriovenous shunts from a dural arterial supply to a dural venous channel, typically supplied by pachymeningeal arteries and located near a major venous sinus.[1] The etiology of these lesions is not fully understood; some are congenital, and others are acquired. DAVFs in the pediatric population are associated with structural venous abnormalities,[2] but most DAVFs are thought to be acquired.[3,4] The development of venous obstruction and hypertension with aberrant angiogenesis[5] can contribute to the pathogenesis of these lesions. This altered angiogenesis occurs within the dura following an inciting event such as trauma, surgery, chronic infection, or sinus thrombosis. As microshunts proliferate in association with venous hypertension, these mature into clinically significant DAVF. The degree of progression or involution determines the significance of the abnormality. This can then result in hemorrhage or other focal manifestations including hemodynamic insufficiency. DAVFs can also cause decreased regional cerebral blood flow in cortical regions where there is retrograde venous drainage.

Department of Neurosurgery, Jefferson Hospital for Neuroscience, Thomas Jefferson University Hospital, 909 Walnut Street, Philadelphia, PA 19107, USA
* Corresponding author. 909 Walnut Street, 2nd Floor, Philadelphia, PA 19107.
E-mail address: Pascal.jabbour@jefferson.edu

Neuroimag Clin N Am 23 (2013) 625–636
http://dx.doi.org/10.1016/j.nic.2013.03.010
1052-5149/13/$ – see front matter © 2013 Elsevier Inc. All rights reserved.

neuroimaging.theclinics.com

At the same time, some cases of DAVF have no clear inciting event or are at a site that is clearly distinct from the presumed inciting event. It is thought that the development of a DAVF in these settings requires a common unclear mechanism as well as a possible anatomic or genetic predisposition.[6,7]

DAVFs have been reported in all age groups, but mainly in the fifth and sixth decades of life.[8–10] The estimated incidence of DAVFs is 0.17 cases per 100,000 population, and they are one-fifth as common as arteriovenous malformations (AVMs).[11,12] They represent 10% to 15% of all intracranial vascular malformations,[11–17] with a higher incidence in women. A female-to-male ratio of 2:1 exists in certain anatomic sites such as the cavernous and transverse–sigmoid sinuses.[4,8,9,18–20] DAVFs are usually solitary, although in 5% of cases, multiple lesions have been described.[12,21,22] The goal of this article is to describe the natural history, clinical presentation, and treatment of dural and pial fistulas with emphasis on the endovascular treatment.

Natural History

An established DAVF may follow 1 of several unpredictable natural courses. Some lesions remain asymptomatic or maintain stable clinical symptomatology and angiographic features over many years. Others undergo spontaneous regression, involution, and resolution with stabilization or improvement of neurologic symptoms.[23–28] Features that may predispose to such spontaneous involution are not known. DAVFs in the region of the cavernous sinus are particularly prone to this phenomenon, with as many as 40% of reported cases having undergone spontaneous involution.

In contrast, some DAVFs may demonstrate an increase in size from either arterial or venous enlargement[1,11,29] or even de novo development of a DAVF.[30] Pachymeningeal arterial feeders may be progressively recruited causing enlargement of the nidus due to unknown mechanisms. This results in hypertrophy of dural arteries and the reappearance of involuted embryonic arteries that may not normally be visible in the adult dura mater. In some DAVFs there is also progression on the venous side. Progressive arterialization of the pathologic dural leaflets results in hypertension in adjacent leptomeningeal venous channels, leading to retrograde leptomeningeal venous drainage. Under arterialized pressures these channels may become tortuous and become varices or aneurysms. The catastrophic consequence that ensues is a cerebral hemorrhage from retrograde cortical venous drainage (CVD).

Clinical Presentation and Assessment

Clinical manifestations of DAVFs are highly variable and are related primarily to the location of the fistula as well as retrograde CVD. These range from minor symptoms to intracranial hemorrhage. The vast majority of symptoms can be attributed to the anatomy of the DAVF.

Patients' symptoms may be sudden or slowly progressive. The degree and type are determined by venous topography, venous flow pattern, and the capacity of surrounding compensatory venous drainage. The most serious neurologic sequelae from DAVFs are associated with retrograde CVD,[11] leading to a propensity to rupture. Focal neurologic deficits likely result from venous hypertension and intracranial hemorrhage from rupture of arterialized leptomeningeal veins.

There are a wide variety of nonhemorrhagic symptoms with which DAVF can present.[31,32] Relatively benign symptoms such as pain, tinnitus, or bruit are related to arteriovenous shunting and flow within the DAVF. Pulsatile tinnitus or other auditory symptoms may occur with or without pain. These symptoms are likely related to high flow through dural vascular channels at the base of the skull. Other more painful complaints may be related to orbital congestion, stretching of dural leaflets by engorged vascular channels, or to direct compression of the trigeminal nerve by arterialized venous structures near the petrous apex.

Various neuro-ophthalmologic manifestations of DAVFs include visual and gaze abnormalities caused by venous hypertension. Orbital or ocular venous hypertension with resulting orbital crowding, venous stasis retinopathy, and glaucoma can also be seen.

Other intracranial DAVFs may present with symptoms of increased intracranial pressure (ICP) or a poorly defined headache.[33,34] While the headaches are nonspecific, there does appear to be an association with the dysplastic changes in meningeal vessels that are often present in DAVFs. There are also a wide spectrum of neurologic symptoms including seizure, hearing loss, cranial nerve palsy, papilledema, vision changes, and motor/sensory deficits that can be seen with intracranial DAVF.

DAVFs may also result in altered cerebrospinal (CSF) flow.[35] Dilated venous structures may act as mass lesions, obstructing the CSF circulation and causing hydrocephalus. In other cases, dural venous hypertension may result in decreased absorption of CSF with secondary intracranial hypertension and papilledema. This latter complication appears to be more common in high-flow lesions draining into large dural venous sinuses in the setting of concomitant sinus outflow obstruction.

Certain clinical presentations are seen with DAVFs in specific locations.[11,29,31,32] DAVFs in the region of the transverse or sigmoid sinus, or near the cavernous sinus, often drain into the associated venous sinuses and may cause a variety of clinical manifestations due to increased flow or local venous engorgement. High-flow lesions in the region of the transverse sigmoid sinus junction often result in pulsatile tinnitus, headache, and bruit. This phenomenon does not lead to intracranial hemorrhage unless there is associated retrograde CVD. Lesions at the anterior cranial fossa or the tentorial incisura rarely drain into a patent dural venous sinus and are more frequently associated with leptomeningeal venous drainage. They are more likely to cause serious clinical sequelae from venous hypertension and hemorrhage.

Imaging Studies and Classification

Dilated or thrombosed venous structures on head computed tomography (CT) and brain magnetic resonance imaging (MRI) may suggest the presence of a DAVF. However, these routine studies are frequently equivocal and do not provide information about the anatomy of the fistula. CT angiography and magnetic resonance angiography (MRA) are important noninvasive diagnostic studies that provide not only anatomic details but may be coupled with perfusion studies as well to evaluate the effect of a DAVF on regional blood flow. Angiography is needed for definitive diagnosis and pretreatment analysis of intracranial DAVFs. Projections usually include the external and internal carotid arteries bilaterally and the vertebral arteries. A thorough study of the arterial supply, anastomoses, and venous anatomy is performed before the use of embolic materials.

Classification of DAVFs has evolved over time to be useful in guiding therapeutic intervention. Initial attempts were simplistic, emphasizing the anatomic location, but lacked meaningful information in regard to predicting the nature or outcome of the abnormality. Subsequent systems incorporated information from diagnostic angiography.[36–38]

Perhaps 1 of the most well recognized classification schemes specific to DAVFs is that developed by Djindjian and colleagues. This system categorizes a lesion into 1 of 4 types. Type I DAVFs are characterized by normal anterograde drainage into a venous sinus or meningeal vein; type II lesions drain into a sinus, with reflux into adjacent sinuses or cortical veins. Type III DAVFs drain directly into cortical veins with resultant retrograde flow into the cerebral venous compartment, and type IV DAVFs have drainage directly into a venous pouch (venous lake or venous ectasia). Djindjian

and colleagues concluded from their study that type I DAVFs were benign, with each sequential type having more aggressive characteristics. Since the introduction of the Djindjian classification, other studies have been published in the literature attempting to correlate certain features of the DAVF with the likelihood of hemorrhage or other neurologic complications.[11,31,39,40]

With the advent of more effective endovascular techniques, a means of predicting lesion risk and management options emerged. Cognard and colleagues developed a classification system derived from a modified version of the Djindjian classification. They defined 5 types of DAVFs that are based on the pattern of venous outflow. Type I DAVFs were characterized by normal antegrade flow into the affected dural sinus. Type II lesions were associated with an abnormal direction of venous drainage within the affected dural sinus. These lesions could be further categorized into 3 subtypes: type IIa, lesions with retrograde flow exclusively into a sinus or sinuses; type IIb, lesions with retrograde venous drainage into the cortical veins only; and type II a + b, lesions with retrograde drainage into sinuses and cortical veins. Type III DAVFs drained directly into a cortical vein or veins without venous ectasia, whereas type IV DAVFs had drainage into cortical veins with the critical component of venous ectasia greater than 5 mm in diameter and 3 times larger than the diameter of the draining vein. A DAVF was considered to be type V when drainage was into spinal perimedullary veins. Correlation with their clinical data yielded the following conclusions.

> Type I DAVFs are considered benign, and treatment is usually not necessary, except possibly for palliation of symptoms.
> Type IIa lesions are best treated with arterial embolization.
> Type IIb and IIa + b lesions usually require both transarterial and transvenous embolization for effective obliteration.

For types III to V, transarterial embolization and occasionally transvenous embolization aimed at complete occlusion of the fistula are necessary and often will need to be combined with surgical techniques to eradicate the threatening cortical venous drainage.

Borden and colleagues[38] also proposed a classification system emphasizing venous anatomy with 3 categories. Type I DAVFs drain directly into dural venous sinuses or pachymeningeal veins. Type II DAVFs drain into dural sinuses or pachymeningeal veins but also have retrograde drainage into subarachnoid (leptomeningeal) veins. Type III DAVFs drain solely into subarachnoid veins and do not have dural sinus or meningeal venous drainage. The validity of both the Cognard and Borden classification systems was confirmed in 102 intracranial DAVFs in 98 patients (**Table 1**).[40]

Regardless of lesion location, clinical presentation, or other symptomatology, the most important factor determining the propensity of a lesion to have an aggressive clinical course appears to be the presence of leptomeningeal venous drainage. Lesions that drain into a large patent venous sinus may have various clinical associations but are less likely to bleed or cause focal neurologic deficits unless associated with retrograde leptomeningeal venous drainage. Lesions without drainage into a patent dural venous sinus are more frequently associated with leptomeningeal venous drainage and prone to serious clinical sequelae such as an intracerebral hemorrhage. The risk of hemorrhage appears to be related directly to the presence of tortuous and aneurysmal leptomeningeal arterialized veins in association with DAVFs.

Treatment and Follow-up

A DAVF may rarely be discovered on imaging studies or digital subtraction angiography performed for other indications. Incidental lesions must be carefully assessed for features predisposing to aggressive clinical behavior. Complete angiographic evaluation is indicated in every case of suspected DAVF unless the patient is a poor candidate for therapeutic intervention or refuses invasive diagnostic studies. Lesions should be evaluated specifically for the presence of leptomeningeal venous drainage, varices (aneurysmal changes in the venous circulation), and venous ectasia. In the absence of these features, the lesion

should be followed expectantly. There is no evidence demonstrating significant benefits to prophylactic treatment of unruptured DAVFs that are not associated with leptomeningeal cortical venous drainage. Expectant follow-up of these lesions should include serial MRI for any evidence of changes in the DAVF anatomy. Angiographic reexamination of the lesion every few years should be considered, especially for DAVFs at the anterior cranial fossa or the tentorial incisura, which commonly harbor leptomeningeal venous drainage.

Definitive prophylactic treatment should be strongly considered for asymptomatic and incidentally discovered DAVFs with leptomeningeal venous drainage. The patient should be given the option of open surgical, radiosurgical, or endovascular interventions as may be appropriate for the specific lesion type and location. If treatment does not succeed at totally eliminating leptomeningeal venous drainage, then further definitive therapy or close follow-up of the lesion is indicated. Anticoagulation is contraindicated in the setting of DAVFs with leptomeningeal venous drainage.

Definitive intervention for DAVFs that behaved aggressively in the past warrants serious thought. The morbidity of a first hemorrhage with DAVFs is substantial, and many patients do not survive or recover to a condition suitable for therapeutic intervention. However, there are numerous documented cases of progression of focal neurologic symptoms resulting in death or major disability unless the DAVF is obliterated. Lesions that have hemorrhaged or caused focal neurologic symptoms due to venous hypertension without retrograde CVD should still undergo definitive treatment in those patients who are clinically stable. Palliative therapy is often inadequate in this setting. Those patients with retrograde CVD with

Table 1
Classification of DAVFs

Type	Djindjian	Cognard	Borden
I	Normal antegrade flow into dural sinus	Normal antegrade flow into dural sinus	Drains directly into venous sinus or meningeal vein
II	Drainage into venous sinus with reflux into adjacent sinus or cortical vein	a. Retrograde flow into sinus(es) b. Retrograde filling of cortical vein(s) c. Retrograde drainage into sinus(es) and cortical vein(s)	Drains into dural sinus or meningeal veins with retrograde drainage into subarachnoid veins
III	Drainage into cortical veins with retrograde flow	Direct drainage into cortical veins without venous ectasia	Drains into subarachnoid veins without dural sinus or meningeal involvement
IV	Drainage into venous pouch (lake)	Direct drainage into cortical veins with venous ectasia >5 mm and 3× larger than diameter of draining vein	
V		Drainage to spinal perimedullary veins	

leptomeningeal spread presenting with hemorrhage clearly need an intervention.

On the other hand, lesions that present with pain or pulsatile tinnitus are evaluated and treated in the same way as incidental lesions. Nonspecific measures aimed at resolving the symptoms are often sufficient. Palliative treatment of the DAVF may be considered for the control of symptomatology. Rarely is definitive treatment indicated solely for pain or pulsatile tinnitus.

Endovascular Neurosurgical Techniques

Transarterial embolization (TAE) has been widely used in the treatment of DAVFs.[1,41,42] The use of flow-guided catheter technology and increased experience with particle and glue embolization, as well as detachable coils have greatly improved the safety and efficacy of this method.[43–45] However, TAE rarely succeeds in totally eliminating a DAVF except in rare instances of limited fistulae with a small number of accessible feeders. More commonly, DAVFs involve a multitude of feeders, which often arise as multiple, small tributaries from major cerebral arteries that are not amenable to TAE. While TAE may obliterate the filling of the lesion after 1 injection, the DAVF often continues to draw feeders from other sources and will reappear on subsequent angiography. DAVFs that are partially treated with TAE may later recur and result in hemorrhage.

TAE can be effective in palliating disabling symptoms even without completely curing the DAVF. Symptomatic palliation may be accomplished by TAE of feeders to the DAVF, although such an intervention is not without risk and not always successful in eliminating the DAVF. Arterial embolization may give a false sense of security that the lesion was treated, while the DAVF may progress to acquire more aggressive features including leptomeningeal venous drainage (even in the absence of recurrent symptoms). DAVFs that are followed expectantly or treated palliatively should be monitored closely with serial diagnostic imaging. TAE also plays an important role in decreasing flow through DAVFs before surgical intervention, transvenous obliteration, or radiosurgery.[46–48] This preparatory use of TAE has greatly enhanced the safety and efficacy of other treatment measures.

Noninvasive imaging methods, including MRI and MRA, may be used for interval studies, although these modalities may miss subtle development of leptomeningeal venous drainage. Depending on the clinical situation and the particular lesion, serial magnetic resonance studies may be performed on a yearly basis, with formal angiography every few years or sooner if symptoms change, or if there is a suggestion of new leptomeningeal venous drainage on MRI.

Transvenous embolization (TVE) of DAVFs has recently been used with good results.[49–51] This modality aims at the thrombosis of the venous side of the lesion, often including the obliteration of the adjacent dural venous sinus. Occlusion of the venous side of DAVFs is usually well tolerated if the pathologic dural sinus is arterialized and does not serve as a site of drainage of normal circulation. Instead, the pathologic dural segment is often associated with harmful retrograde leptomeningeal venous drainage, and these channels are secondarily obliterated with thrombosis of the venous side of DAVFs. This strategy has been used most successfully in the treatment of DAVFs with accessible venous drainage. TVE is particularly effective in the treatment of cavernous sinus DAVFs (via the inferior petrosal sinus), although these lesions frequently do not require any therapeutic intervention because of their benign clinical symptomatology and tendency toward spontaneous regression.

TVE has also been used in cases of transverse sigmoid sinus DAVFs, and may be substantially safer than open surgical approaches to these lesions. However, there may be no accessible transvenous route for many DAVFs, including tentorial incisura DAVFs and anterior cranial fossa DAVFs, which frequently behave aggressively. Transvenous obliteration may occasionally be performed after open surgical exposure, through puncture of the dural venous sinus or the arterialized venous varix with the injection of coils or glue.[52–54] Rarely, TVE may result in propagating venous thrombosis or altered hemodynamic patterns with paradoxic clinical deterioration or hemorrhage.

Various embolic materials have been used, including particles, liquid silicone, ethyl alcohol, platinum microcoils, and cyanoacrylates for endovascular therapy. N-butyl cyanoacrylate (NBCA) has a fast polymerization rate and binding properties, making it somewhat difficult to use. Both preparation and delivery of NBCA require an experienced user. NBCA is injected until it reaches the proximal draining vein, and then the microcatheter is then removed promptly to prevent its adhesion to the NBCA; the D5W push technique has been used to try to push, then glue distally in the fistula to the venous side, and the use of glacial acetic acid has been also described to delay the polymerization of the glue, enabling the glue to travel distally.

Onyx liquid embolic system is an ethylene vinyl alcohol polymer dissolved in dimethyl sulfoxide (DMSO). Injection of onyx in blood results in solvent diffusion, allowing the polymer to precipitate and mechanically occlude the vessel. Injection of larger amounts of onyx can result in filling of the fistulous network and allow for reflux into other arterial feeders. At the same time, there have been theories that onyx can leave microchannels within the cast that allow small amounts of flow through the fistula, resulting in recurrence of the fistula or possibly residual fistula despite angiographic embolization.

In addition, onyx has been known to cause significant inflammation within the vasculature. This can be seen in the treatment of cavernous carotid fistulas in which the surrounding cranial nerves are often irritated, resulting in various cranial nerve palsies. The significance of this inflammation in other areas remains to be seen. Others report that theoretically there should be less inflammation than NBCA, since there is no protein denaturation, which has been demonstrated in animal models. Regardless, onyx remains an important and effective modality in the armamentarium against fistulas and other vascular anomalies.

Occasionally a DAVF will recur adjacent to an endovascularly occluded venous sinus, and this could represent reconstitution of arteriovenous channels within the walls of the occluded sinus, or in the organized thrombus within the sinus channel. These cases are amenable to surgical excision of the segment of occluded sinus with disconnection of associated arterialized leptomeningeal veins.

The Jefferson Hospital for Neuroscience Experience

Methods

Thirty-nine patients (22 men and 17 women) underwent endovascular treatment of DAVFs at the authors' institution from 2001 to 2009 (**Table 2**). Ages ranged from 39 to 71 (mean 48). Seventy-nine percent of patients had retrograde CVD. Upon completion of diagnostic angiography, transarterial embolization was attempted first with either NBCA or onyx. The number of arterial embolizations and need for transvenous embolization, open surgery, or radiosurgery were assessed. Normalization of retrograde CVD was also assessed. Finally, postoperative complications were addressed.

Results

Obliteration of DAVF The average number of embolizations in all patients was 2.1. Patients were considered completely treated when there was a greater than 95% reduction in DAVF flow based on the angiographer's radiographic assessment. Seventy-one percent (28 of 39) of patients had

Table 2 DAVF demographics and treatment summary	
Characteristics	**n (%)**
Time period	2001–2009
Number of patients	39
Age range	39–71
Median age, y	48
Number of treatments	
Onyx	12
NBCA	11
Coils	5
Craniotomy	2
Radiosurgery	7
Median volume, cc	2.5
Median dose, Gy	22
Cortical venous drainage	18
Complete treatment	28 (71)
Endovascular alone	21
Endovascular followed by resection	7
Transvenous approach	5
Transarterial approach	25

complete treatment of the fistula: 21 by purely endovascular treatment and 7 with endovascular therapy followed by craniotomy.

Of the 11 patients who did not have complete treatment of the fistula, 7 (64%) had at least 90% obliteration with only 1 feeding pedicle remaining. Three of those with incomplete treatment (but absent CVD) underwent radiosurgery as the final approach for treatment. The average dose for treatment of the DAVF was 22 Gy in single fraction; follow-up in this subgroup is ongoing.

Use of onyx in DAVF embolization Forty treatments were made for 12 patients (**Table 3**). There were 3.33 treatments per patient, with a complete

Table 3 Summary of onyx transarterial emoblization results	
	n (%)
Treatments	40
Number of patients	12
Complete obliteration of fistula	8 (75)
Median treatments per patient	3.33
Morbidity	3 (7.5)
Mortality	0
Reversal of cortical venous drainage	30 (85)

obliteration rate of 75% at the end of the follow-up period. The cessation of CVD was seen in 85% of patients at end of follow-up for patients with onyx treatment.

Normalization of retrograde CVD Of those patients with retrograde CVD, 87% (26 of 30) had resolution with treatment. Of these 26 patients, 69% (18 of 26) patients had obliteration by endovascular means alone, while the rest required open surgical clipping of the fistula following embolization.

In 5 of the 18 patients who had CVD treated via embolization, success was only obtained when a transvenous approach was performed, due to difficulty with catheterization of feeding vessels. Three of the 5 patients received coils in addition to onyx for transvenous embolization.

Postoperative complications Epidural infection after craniotomy, postembolization intracranial hemorrhage not requiring surgery, and need for femoral artery repair after embolization were all encountered (**Table 4**). All complications were diagnosed and treated expeditiously.

Fig. 1 shows a case illustration of a DAVF treated with onyx.

Summary

Much has been learned in recent years about the pathoanatomy, pathophysiology, natural history and therapeutic options for DAVFs. A better understanding of these lesions has allowed more prompt and precise diagnosis, and a realistic assessment of features predisposing to aggressive clinical course. Clinical symptoms other than hemorrhage and progressive neurologic deficits rarely warrant aggressive treatment of a DAVF, unless the lesion is particularly accessible or is associated with features predisposing to subsequent aggressive clinical behavior. Patient reassurance, symptomatic treatment, and palliative therapy are frequently sufficient. In DAVFs with features predisposing to an aggressive clinical course, a

more definitive treatment strategy should be adopted. It is obvious that the myriad of clinical manifestations of DAVFs and the wide spectrum of possible angiographic and pathophysiologic scenarios call for highly individualized management strategies. Diagnostic investigation should be thorough so as to identify DAVFs with features predisposing to aggressive clinical behavior such as retrograde and leptomeningeal CVD, associated aneurysms, or venous ecstasia.

The therapeutic armamentarium to treat DAVFs includes a number of options with varying risk and effectiveness for individual lesions. TAE, TVE, open surgical therapy, and radiosurgery can be used alone or in various combinations as required for individual clinical scenarios. Endovascular management of DAVFs is a safe and effective method of treating these complex lesions. Based on our data, endovascular embolization should be the primary modality for treating DAVFs with modalities such as surgery and radiosurgery as secondary options. Regardless, the treatment of DAVFs should be entrusted to a multidisciplinary team with expertise in the recognition and management of these lesions and with experience in a variety of treatment options approaches.

PIAL ARTERIOVENOUS FISTULA

PAVF is a rare vascular abnormality that accounts for only 1.6% of all intracranial vascular malformations.[55] It is composed of 1 or more arterial feeders with a single venous channel. The lack of an intervening nidus or capillary bed differentiates this lesion from the arteriovenous malformation. It also differs from DAVF in that its arterial supply derives from pial and cortical arteries and is not located within the leaflets of the dura.[56] The direct arteriovenous shunt results in high venous blood flow and varix formation with the subsequent risk of hemorrhage. PAVF can be congenital or result from iatrogenic or traumatic injury. Congenital PAVFs develop in childhood as part of syndromes such as Rendu-Osler-Weber,[57] Klippel-Trenaunay-Weber,[58] Ehlers-Danlos,[59] and neurofibromatosis type 1.[60]

Natural History

The natural history of PAVF is largely unknown due to the restricted number of cases. There is only 1 reported case of spontaneous closure in the literature.[61] The direct arteriovenous shunt results in high venous blood flow and huge varices formation with the subsequent risk of hemorrhage.[62] One study reported that 5 out of 8 symptomatic patients with PAVF who were treated conservatively died.[63] Another study reported good

Table 4 Complications of Onyx-18 transarterial embolizations of DAVFs	
Complication	**n (%)**
Stroke	1
Femoral dissection	1
Retroperitoneal hematoma	0
Postembolization-associated hemorrhage	1
Renal failure	0

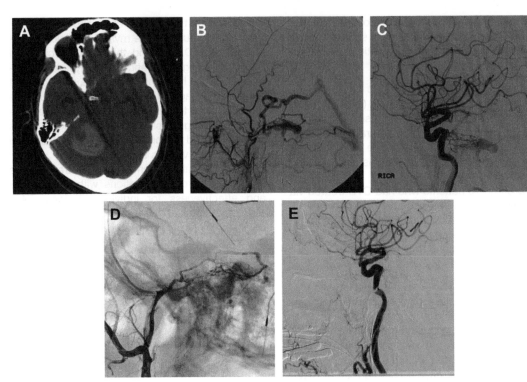

Fig. 1. A 60-year-old woman presented with a worsening headache. (*A*) Axial noncontrast CT scan of the head shows an intraparenchymal hemorrhage within the right cerebellar hemisphere. (*B*) Lateral view of a right external carotid artery angiogram shows a DAVF fed by multiple branches of the middle meningeal artery and ascending pharyngeal artery draining in the transverse and sigmoid sinus with dysplastic a venous varix. (*C*) Lateral view of a right internal carotid artery angiogram shows contribution of multiple meningeal feeders from the cavernous carotid artery feeding the DAVF. (*D*) Lateral spot fluoroscopic image shows the onyx cast in the arterial feeders and venous varix. (*E*) Postembolization lateral view of a right common carotid artery angiogram shows occlusion of the DAVF.

outcome with flow disconnection either by surgery or endovascular means.[56]

Clinical Presentation

PAVFs can present with headaches, hemorrhage, seizures, focal neurologic deficits, and raised intracranial pressure. Some of these manifestations can be explained by the mass effect exerted by the giant varices on the surrounding structures and the impairment of CSF pathway. In neonates and infants, these malformations can present with high-output cardiac failure, increased head circumference, and skull erosion.[64]

Endovascular Treatment

PAVFs are associated with a high morbidity and mortality and should be treated in most cases. Because of the absence of an intervening nidus (as in AVM), flow disconnection can obliterate the fistula without the necessity for lesion or varix resection.[56] This can be achieved by microsurgery (clip placement or vessels cauterization) or by

endovascular means. Because of the deep localization of these lesions or their presence in eloquent areas, surgery can be challenging and may require the use of a cardiopulmonary bypass.[65] Furthermore, the arterialized and thickened nature of the draining veins makes identification of the fistula difficult. Endovascular techniques offer a safe and effective approach to the treatment of PAVFs. In the authors' institution, we treat almost all patients with PAVF by endovascular techniques. The goal of therapy is to occlude all arterial feeders as close as possible to the site of the fistula using embolic materials. The 2 types of embolic materials that have been used are NBCA and onyx. NBCA is an adhesive agent that is delivered in a single injection. Onyx offers the ability to redirect flow during the course of delivery, which allows for a more precise targeting of the material into the fistula. Because of the high flow nature of these lesions, application of the embolic material can be challenging, and distal migration can be seen. A balloon can be inflated proximally in the feeding artery to block the flow, which allows enough time for the embolic plug to form. Coils have also been used to treat PAVF with good results.[56] However, these should be reserved for single-artery–single-vein PAVF.

Regardless of the embolic material being used, PAVFs are high-flow lesions, and therefore the risk of migration of the material into the draining vein,[66] lung, or elsewhere in the cerebral vasculature should be considered.[57] Embolizing the draining vein in the presence of a nonoccluded fistula can lead to a massive brain hemorrhage, and a venous infarct can also result if a normal cerebral vein is occluded. Bleeding and edema after successful obliteration of the PAVF have also been reported by several authors and attributed to the normal perfusion pressure breakthrough phenomenon.[64,67] Finally, if embolization is too proximal in the arterial pedicle, new arterial recruitment and fistula recurrence can occur.[56] **Fig. 2** shows a case illustration of PAVF.

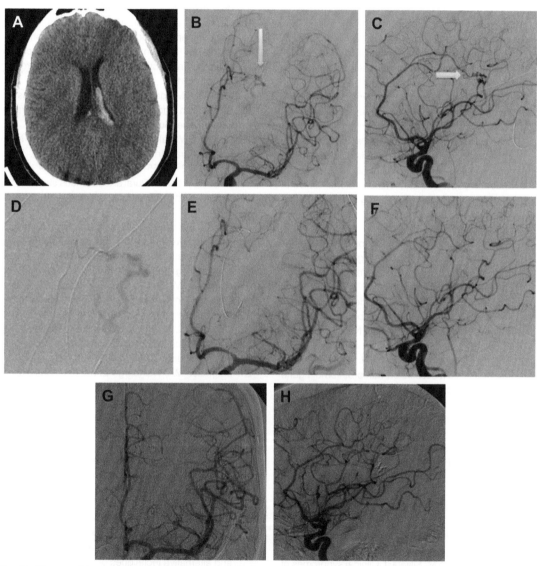

Fig. 2. 45-year-old man who presented with headache and vomiting. (*A*) Axial noncontrast CT scan of the head shows intraventricular hemorrhage. (*B*) Frontal projection of a left internal carotid artery angiogram shows filling of the PAVF (*arrow*). (*C*) Lateral projection of a left internal carotid artery angiogram shows a PAVF fed from distal pericallosal branches off the anterior cerebral artery (*arrow*). (*D*) Frontal projection of an angiogram performed by injecting contrast through the microcatheter in the arterial feeder shows filling of the PAVF. (*E, F*): Postembolization, left internal carotid angiogram in the frontal (*E*) and lateral projection (*F*) shows complete occlusion of the PAVF with NBCA. (*G, H*) At 7-month follow-up, left internal carotid angiogram in the frontal (*G*) and lateral projection (*H*) shows continued complete occlusion of the PAVF with NBCA.

Summary

PAVF is a rare vascular malformation that leads to a high morbidity and mortality. Adequate treatment with flow disconnection is associated with good clinical outcome. Endovascular treatment with liquid embolics seems to be efficacious, with a reasonable morbidity related to the procedure, compared with the natural history of this disease.

REFERENCES

1. Lasjaunias P, Lopez-Ibor L, Abanou A, et al. Radiological anatomy of the vascularization of cranial dural arteriovenous malformations. Anat Clin 1984;6: 87–99.
2. Jafar J, Awad I, Huang P. Intracranial vascular malformations: clinical decisions and multimodality management strategies. In: Jafar J, Awad I, Rosenwasser R, editors. Vascular malformations of the central nervous system. Philadelphia: Lippincott Williams & Wilkins; 1999. p. 219–32.
3. Chaudhary MY, Sachdev VP, Cho SH, et al. Dural arteriovenous malformation of the major venous sinuses: an acquired lesion. AJNR Am J Neuroradiol 1982;3:13–9.
4. Houser OW, Campbell JK, Campbell RJ, et al. Arteriovenous malformation affecting the transverse dural venous sinus—an acquired lesion. Mayo Clin Proc 1979;54:651–61.
5. Lawton MT, Jacobowitz R, Spetzler RF. Redefined role of angiogenesis in the pathogenesis of dural arteriovenous malformations. J Neurosurg 1997; 87:267–74.
6. Singh V, Meyers PM, Halbach VH, et al. Dural arteriovenous fistula associated with prothrombin gene mutation. J Neuroimaging 2001;11:319–21.
7. Yassari R, Jahromi B, Macdonald R. Dural arteriovenous fistula after craniotomy for pilocytic astrocytoma in a patient with protein S deficiency. Surg Neurol 2002;58:59–64 [discussion: 64].
8. Chaloupka J, Putman C, Roth T. Diagnostic evaluation. In: Batjer, editor. Techniques in neurosurgery. Philadelphia: Lippincott-Raven; 1996. p. 5–25.
9. Fermand M, Reizine D, Melki JP, et al. Long-term follow-up of 43 pure dural arteriovenous fistulae (AVF) of the lateral sinus. Neuroradiology 1987; 29:348–53.
10. Obrador S, Soto M, Silvela J. Clinical syndromes of arteriovenous malformations of the transverse-sigmoid sinus. J Neurol Neurosurg Psychiatry 1975;38:436–51.
11. Awad IA, Little JR, Akarawi WP, et al. Intracranial dural arteriovenous malformations: factors predisposing to an aggressive neurological course. J Neurosurg 1990;72:839–50.
12. Flemming K, Brown R. Natural history of intracranial vascular malformations. In: Winn R, editor. Neurological surgery. Philadelphia: Elsevier; 2004. p. 2159–83.
13. Luessenhop A. Dural arteriovenous malformations. In: Rengachary R, editor. Neurosurgery. New York: McGraw-Hill; 1986. p. 1473–7.
14. Grady MS, Pobereskin L. Arteriovenous malformations of the dura mater. Surg Neurol 1987;28: 135–40.
15. Aminoff MJ. Vascular anomalies in the intracranial dura mater. Brain 1973;96:601–12.
16. Brown RD Jr, Wiebers DO, Nichols DA. Intracranial dural arteriovenous fistulae: angiographic predictors of intracranial hemorrhage and clinical outcome in nonsurgical patients. J Neurosurg 1994;81:531–8.
17. Malik GM, Morgan JK, Boulos RS, et al. Venous angiomas: an underestimated cause of intracranial hemorrhage. Surg Neurol 1988;30:350–8.
18. Houser OW, Baker HL Jr, Rhoton AL Jr, et al. Intracranial dural arteriovenous malformations. Radiology 1972;105:55–64.
19. Newton T, Hoyt W. Dural arteriovenous shunts in the region of the cavernous sinus. Neuroradiology 1970;1:71–81.
20. Toya S, Shiobara R, Izumi J, et al. Spontaneous carotid–cavernous fistula during pregnancy or in the postpartum stage. Report of two cases. J Neurosurg 1981;54:252–6.
21. Nakamura M, Tamaki N, Hara Y, et al. Two unusual cases of multiple dural arteriovenous fistulas. Neurosurgery 1997;41:288–92 [discussion: 92–3].
22. Ushikoshi S, Kikuchi Y, Miyasaka K. Multiple dural arteriovenous shunts in a 5-year-old boy. AJNR Am J Neuroradiol 1999;20:728–30.
23. Magidson MA, Weinberg PE. Spontaneous closure of a dural arteriovenous malformation. Surg Neurol 1976;6:107–10.
24. Hansen JH, Sogaard I. Spontaneous regression of an extra- and intracranial arteriovenous malformation. Case report. J Neurosurg 1976;45:338–41.
25. Luciani A, Houdart E, Mounayer C, et al. Spontaneous closure of dural arteriovenous fistulas: report of three cases and review of the literature. AJNR Am J Neuroradiol 2001;22:992–6.
26. Kiyosue H, Hori Y, Okahara M, et al. Treatment of intracranial dural arteriovenous fistulas: current strategies based on location and hemodynamics, and alternative techniques of transcatheter embolization. Radiographics 2004;24:1637–53.
27. Bitoh S, Sakaki S. Spontaneous cure of dural arteriovenous malformation in the posterior fossa. Surg Neurol 1979;12:111–4.
28. Olutola PS, Eliam M, Molot M, et al. Spontaneous regression of a dural arteriovenous malformation. Neurosurgery 1983;12:687–90.

29. Awad IA, Barrow D. Dural arteriovenous malformations. Park Ridge (IL): American Association of Neurological Surgeons; 1993.

30. Friedman JA, Pollock BE, Nichols DA. Development of a cerebral arteriovenous malformation documented in an adult by serial angiography. Case report. J Neurosurg 2000;93:1058–61.

31. Lasjaunias P, Chiu M, ter Brugge K, et al. Neurological manifestations of intracranial dural arteriovenous malformations. J Neurosurg 1986;64:724–30.

32. Vinuela F, Fox AJ, Pelz DM, et al. Unusual clinical manifestations of dural arteriovenous malformations. J Neurosurg 1986;64:554–8.

33. Chimowitz MI, Little JR, Awad IA, et al. Intracranial hypertension associated with unruptured cerebral arteriovenous malformations. Ann Neurol 1990;27:474–9.

34. Cognard C, Casasco A, Toevi M, et al. Dural arteriovenous fistulas as a cause of intracranial hypertension due to impairment of cranial venous outflow. J Neurol Neurosurg Psychiatry 1998;65:308–16.

35. Gelwan MJ, Choi IS, Berenstein A, et al. Dural arteriovenous malformations and papilledema. Neurosurgery 1988;22:1079–84.

36. Djindjian R, Merland JJ, Theron J. Superselective arteriography of the external carotid artery. New York: Springer-Verlag; 1977. p. 606–28.

37. Cognard C, Gobin YP, Pierot L, et al. Cerebral dural arteriovenous fistulas: clinical and angiographic correlation with a revised classification of venous drainage. Radiology 1995;194:671–80.

38. Borden JA, Wu JK, Shucart WA. A proposed classification for spinal and cranial dural arteriovenous fistulous malformations and implications for treatment. J Neurosurg 1995;82:166–79.

39. Malik GM, Pearce JE, Ausman JI, et al. Dural arteriovenous malformations and intracranial hemorrhage. Neurosurgery 1984;15:332–9.

40. Davies MA, TerBrugge K, Willinsky R, et al. The validity of classification for the clinical presentation of intracranial dural arteriovenous fistulas. J Neurosurg 1996;85:830–7.

41. Hardy RW, Costin JA, Weinstein M, et al. External carotid cavernous fistula treated by transfemoral embolization. Surg Neurol 1978;9:255–6.

42. Vinuela FV, Debrun GM, Fox AJ, et al. Detachable calibrated-leak balloon for superselective angiography and embolization of dural arteriovenous malformations. J Neurosurg 1983;58:817–23.

43. Nesbit GM, Barnwell SL. The use of electrolytically detachable coils in treating high-flow arteriovenous fistulas. AJNR Am J Neuroradiol 1998;19:1565–9.

44. Jansen O, Dorfler A, Forsting M, et al. Endovascular therapy of arteriovenous fistulae with electrolytically detachable coils. Neuroradiology 1999;41:951–7.

45. Liu HM, Huang YC, Wang YH, et al. Transarterial embolisation of complex cavernous sinus dural arteriovenous fistulae with low-concentration cyanoacrylate. Neuroradiology 2000;42:766–70.

46. Goto K, Sidipratomo P, Ogata N, et al. Combining endovascular and neurosurgical treatments of high-risk dural arteriovenous fistulas in the lateral sinus and the confluence of the sinuses. J Neurosurg 1999;90:289–99.

47. Collice M, D'Aliberti G, Arena O, et al. Surgical treatment of intracranial dural arteriovenous fistulae: role of venous drainage. Neurosurgery 2000;47:56–66 [discussion: 7].

48. Friedman JA, Pollock BE, Nichols DA, et al. Results of combined stereotactic radiosurgery and transarterial embolization for dural arteriovenous fistulas of the transverse and sigmoid sinuses. J Neurosurg 2001;94:886–91.

49. Halbach VV, Higashida RT, Hieshima GB, et al. Transvenous embolization of dural fistulas involving the cavernous sinus. AJNR Am J Neuroradiol 1989;10:377–83.

50. Halbach VV, Higashida RT, Hieshima GB, et al. Transvenous embolization of dural fistulas involving the transverse and sigmoid sinuses. AJNR Am J Neuroradiol 1989;10:385–92.

51. Roy D, Raymond J. The role of transvenous embolization in the treatment of intracranial dural arteriovenous fistulas. Neurosurgery 1997;40:1133–41 [discussion: 41–4].

52. Endo S, Kuwayama N, Takaku A, et al. Direct packing of the isolated sinus in patients with dural arteriovenous fistulas of the transverse-sigmoid sinus. J Neurosurg 1998;88:449–56.

53. Steiger HJ, Hanggi D, Schmid-Elsaesser R. Cranial and spinal dural arteriovenous malformations and fistulas: an update. Acta Neurochir Suppl 2005;94:115–22.

54. Duffau H, Lopes M, Janosevic V, et al. Early rebleeding from intracranial dural arteriovenous fistulas: report of 20 cases and review of the literature. J Neurosurg 1999;90:78–84.

55. Halbach VV, Higashida RT, Hieshima GB, et al. Transarterial occlusion of solitary intracerebral arteriovenous fistulas. AJNR Am J Neuroradiol 1989;10:747–52.

56. Hoh BL, Putman CM, Budzik RF, et al. Surgical and endovascular flow disconnection of intracranial pial single-channel arteriovenous fistulae. Neurosurgery 2001;49:1351–63 [discussion: 63–4].

57. Kikuchi K, Kowada M, Sasajima H. Vascular malformations of the brain in hereditary hemorrhagic telangiectasia (Rendu-Osler-Weber disease). Surg Neurol 1994;41:374–80.

58. Oyesiku NM, Gahm NH, Goldman RL. Cerebral arteriovenous fistula in the Klippel-Trenaunay-Weber syndrome. Dev Med Child Neurol 1988;30:245–8.

59. Oya S, Shigeno T, Kumai J, et al. A case of pial single-channel cerebral arteriovenous fistula. No Shinkei Geka 2004;32:67–72 [in Japanese].

60. Kubota T, Nakai H, Tanaka T, et al. A case of intracranial arteriovenous fistula in an infant with neurofibromatosis type 1. Childs Nerv Syst 2002;18: 166–70.

61. Santosh C, Teasdale E, Molyneux A. Spontaneous closure of an intracranial middle cerebral arteriovenous fistula. Neuroradiology 1991;33: 65–6.

62. Wang YC, Wong HF, Yeh YS. Intracranial pial arteriovenous fistulas with single-vein drainage. Report of three cases and review of the literature. J Neurosurg 2004;100:201–5.

63. Nelson K, Nimi Y, Lasjaunias P, et al. Endovascular embolization of congenital intracranial pial arteriovenous fistulas. Neuroimaging Clin N Am 1992;2:309–17.

64. Tomlinson FH, Rufenacht DA, Sundt TM Jr, et al. Arteriovenous fistulas of the brain and the spinal cord. J Neurosurg 1993;79:16–27.

65. Halbach VV, Dowd CF, Higashida RT, et al. Endovascular treatment of mural-type vein of Galen malformations. J Neurosurg 1998;89:74–80.

66. Giller CA, Batjer HH, Purdy P, et al. Interdisciplinary evaluation of cerebral hemodynamics in the treatment of arteriovenous fistulae associated with giant varices. Neurosurgery 1994;35:778–82 [discussion: 82–4].

67. Aoki N, Sakai T, Oikawa A. Intracranial arteriovenous fistula manifesting as progressive neurological deterioration in an infant: case report. Neurosurgery 1991;28:619–22 [discussion: 22–3].

Endovascular Treatment of Carotid Occlusive Disease

William Stetler, MD[a], Joseph J. Gemmete, MD, FSIR[b,*],
Aditya S. Pandey, MD[c], Neeraj Chaudhary, MD, MRCS, FRCR[c]

KEYWORDS

- Carotid arteries • Atherosclerosis • Carotid endarterectomy • Carotid stent placement • Stroke
- Transient ischemic attack

KEY POINTS

- Patients who have severe (>70%) symptomatic carotid stenosis have up to a 20% risk of an ipsilateral stroke over the following 3-month time period, with 30% to 35% risk of ipsilateral stroke over 2 to 3 years' time when treated with optimum medical management.
- The degree of carotid stenosis by ultrasound should be reported based on the Society of Radiologists in Ultrasound's consensus conference in 2003.
- Carotid artery balloon angioplasty and stent placement (CAS) has a higher incidence of perioperative stroke when compared with carotid endarterectomy (CAE); however, there is a decreased incidence of myocardial infarction, infection, and cranial nerve injury.
- Patients that are ideal for CAS include patients that have a high surgical risk, such as patients with prior neck irradiation, aberrant neck anatomy, contralateral recurrent laryngeal nerve injury, prior ipsilateral CEA, significant coronary artery disease, high cervical stenotic lesion location, and tracheostomy.
- Patients with type II and III aortic arches, tortuous common carotid artery (CCA), or young patients with otherwise normal anatomy and a low-lying cervical lesion location precluding mandibular disarticulation are best served with CEA.

INTRODUCTION

In the United States, 150,000 patients die and 600,000 suffer significant morbidity each year as a result of a cerebrovascular accident (CVA), making stroke the second most common cause of death in the United States.[1–7] An estimated 88% of these are ischemic strokes, with 15% attributed to extracranial carotid occlusive disease.[8–11] Endovascular therapy for the treatment of carotid atherosclerotic disease has advanced over the last decade and is now considered to be a viable alternative to carotid endarterectomy (CEA) in appropriately selected patients.[11–16] Carotid artery balloon angioplasty and stent placement (CAS) during its infancy was associated with higher rates of perioperative ischemic complications when compared with CEA. However, lower rates of other perioperative complications were noted, including myocardial infarctions and infection.[13,14] As a result of increased experience with the procedure and improvements in technology specifically designed for CAS, the rates of periprocedural ischemic complications have diminished. Today, the rate of complications from CEA versus CAS are nearly equivocal, making the choice of therapy based more on clinical presentation, medical

[a] Department of Neurosurgery, University of Michigan Hospitals, 1500 East Medical Center Drive, Ann Arbor, MI 48109, USA; [b] Division of Interventional Neuroradiology and Cranial Base Surgery, Departments of Radiology, Neurosurgery, and Otolaryngology, University of Michigan Hospitals, UH B1 D328, 1500 East Medical Center Drive, Ann Arbor, MI 48109–5030, USA; [c] Division of Interventional Neuroradiology, Departments of Neurosurgery and Radiology, University of Michigan Hospitals, 1500 East Medical Center Drive, Ann Arbor, MI 48109, USA
* Corresponding author.
E-mail address: gemmete@med.umich.edu

Neuroimag Clin N Am 23 (2013) 637–652
http://dx.doi.org/10.1016/j.nic.2013.03.011
1052-5149/13/$ – see front matter © 2013 Elsevier Inc. All rights reserved.

neuroimaging.theclinics.com

comorbidities, and carotid artery anatomy.[14,15] In this review, the authors concentrate their discussion on the treatment of carotid atherosclerotic disease with particular attention on the endovascular treatment.

CLINICAL PRESENTATION

Carotid artery stenosis in patients is usually discovered after an ischemic event (either a transient ischemic attack [TIA] or a permanent stroke).[17] The remainder of carotid artery occlusive disease is usually discovered after an initial abnormality is revealed on physical examination (ie, carotid bruit), which is then confirmed on imaging studies.[18] The most common ischemic stroke syndrome is a middle cerebral artery occlusion resulting in contralateral hemiparesis (arm more than leg) and hemisensory loss as well as aphasia depending on hemispheric dominance.[19] Other TIA symptoms can include ocular symptoms, such as amaurosis fugax, which is most commonly described as a shade being pulled over one's eye on the ipsilateral side. Unfortunately, in many patients', carotid atherosclerotic disease is discovered after a large stroke has occurred.[9,10,20]

EPIDEMIOLOGY AND NATURAL HISTORY

Approximately 88% of strokes have an ischemic cause, with approximately 15% being secondary to carotid occlusive disease.[1–7,21–24] Risk factors for stroke of all types include increasing age, male sex, hypertension, smoking history, diabetes, obesity, hypercoagulable states, African American race, and presence of carotid artery atherosclerosis.[20] The prevalence of carotid stenosis (>50%) in patients 65 years of age or older is estimated at 5% to 9%. In patients without symptoms of cerebral ischemia (TIA, stroke, amaurosis fugax) with carotid stenosis (>60%), the risk of stroke has been cited between 2% and 5% annually, with a 2.2% per year risk of ipsilateral stroke when treated with maximum medical management.[25] Alternatively, patients who have severe (>70%) symptomatic carotid stenosis have up to a 20% risk of an ipsilateral stroke over the following 3-month time period, with a 30% to 35% risk of ipsilateral stroke over 2 to 3 years time when treated with optimum medical management. For symptomatic patients with moderate stenosis (50%–69%), the risk of stroke on medical management is 15% to 20% over a period of 3 years.[18,25–27]

The likelihood of stroke has more recently been shown to be higher in patients with an echolucent plaque on ultrasound, suggesting that plaque morphology in addition to the degree of stenosis plays a role in the risk of stroke.[28] An ulcerated atherosclerotic plaque on imaging studies also has been shown to have a higher likelihood of becoming symptomatic when compared with a nonulcerated, smooth atherosclerotic plaque.[29] Furthermore, patients who have suffered a stroke of any cause are also 2 to 3 times as likely to have a myocardial infarction.[27] It has also been shown that the degree of carotid stenosis is directly related to the amount of cerebral collateralization. This finding implies that a hemodynamically significant carotid lesion causing cerebral hypoperfusion recruits arterial collateral vessels to the territory affected.[30] The annual risk of a subsequent stroke in any cerebral territory following an occlusion of the carotid artery is high at 5.5% according to a meta-analysis of 20 follow-up studies in patients with TIA or a minor ischemic stroke; however, interestingly, the risk of subsequent ipsilateral stroke following such an occlusion is only 2.1% per year.[31] The hypothesis being that the development of collaterals in the ipsilateral hemisphere is facilitated by worsening vessel stenosis caused by the incriminating carotid plaque over a period of time, which then offers protection against further ischemia once the carotid artery becomes occluded. Recent long-term data have shown that this risk of stroke is highest in the first 18 months following occlusion and then drops off dramatically to an average annual rate of only 2.4% for all types of stroke at the 10-year follow-up. Interestingly, cerebral leptomeningeal collateralization increased the risk of recurrent ipsilateral ischemic events.[32] The implication being that in the first 18 months following carotid vessel occlusion, the collateral circulation is not completely established and any hypoperfusion episode can potentially precipitate an ischemic event; however, beyond this period the risk drops off significantly because of the establishment of a new equilibrium in the cerebral perfusion. The apparent fallacy demonstrated in the long-term follow-up study from Netherlands showing leptomeningeal collateral presence predicting increased risk of subsequent ischemia merely reveals the delicate balance of cerebral perfusion in the midst of progressively occluding carotid vessel.[32]

ANATOMY AND PATHOPHYSIOLOGY

In most patients, the right common carotid artery (CCA) arises from the brachiocephalic artery, whereas the left CCA typically arises directly from the aortic arch. At approximately the level of the superior border of the thyroid cartilage or the inferior edge of the hyoid bone, the carotid artery bifurcates into the internal carotid artery (ICA) and the external carotid artery (ECA). In one cadaveric study, 73% of specimens' bifurcations were above the thyroid cartilage and 63% were below the hyoid bone,[33] which typically correlates to approximately the midportion of the vertebral body of C3.[34] At the bifurcation, there is a dilation referred to as the carotid bulb.[35] On average, the outer diameter of the proximal ICA is 8.1 mm, whereas the carotid bulb is 12.8 mm. Distal to the bifurcation, the ICA then narrows to an average diameter of 6.1 mm.[34] These average numbers are helpful when choosing stent and balloon sizes during endovascular cases as well as when using Fogarty balloons and shunts in CEA.

The cervical ICA proceeds into the carotid foramen, entering the petrous portion of the temporal bone. After exiting the petrous temporal bone, the ICA swings anteriorly in the cavernous sinus before then bending posteriorly as it exits the cavernous sinus to become an intracranial vessel. The ICA then continues to terminate into the middle cerebral artery and the anterior cerebral artery.

Atherosclerotic changes of the carotid artery typically extend from the carotid bulb into the ICA. There is a dramatic change in vessel diameter from approximately 8 mm in the CCA to a 4–5 mm ICA.

Atherosclerotic lesions tend to occur at areas experiencing low endothelial shear stress which are local wall stresses that are generated by patterns of blood flow, such as the carotid bifurcation region.[36] Low shear stress promotes atherosclerosis by a variety of mechanisms, including impairment of endothelial function by downregulation of the endothelial isoform of nitric oxide synthase (e-NOS) and upregulation of endothelin-1, increased endothelial uptake of low-density lipoprotein (LDL), promotion of oxidative stress, and increased plaque thrombogenicity.[37–40] Low endothelial shear stress also enhances the proatherogenic effect of chronic inflammation because it allows for the attachment and infiltration of inflammatory cells via the activation of nuclear factor kappa-light-chain-enhancer of activated B cells (NF-kB) and subsequent upregulation of adhesion molecules, chemokines, and proinflammatory cytokines.[41–43] Low endothelial shear stress has also been implicated in the transition of stable atherosclerotic lesions to vulnerable plaques resulting in acute coronary syndromes.[44] As the diameter of the vessel narrows because of plaque buildup, it can cause reduction of blood flow and, hence, ischemic changes. However, more importantly, most TIAs and stroke occur from ulceration of the atherosclerotic plaque with distal embolization into the intracranial circulation. Finally, with plaque rupture, a vigorous local coagulation cascade may be initiated and a platelet plug may form and occlude the entire ICA at the area of the lesion or send distal emboli into the intracranial circulation.

DIAGNOSTIC IMAGING FEATURES

Many diagnostic imaging modalities may be used to help confirm the diagnosis of carotid occlusive disease. Carotid duplex ultrasonography is often the first test performed when the clinician suspects carotid stenosis. The duplex ultrasound examination includes a quantitative measurement of the degree of arterial narrowing using a brightness mode (B-mode technique) as well as a spectral analysis to determine the measurement of blood flow velocity across the lesion. This examination provides 2 pieces of information for the ultrasonographer to interpret. The degree of carotid stenosis should be reported based on the Society of Radiologists in Ultrasound's consensus conference in 2003:

- Normal: ICA peak systolic velocity (PSV) less than 125 cm/s and no plaque or intimal thickening is visible
- Less than 50% stenosis: ICA PSV less than 125 cm/s and plaque or intimal thickening is visible
- 50% to 69% stenosis: ICA PSV is 125 to 230 cm/s and plaque is visible
- Greater than 70% stenosis to near occlusion: ICA PSV greater than 230 cm/s and visible plaque and lumen narrowing are seen[45]

Ultrasound is, however, a limited assessment of only the extracranial carotid vessels and results can vary based on artifact induced by calcific plaque within the lesion.[8,45] Carotid ultrasound has been shown to often overestimate the degree of stenosis when compared with the gold standard measurements of diagnostic carotid angiography.[46,47] Ultrasound technology has continued to improve over the last 30 years; however, it remains inferior to computed tomography angiography (CTA) and magnetic resonance angiography (MRA). Therefore, after this noninvasive study is performed, a confirmatory study, such as a CTA or MRA, is needed to determine the further management of patients.

CTA is performed by intravenous injection of iodinated contrast. Axial images are obtained as the contrast density peaks in the arterial phase. Sagittal, coronal, and multiplanar 3-dimensional (3D) images can be formatted based on the axial images obtained to help measure the intraluminal diameter at the narrowest portion of the proximal ICA and across the area of the ICA that is above the stenosis that is thought to be normal. The degree of stenosis is then calculated based on the

North American Surgical Carotid Endarterectomy Trial (NASCET) criteria as a percentage. CTA accuracy exceeds 95% and is limited largely by technical factors alone.[26,48,49] Patient motion and poor cardiac function can decrease the accuracy of CTA because of the motion artifact and suboptimal luminal contrast related to compromised cardiac function. Furthermore, any venous contrast contamination can make the images more difficult to interpret. Additionally, the contrast load administered is not insignificant and must be taken into consideration in patients with renal insufficiency or those on hemodialysis. Patients with iodinated contrast allergies may also require special consideration and might need a steroid preparation before the administration of contrast.

MRA offers another noninvasive approach to measure the degree of carotid stenosis. The 2 main MRA techniques to assess carotid stenosis are (1) 2-dimensional and 3D multiple overlapping thin slab angiography (MOTSA) time-of-flight (TOF) without the use of gadolinium contrast and (2) contrast-enhanced MRA with rapid injection of gadolinium to produce axial images through the neck from the aortic arch to include the circle of Willis. These images, much like CTA, can then be formatted into 3D images and the stenosis can be calculated in a similar manner according to NASCET criteria as described later. MR using TOF sequences is especially useful in patients with either contrast allergies or renal insufficiency because contrast (gadolinium) is not required to obtain these images with the caveat that flow-dependent TOF MRA readily lends itself to artifacts related to flow phenomena exaggerating stenosis. Turbulence can create artifacts on the TOF images that can overestimate stenotic lesions.[8,45,50] Additionally, intracranial images can be obtained at the same time to assess for prior cerebral vascular accident (CVA) or additional intracranial pathologies; the intracranial (as well as the extracranial) circulations can also be assessed, making it a superior test to carotid ultrasound. However, MR is contraindicated in patients with metal implants, such as pacemakers. The sensitivity and accuracy of MRA is up 92% to 97%, making it an acceptable and sensitive noninvasive test.[47]

Diagnostic cerebral angiography remains the gold standard to determine the degree of carotid artery stenosis of both the extracranial and intracranial circulation and to determine the optimal method of treatment.[8,46,47,51,52] This invasive study carries an approximately 0.5% risk of significant morbidity and mortality, with the most notable complications being arterial dissection, stroke, and retroperitoneal hematoma.[51] Additionally, the amount of iodinated contrast used varies but could represent a relative contraindication in patients with renal insufficiency, much like with CTA.

The degree of stenosis can be calculated in 2 ways: (1) using the maximal ICA stenosis/ICA normal caliber above the stenosis ratio or (2) using the maximal ICA stenosis/ICA outer to outer wall caliber ratio at the site of the stenosis. The former was used in the NASCET criteria and the latter in the European Carotid Surgery Trial (ECST) criteria.[25,26] The other 2 methods are the common carotid criteria (CC) and the Carotid Stenosis Index (CSI) method (Fig. 1).[53,54] There are some discrepancies and inconsistencies in the measurements obtained by the NASCET and ECST criteria. The criteria are based on indirect ratios where there is estimation of the outer wall diameter of the ICA at the level of the stenosis. Both the above methods are based on angiographic measurements, which make it impossible to directly measure the outer wall of the ICA at the level of the stenosis. These variables in the measurements result in wide disparity in stenosis estimates by NASCET or ECST criteria. Studies show that measurement of 50% stenosis by NASCET is equivalent to 70% by ECST.[55,56] The numerator both in NASCET and ECST is the direct measurement of the stenosis at its narrowest location. As for the denominator NASCET uses the diameter of the normal distal ICA, while ECST estimates the unseen outer wall diameter of the ICA at the carotid bulb stenosis. The diameter of the carotid bulb is usually double that of the normal ICA. This is the main reason for a different percentage stenosis measurement of the same carotid lesion using the two criteria.[57,58] The CSI method of stenosis measurement is based on multiplying the CCA measurement with a factor of 1.2. The factor of 1.2 was based on studies of anatomic estimates of the ICA diameter from the CCA diameter, which was found to be 1:1.19 ($\pm$0.09).[53] Percent stenosis is then calculated as in the other methods by comparing this with the diameter of the ICA stenosis (D) using the formula $(1 - D/N) \times 100\%$, with $N = 1.2 \times$ CCA diameter. With the advent of improved CTA technology, there have been studies that have validated a more direct estimation of the stenosis by using better visualization of the vessel wall and the contrast opacified lumen of the ICA stenosis.[59] Most clinicians favor using the NASCET criteria for determining the degree of stenosis as a more accurate representation of actual ICA stenosis because the ICA often has a smaller caliber from the CCA at baseline.[8,25,26,52] The reason the common carotid method is advocated by some investigators is that CCA and CSI criteria were created to preclude certain

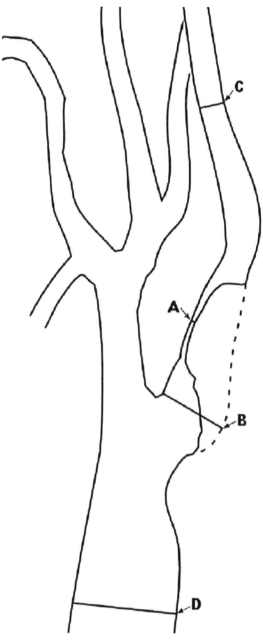

MEASUREMENT of STENOSIS

NASCET

$$1-\frac{A}{C} \times 100 = \% \text{ Stenosis}$$

ECST

$$1-\frac{A}{B} \times 100 = \% \text{ Stenosis}$$

CC

$$1-\frac{A}{D} \times 100 = \% \text{ Stenosis}$$

Fig. 1. Diagram shows the NASCET, ECST, and common CC to calculated stenosis. A, narrowest diameter of the internal carotid artery; B, expect diameter of the carotid bulb; C, normal diameter of the internal carotid artery; D, normal diameter of the common carotid artery.

ambiguities in the NASCET and the ECST criteria. This calculation is based on the use of CCA as a denominator and the relative ease of determining the precise diameter on angiographic images without superimposed vessels or branches and its alleged disease-free state.[53,54,58] The reader is advised to have a detailed understanding of the background of the various methods of estimating carotid stenosis to make an informed

decision in selecting patients for the treatment of either CAS or CEA.

Treatment options are considered based on patients' medical comorbidities, if they are symptomatic or asymptomatic, and the percent of ICA stenosis. At the authors' institution, symptomatic patients with a stenosis of greater than 70% are offered treatment. Symptomatic patients with a 50% to 65% stenosis are also considered for treatment. The authors currently only consider treatment in patients who are asymptomatic if the operator has a less than 3% complication rate, the degree of stenosis is greater than 80%, and patients have a life expectancy of greater than 3 years. Currently, the treatment options include CAS and CEA. CEA is the traditional treatment approach; however, CAS has gained some acceptance based on the results of the Carotid Revascularization Endarterectomy Versus Stenting Trial (CREST).[16,60–62] In the next few paragraphs, the authors discuss the technical details of CAS followed by CEA. Finally, the authors discuss the pros and cons of both techniques.

ENDOVASCULAR TECHNIQUE
Technique

The procedure is performed under conscious sedation. A radial arterial line is placed to monitor patients' blood pressure during and after the procedure. To minimize thromboembolic complication during stent placement and subsequent in-stent thrombosis caused by platelet aggregation, patients are placed on dual antiplatelet agents before the procedure. There is a lack of consensus on the standard dose regime. The authors recommend a loading dose of 325 mg aspirin with 300 mg clopidogrel bisulfate (Plavix) followed by a daily dose of 81 mg aspirin and 75 mg clopidogrel bisulfate (Plavix) for one week before the procedure. Aspirin function and P2Y12 inhibition assays are checked to ensure adequate platelet inhibition before the procedure. If patients are found to have inadequate platelet inhibition, the administration of an alternative antiplatelet agent, such as prasugrel (Effient), tricagrelor (Brilinta), or ticlopidine (Ticlid), should be considered.

Patients are placed supine on the angiographic table. Both groins are prepped and draped in the usual sterile fashion. The right common femoral artery is punctured retrograde under ultrasound guidance with a micropuncture kit using a modified Seldinger technique. The authors perform a complete cerebral angiogram with contrast injection in both common carotid arteries and one vertebral artery with projections over the neck and head before treatment. This procedure is to evaluate the intracranial vasculature and to assess the collateral circulation of the circle of Willis.

An 8F sheath is then placed at the arteriotomy site if the procedure is performed using a guide catheter. If the GORE flow reversal device (Gore Medical, Flagstaff, AZ) is used, a 9F sheath must be placed in the artery and a 6F sheath placed in the opposite common femoral vein. The Cook shuttle system (Cook Medial, Bloomington, IN)

uses a 6F 90- or 100-cm length sheath directly introduced through the arteriotomy. After adequate femoral access is secured, patients are given a bolus of heparin (70–100 mg/kg) to achieve activated clotting times of approximately 250 to 300 (or 1.5–2.0 × baseline). The brachial artery or common carotid artery can be accessed in a similar fashion, if there is a contraindication to using the femoral artery. The details of these techniques are beyond the scope of this article.

The 8F guide catheter can be directly advanced through the sheath over a 0.035 inch Terumo Glidewire (Terumo Medical, Somerset, NJ) or coaxially over a 125-cm 6.5F Cook vertebral artery catheter (Cook Medical, Bloomington, IN) into the common carotid artery under biplane fluoroscopy. A digital subtraction angiogram (DSA) is obtained in the standard projection. A 30° right or left anterior oblique angulation in the anterior posterior (AP) plane is often beneficial to splay out the bifurcation of the respective CCA.

Under road map guidance, the guide catheter is navigated over the wire just proximal to the lesion, while taking care not to cross the stenotic lesion with the wire. If additional wire purchase is required to navigate the CCA, the wire should be placed into the ECA and not the ICA to avoid any disruption of the plaque. The lesion is then crossed with an umbrella type of cerebral protection device placed into the distal cervical segment of the ICA.

There are various cerebral protection devices commercially available, but they all use 1 of 2 principles: (1) proximal flow reversal or (2) a distal embolic protection umbrella to arrest any platelet aggregates/thromboemboli from transgression into the intracranial circulation. Table 1 is a list of all the currently available protection devices.

The proximal flow reversal system is used as follows: the balloon catheter integrated with the 8F sheath is positioned proximal to the CCA bifurcation, the small microcatheter with a distal balloon is advanced through the sheath and positioned in the proximal ECA, the balloon is inflated to the occluded follow within the ECA, then the balloon on the sheath in the CCA is inflated to the occluded flow, and a small injection of contrast is performed to confirm the flow reversal. Connecting the 8F sheath with the sheath placed in the contralateral common femoral vein creates an arterial venous shunt (Fig. 2). A complete circle of Willis is a prerequisite for the use of the flow reversal device; this ensures a reversal of flow into the ipsilateral ICA. Once the reversal of flow is confirmed with a DSA, the lesion is crossed with the operator's wire of preference.

Alternatively, a distal embolic protection umbrella can be placed distal to the stenotic lesion,

Table 1
Comparison of protection devices

Device	Company	Type	Crossing Profile (F)	Guiding Catheter (F)	Diameter (mm)
GuardWire	Medtronic Vascular, Santa Rosa, CA	Distal balloon	2.1–2.7	6	2.5–6.0
Angioguard XP	Cordis Corp, Bridgewater, NJ	Filter	3.2–3.7	7–8	3.0–7.5
Spider	Ev3, Plymouth, MN	Filter	2.9	6–7	3.0–7.0
FilterWire EZ	Boston Scientific Corp, Natick, MA	Filter	3.2	6	3.5–5.5
EmboShield Nav6	Abbott Vascular, Santa Clara, CA	Filter	2.9–3.3	6	2.5–7.0
RX Accunet	Abbott	Filter	3.5–3.7	7–8	3.25–7.0
FiberNet	Medtronic	Filter	2.4–2.7	6–7	3.5–7.0
Mo.Ma Ultra	Medtronic	Proximal Balloon	na	9	6.0 ECA 13.0 CCA
Flow Reversal	W.L. Gore & Associates, Flagstaff, AZ	Proximal Balloon	na	9	<6.0 ECA 12.0 CCA

Abbreviation: na, not applicable.

usually in the high cervical portion of the ICA; this consists of a small permeable embolic umbrella on a torqueable wire that is house in a small sheath (Fig. 3). The system is navigated beyond the stenotic lesion and the basket is unsheathed to open. Care must be taken during this maneuver to keep the wire (on which the basket is attached) fixed in one position to prevent the basket from being pulled into the atherosclerotic lesion. All particles are not captured by the filter (Fig. 4).

After successful deployment of the flow reversal system or the distal embolic protection device, the lesion is usually predilated with a 3-mm diameter angioplasty balloon corresponding to the length of the lesion; to allow for easy navigation of the stent across the stenosis. A carotid stent is chosen based on the tortuosity of the blood vessel, calcification within the blood vessel wall, and composition of the plaque. Again, there are many commercially available carotid stents. The authors usually choose a closed-cell system for symptomatic lesions and an open-cell nitinol stent for a tortuous ICA (Box 1, Fig. 5). The stent should be slightly longer than the length of the lesion, and the diameter chosen should correspond to the largest diameter of the artery where stent placement is anticipated. For a lesion extending from the ICA into the distal common carotid artery, the authors use the diameter of the normal-appearing segment of the common carotid artery to size the diameter of the stent. The stent is then navigated over a standard 0.014 inch wire (proximal flow reversal) or the wire of the distal

embolic protection device and placed to cover the lesion. The length of the stent should cover 5 to 10 mm distal and proximal to the area of narrowing. If the distal common carotid artery is involved, the stent should extend from the distal portion of the lesion in the ICA to the proximal CCA, covering the stenotic area entirely and jailing the ECA from the CCA. After navigation of the stent in the desired location, deployment should proceed in a smooth and continuous motion of unsheathing of the stent. An angiogram should be performed after stent placement to ensure there is no evidence of an arterial dissection or vasospasm and to confirm the placement of the stent.

The authors then usually perform balloon angioplasty after stent placement. The balloon is sized slightly smaller than the diameter of the distal ICA lumen. The length of the balloon should be slightly shorter than the length of the deployed stent. The balloon should be placed within the stent to avoid dissection of the blood vessel. The balloon should be gently inflated to the pressure corresponding to the size of the lumen desired. A profound vagal response may occur during this step of the procedure. Some clinicians choose to administer intravenous glycopyrrolate (Robinul) or atropine just before inflating the balloon, whereas others only use medications if patients become bradycardic. This response may also occur while deploying the stent, but it is much more common with post dilatation with the angioplasty balloon.

After postdilatation, another angiogram is obtained to confirm adequate antegrade flow through

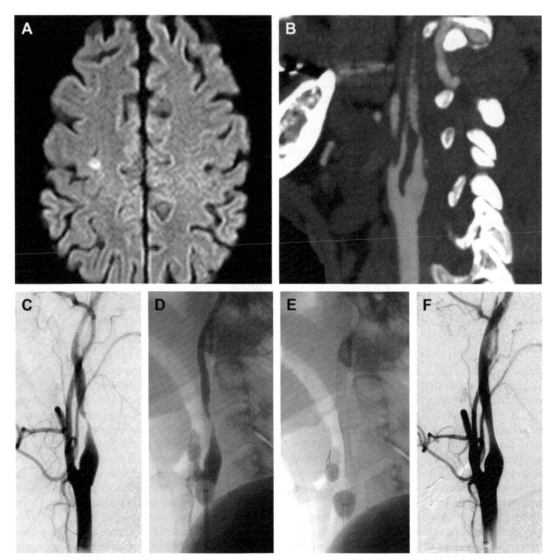

Fig. 2. A 64-year-old man with a history of a symptomatic right internal carotid artery (RICA) stenosis; based on the location of the stenotic lesion, it was thought that the mandible would have to be disarticulated to get proximal control of the ICA for a carotid endarterectomy (CEA). (*A*) Axial diffusion-weighted MR image shows a focal area of high signal within the right frontal lobe. (*B*) Sagittal maximum intensity projection (MIP) MR image of the RICA shows a severe stenosis approximately 2 cm above the carotid bifurcation. Note how the stenosis extends to C3. (*C*) Lateral right common carotid artery (RCCA) angiogram shows a severe stenosis approximately 2 cm above the carotid bifurcation. (*D*) Lateral spot fluoroscopic image of the neck shows the Gore flow reversal system in the right external carotid artery (RECA) and RCCA with flow reversal. (*E*) Lateral spot fluoroscopic image of the neck shows a stent with the RICA. (*F*) After carotid stent placement (CAS), RCCA shows a patent RICA with mild residual stenosis.

the vessel without evidence of again an arterial dissection or vasospasm. If good antegrade flow is identified and the radiopaque dots on the filter are open, the device is captured. This process is completed by running the retrieval catheter over the wire and capturing the device by pulling it into the sheath. The catheter is then removed with the device safely within the lumen of the retrieval catheter. If poor antegrade flow is identified in the ICA, the operator must determine if this is related to vasospasm from the distal protection device or caused by a large embolic load overwhelming the filter. To determine this, the operator looks at the embolic dots on the filter. If they are closed, this is caused by vasospasm from the filter. If they are open, then the most likely cause is from the embolic load overwhelming the filter. In the case of vasospasm, the operator can

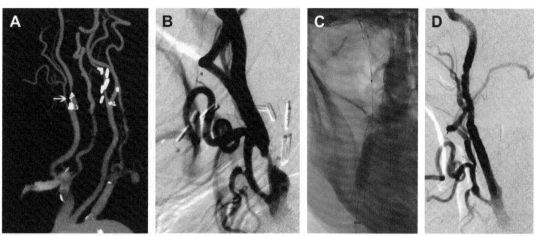

Fig. 3. A 65-year-old man with a symptomatic right internal carotid artery (RICA) stenosis with a prior history of neck dissection and radiation for squamous cell carcinoma. (*A–D*) Maximum intensity projection (MIP) image of a CTA demonstrates a severe calcified stenosis in the RICA (*white arrow*). (*B*) Lateral right common carotid artery (RCCA) angiogram shows a severe focal stenosis within the proximal RICA, note multiple surgical clips from the radial neck dissection. (*C*) Spot anterior-posterior (AP) fluoroscopic image shows a distal protection device just below the skull base with a stent and angioplasty balloon in the RICA. (*D*) After carotid stent placement (CAS), RCCA angiogram shows a widely patent RICA with middle vasospasm within the distal RICA.

administer intra-arterial vasodilators and this will usually resolve. In the latter case, the operator must advance a catheter over the wire and perform suction to remove the debris from the filter before removal. A final angiogram is performed to verify adequate angiographic flow within the stented segment and to determine that there is no evidence of distal emboli to the brain. A common femoral arteriogram is performed to ensure that the vessel is of adequate caliber to place a closure device; if so, a closure device is placed according to manufacturer guidelines. If the artery is not of sufficient diameter, then the sheath is removed and manual pressure is held at the puncture site to achieve hemostasis.

Throughout the procedure, patients are maintained under light conscious sedation. The authors place a rubber squeeze toy in the patients' hand on the contralateral side of the lesion and periodically ask the patient to squeeze the toy to ensure adequate function of the contralateral hand. If at any time the patient is unable to squeeze the toy, a neurologic assessment is performed; if there is a change from baseline, attention is immediately turned to the intracranial circulation, and DSA of the carotid circulation is performed to assess for any thromboemboli. If this is confirmed, either mechanical thrombectomy or intra-arterial lysis can be performed.

SURGICAL TREATMENT

CEA is still considered the gold standard for treatment of symptomatic carotid stenosis.[11,18,26] This operation involves exposing the CCA bifurcation, ECA, and ICA from a curvilinear incision adjacent to the anterior border of the sternocleidomastoid. After clamp placement on the ECA, ICA, and CCAs, an arteriotomy is made in the CCA below the bulb, which is carried into the ICA. The plaque is identified and is bluntly dissected free from the arterial media and the artery is closed either primarily or with a patch graft to increase the caliber of the ICA lumen. The field is then irrigated copiously, and the arteries are flushed via retrograde fill by opening the ECA clamp before opening the ICA allowing for any small plaques dislodged in

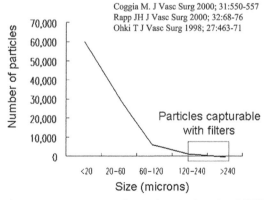

Size and Number of embolic particles produced during Carotid PTA

Coggia M. J Vasc Surg 2000; 31:550-557
Rapp JH J Vasc Surg 2000; 32:68-76
Ohki T J Vasc Surg 1998; 27:463-71

Number of particles — 70,000, 60,000, 50,000, 40,000, 30,000, 20,000, 10,000, 0

Particles capturable with filters

Size (microns): <20, 20–60, 60–120, 120–240, >240

Fig. 4. Percutaneous transluminal angioplasty (PTA).[63–65]

> **Box 1**
> **Stent of choice in certain carotid lesions**
>
> **Vulnerable plaque**
>
> Closed cell
>
> Wallstent (Boston Scientific, Natick, MA)
>
> Xact (Abbott Vascular, Santa Clara, CA)
>
> **Calcified plaque**
>
> Closed cell
>
> Xact (Abbott Vascular)
>
> Open cell nitinol for conformability
>
> **Tortuous or mismatched diameter**
>
> Open cell nitinol
>
> Precise (Cordis Corp, Bridgewater, NJ)
>
> Acculink (Abbott Vascular)
>
> Protégé (ev3, Plymouth, MN)
>
> Vivexx (C. R. Bard, Inc, Murray Hill, NJ)
>
> Exponenent (Medtronic Vascular, Santa Rosa, CA)

patients, it has been shown to offer a 16% to 22% absolute risk reduction over best medical therapy for patients with severe (>70%) stenosis.[11,25,26] CEA has also been shown to have fewer early CVA/stroke complications when compared with carotid stenting using cerebral embolic protection; however, it has more cardiac complications, namely, myocardial infarction, than CAS.[14] CEA has a higher rate of infectious complications by virtue of being an open surgical procedure. Although the durability of carotid stenting still remains controversial to some investigators, it is thought that the ischemic stroke complications of stenting versus CEA are comparable at the 2- and 4-year follow-up.

The main advantage that CEA has over CAS is that CEA has a direct approach to the carotid artery. One of the most challenging and risky maneuvers of CAS is not necessarily crossing a tight stenosis but is navigating a tortuous aortic arch. Type II and type III aortic arches can be challenging to navigate the guide or sheath far enough into the CCA to obtain robust support for the CAS system being used. If this is the case, there is significant risk of dislodging plaque from the arch and CCA origin, which can cause distal embolization before cerebral protection can be established. In these patients, an open surgical approach is more desirable. Additionally, extremely tight stenotic lesions or lesions with an ulcerated plaque may be a higher risk to cross and will increase the risk of plaque disruption, distal embolization, and stroke. Again, in these cases, CEA might be considered as a more favorable option.[66]

the operation to wash into the ECA as opposed to into the ICA.

COMPLICATIONS
CAS Versus CEA

CEA carries a 2% to 7% percent risk of major perioperative stroke or death. In symptomatic

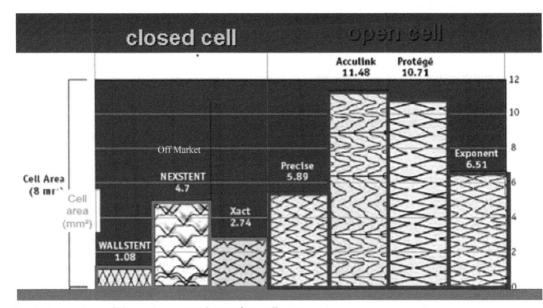

Fig. 5. Comparison of the various carotid stent free cell areas.

It is logical that CAS could be superior to CEA in patients that are poor surgical candidates because CAS is a less invasive procedure, although both can be performed without general anesthesia. A poor surgical candidate could be either secondary to poor functional status overall with significant medical comorbidities or, even more importantly, secondary to poor anatomic dissection planes surrounding the carotid artery. Patients with prior neck irradiation, prior CEA, head/neck cancer, or with contralateral recurrent laryngeal nerve palsy are high-risk open CEA candidates, and CAS should be considered. The risk of general anesthetic in patients with poor functional status is a relative contraindication of CEA because there are reports of the procedure being performed in a patient awake under regional anesthesia. The increased risk of myocardial infarction following CEA makes CAS a more attractive option in patients with severe ischemic cardiomyopathy or coronary artery disease.[11]

CLINICAL OUTCOMES OF TREATMENT OPTIONS

Earlier CAS trials are difficult to apply in current practice, given the rapid advancements in endovascular technology. The 4 most recent randomized prospective CAS trials (Protected Carotid-Artery Stenting versus Endarterectomy in High-Risk Patients (SAPPHIRE), Endarterectomy Versus Angioplasty in Patients With Severe Symptomatic Carotid Stenosis (EVA-3S), CREST, International Carotid Stenting Study [ICSS] have compared CEA with CAS with the use of cerebral protection devices (Table 2). Although the results of three of these trials are similar, the conclusions drawn by the respective investigators differ, making the selection of CAS or CEA for patients with carotid occlusive disease controversial.

In the SAPPHIRE trial, 747 high-risk surgical patients with carotid stenosis (both symptomatic and asymptomatic) were randomized to CAS versus CEA. The 30-day risk of stroke, death, and myocardial infarction was found to be lower in the CAS group than the CEA group (4.8% vs 9.8%). However, after 3 years, the rate of stroke, death, and myocardial infarction approach one another for both groups (8.4% for CAS and 9.0% for CEA). The investigators concluded that there is noninferiority of CAS to CEA in the patient population with a higher risk for CEA.[14]

The EVA-3S trial was stopped early for reasons of both safety and futility. The 30-day risk of any stroke or death was significantly higher after stent placement (9.6%) vs endarterectomy (3.9%), resulting in a relative risk of 2.5 (95% confidence interval, 1.2–5.1).[67] At 6 months, the incidence of any stroke or death was 6.1% after endarterectomy and 11.7% after stent placement ($P = .02$). This trial showed overwhelming favor for CEA in patients with symptomatic carotid stenosis of 60% or more.

The CREST trial analyzed both asymptomatic and symptomatic patients with carotid stenosis but in patients of all surgical risk stratification. In total, 2522 patients were enrolled in the study, with a primary end point of stroke, death, and myocardial infarction in both the immediate postoperative period and at the 4-year follow-up. The study found that the immediate postoperative stroke rate was nearly twice as high for CAS than CEA (4.1% vs 2.3%), whereas the postoperative rate of myocardial infarction was nearly twice as high in the CEA group than the CAS group (2.3% vs 1.1%). At the 4-year follow-up, the combined primary end points of death/stroke/myocardial infarction were similar at 6.8% for CEA and 7.1% for CAS. Paradoxically, the results were better for CEA over CAS for patients more than 70 years of age, and the results for CAS were better in younger patients. The investigators concluded that CEA and CAS were overall equally effective and safe.[16]

The most recent CAS versus CEA trial is the ICSS, which randomized patients with symptomatic carotid stenosis to CEA or CAS with the same primary end points as prior trials (stroke, death, and myocardial infarction). Although the long-term data are still pending, the preliminary data show a higher rate of periprocedural myocardial infarction and stroke in the CAS group when compared with the CEA group. At 120 days, the primary end point of stroke or death in the CAS group was 4% and that of the CEA group was 3.4%. The investigators, therefore, concluded that CEA is the treatment of choice for symptomatic patients.[13]

Much of the controversy surrounding CAS is the fact that SAPPHIRE and CREST included both symptomatic and asymptomatic patients. Additionally, both trials are criticized for using asymptomatic elevations of troponin-I as a surrogate for myocardial infarction as a complication in the perioperative period. Furthermore, the studies do not have a best medical management treatment arm, which might show benefit over CAS or CAE.

The Carotid Revascularization Using Endarterectomy or Stenting Systems (CARESS) trial is a nonrandomized trial designed to offer real-world data for CAS versus CEA because clinicians often take multiple factors into account when deciding on which treatment modality. Therefore, the type of aortic arch, risk of anesthesia, surgical risk, and neck anatomic considerations (and any other

Table 2
Key landmark articles

Study	Comparison	Symptomatic vs Asymptomatic Patients	Number of Patients	Follow-up	Primary Outcomes	Results	Conclusions
NASCET[26]	CEA vs BMT	Symptomatic	659	5 y	Stroke, death	Absolute risk reduction of 16.5% in patients with 70%–99% stenosis when compared with BMT	CEA is highly beneficial to symptomatic patients with high-grade carotid stenosis
ECST[25]	CEA vs BMT	Symptomatic	3018	6 y	Major stroke, death	Absolute risk reduction of 21% in patients with 70%–99% stenosis when compared with BMT	CEA is indicated for patients with recent nondisabling cerebral ischemic event and ipsilateral severe stenosis
ACAS[17]	CEA vs BMT	Asymptomatic	1662	5 y	Stroke, death	Aggregate risk reduction of 53% in patients with stenosis >60% when compared with BMT	CEA is indicated in low-risk patients with 60% stenosis
ACST[69]	CEA vs BMT	Asymptomatic	3120	5 y	Stroke, death	5-y stroke rate 11.0% for BMT and 3.8% for CEA	CEA is indicated in low-risk patients with 70% stenosis
SAPPHIRE[14]	CAS vs CEA	Both	747	3 y	Stroke, death, MI	30-d Stroke/death/MI 4.8% in CAS vs 9.8% CEA; 3-y stroke/death/MI 8.4% CAS vs 9.0% CEA	CAS is not inferior to CEA in high-risk patients with severe stenosis when using embolic protection
CARESS[68]	CAS vs CEA	Both	439	1 y	Stroke, death, MI	30-d Stroke/death/MI 2.1% in CAS vs 3.6% CEA; 1-y stroke/death/MI 10.0% CAS vs 13.6% CEA	CAS with embolic protection is equivalent to CEA in broad-risk population with moderate to severe carotid stenosis
CREST[16]	CAS vs CEA	Both	2522	4 y	Stroke, death, MI	30-d Stroke/death/MI 4.1% in CAS vs 2.3% CEA; 4-y stroke/death/MI 7.2% CAS vs 6.8% CEA	CAS has higher risk of early stroke, whereas CEA has higher risk of early MI, but no significant difference at 4 y
ICSS[13]	CAS vs CEA	Symptomatic	1713	120 d	Stroke, death, MI	30-d Stroke/death/MI 8.5% in CAS vs 5.2% CEA; 120-d stroke/death/MI 4.0% CAS vs 3.4% CEA	CEA remains treatment of choice for patients with moderate to severe stenosis in patients suitable for surgery
EVA-3S[67]	CAS vs CEA	Symptomatic	527	6 mo	Stroke, death within 30 d of treatment	30-d Stroke/death 3.9% in CAE vs 9.6% CAS; 6 mo stroke/death 6.1% CEA vs 11.7% CAS	CEA remains treatment of choice for a symptomatic carotid stenosis of 60% or greater

Abbreviations: ACAS, Asymptomatic Carotid Atherosclerosis Study; ACST, Asymptomatic Carotid Surgery Trial; BMT, best medical therapy; MI, myocardial infarction.

common factor clinicians use to help determine treatment) could be measured by the clinician to determine the best treatment modality. This study showed the 30-day and 1-year rate of death and stroke to be not statistically different between CAS and CEA (2.1% for CAS vs 3.6% for CEA at 30 days and 10.0% for CAS vs 13.6% for CEA at 1 year).[68]

Patients with symptomatic, moderate to severe carotid stenosis warrant an intervention in addition to the best medical therapy to reduce the risk of stroke.[11,25,26] In asymptomatic patients with moderate to severe stenosis, the risk of intervention compared with the best medical therapy should be weighed closely and considered on a case-by-case basis in the authors' opinions. In these cases, the absolute risk reduction is much less than in symptomatic patients, but a carotid intervention is still a very reasonable treatment option in addition to the best medical therapy.[17] Despite recent preliminary data from the ICSS trial, it seems that CAS does offer a safe and effective alternative to CEA in the appropriately selected high-risk patient population. The CARESS trial seems to offer proof that CAS and CEA, when performed on appropriate patients, are equally effective and safe. Patients that are ideal for CAS include patients that have high surgical risk, such as patients with prior neck irradiation, aberrant neck anatomy, contralateral recurrent laryngeal nerve injury, prior ipsilateral CEA, significant coronary artery disease, high cervical stenotic lesion location, and tracheostomy. Relative contraindications to CAS include patients with type II and III aortic arches, tortuous CCA, or young patients with otherwise normal anatomy and a low-lying cervical lesion location precluding mandibular disarticulation; CEA should be more heavily considered in these cases. Patients should be informed of the potential for a higher risk of asymptomatic myocardial ischemia if CEA is chosen and the higher up-front risk of early stroke if CAS is chosen. In the end, the clinician must weigh the overall medical, surgical, and anatomic risks of each patient with respect to the proposed intervention to recommend the safest treatment option (CAS vs CEA vs best medical therapy).

SUMMARY

A carotid intervention is warranted in symptomatic patients with moderate to severe carotid stenosis to reduce the risk of ischemic stroke. CAS is a safe and effective alternative to CEA in select patient populations. Anatomic considerations of the aortic arch and tortuosity of the CCA and ICA must be considered when choosing CAS versus

CEA. A multidisciplinary consensus approach should be applied to individual patients to determine the preferred treatment option. The team must weigh the risks and benefits of the best medical therapy versus CEA versus CAS when considering which intervention would achieve optimal stroke risk reduction.

REFERENCES

1. Bogousslavsky J, Van Melle G, Regli F. The Lausanne Stroke Registry: analysis of 1,000 consecutive patients with first stroke. Stroke 1988;19: 1083–92.
2. Longstreth WT Jr, Shemanski L, Lefkowitz D, et al. Asymptomatic internal carotid artery stenosis defined by ultrasound and the risk of subsequent stroke in the elderly. The Cardiovascular Health Study. Stroke 1998;29:2371–6.
3. Petty GW, Brown RD Jr, Whisnant JP, et al. Ischemic stroke subtypes: a population-based study of incidence and risk factors. Stroke 1999; 30:2513–6.
4. Rosamond WD, Folsom AR, Chambless LE, et al. Stroke incidence and survival among middle-aged adults: 9-year follow-up of the Atherosclerosis Risk in Communities (ARIC) cohort. Stroke 1999;30:736–43.
5. Schneider AT, Kissela B, Woo D, et al. Ischemic stroke subtypes: a population-based study of incidence rates among blacks and whites. Stroke 2004;35:1552–6.
6. Sacco RL, Kargman DE, Gu Q, et al. Race-ethnicity and determinants of intracranial atherosclerotic cerebral infarction. The Northern Manhattan Stroke Study. Stroke 1995;26:14–20.
7. Wityk RJ, Lehman D, Klag M, et al. Race and sex differences in the distribution of cerebral atherosclerosis. Stroke 1996;27:1974–80.
8. U-King-Im JM, Young V, Gillard JH. Carotid-artery imaging in the diagnosis and management of patients at risk of stroke. Lancet Neurol 2009;8: 569–80.
9. Donnan GA, Fisher M, Macleod M, et al. Stroke. Lancet 2008;371:1612–23.
10. van der Worp HB, van Gijn J. Clinical practice. Acute ischemic stroke. N Engl J Med 2007;357: 572–9.
11. Ricotta JJ 2nd, Piazza M. Carotid endarterectomy or carotid artery stenting? Matching the patient to the intervention. Perspect Vasc Surg Endovasc Ther 2010;22:124–36.
12. Ederle J, Bonati LH, Dobson J, et al. Endovascular treatment with angioplasty or stenting versus endarterectomy in patients with carotid artery stenosis in the Carotid and Vertebral Artery Transluminal Angioplasty Study (CAVATAS): long-term follow-up

of a randomised trial. Lancet Neurol 2009;8:898–907.

13. Ederle J, Dobson J, Featherstone RL, et al. Carotid artery stenting compared with endarterectomy in patients with symptomatic carotid stenosis (International Carotid Stenting Study): an interim analysis of a randomised controlled trial. Lancet 2010; 375:985–97.

14. Yadav JS, Wholey MH, Kuntz RE, et al. Protected carotid-artery stenting versus endarterectomy in high-risk patients. N Engl J Med 2004;351: 1493–501.

15. Hopkins LN, Myla S, Grube E, et al. Carotid artery revascularization in high surgical risk patients with the NexStent and the Filterwire EX/EZ: 1-year results in the CABERNET trial. Catheter Cardiovasc Interv 2008;71:950–60.

16. Brott TG, Hobson RW 2nd, Howard G, et al. Stenting versus endarterectomy for treatment of carotid-artery stenosis. N Engl J Med 2010;363:11–23.

17. Endarterectomy for asymptomatic carotid artery stenosis. Executive Committee for the Asymptomatic Carotid Atherosclerosis Study. JAMA 1995; 273:1421–8.

18. Lanzino G, Tallarita T, Rabinstein AA. Internal carotid artery stenosis: natural history and management. Semin Neurol 2010;30:518–27.

19. Paciaroni M, Silvestrelli G, Caso V, et al. Neurovascular territory involved in different etiological subtypes of ischemic stroke in the Perugia Stroke Registry. Eur J Neurol 2003;10:361–5.

20. Tegos TJ, Kalodiki E, Daskalopoulou SS, et al. Stroke: epidemiology, clinical picture, and risk factors–part I of III. Angiology 2000;51:793–808.

21. Brott TG, Halperin JL, Abbara S, et al. 2011 ASA/ACCF/AHA/AANN/AANS/ACR/ASNR/ CNS/SAIP/SCAI/SIR/SNIS/SVM/SVS guideline on the management of patients with extracranial carotid and vertebral artery disease: executive summary: a report of the American College of Cardiology Foundation/American Heart Association Task Force on Practice Guidelines, and the American Stroke Association, American Association of Neuroscience Nurses, American Association of Neurological Surgeons, American College of Radiology, American Society of Neuroradiology, Congress of Neurological Surgeons, Society of Atherosclerosis Imaging and Prevention, Society for Cardiovascular Angiography and Interventions, Society of Interventional Radiology, Society of NeuroInterventional Surgery, Society for Vascular Medicine, and Society for Vascular Surgery. Vasc Med 2011;16:35–77.

22. Brott TG, Halperin JL, Abbara S, et al. 2011 ASA/ACCF/AHA/AANN/AANS/ACR/ASNR/ CNS/SAIP/SCAI/SIR/SNIS/SVM/SVS Guideline on the management of patients with extracranial carotid and vertebral artery disease: executive summary. A report of the American College of Cardiology Foundation/American Heart Association Task Force on Practice Guidelines, and the American Stroke Association, American Association of Neuroscience Nurses, American Association of Neurological Surgeons, American College of Radiology, American Society of Neuroradiology, Congress of Neurological Surgeons, Society of Atherosclerosis Imaging and Prevention, Society for Cardiovascular Angiography and Interventions, Society of Interventional Radiology, Society of NeuroInterventional Surgery, Society for Vascular Medicine, and Society for Vascular Surgery Developed in Collaboration With the American Academy of Neurology and Society of Cardiovascular Computed Tomography. J Am Coll Cardiol 2011;57:1002–44.

23. Brott TG, Halperin JL, Abbara S, et al. 2011 ASA/ACCF/AHA/AANN/AANS/ACR/ASNR/ CNS/SAIP/SCAI/SIR/SNIS/SVM/SVS guideline on the management of patients with extracranial carotid and vertebral artery disease: executive summary. A report of the American College of Cardiology Foundation/American Heart Association Task Force on Practice Guidelines, and the American Stroke Association, American Association of Neuroscience Nurses, American Association of Neurological Surgeons, American College of Radiology, American Society of Neuroradiology, Congress of Neurological Surgeons, Society of Atherosclerosis Imaging and Prevention, Society for Cardiovascular Angiography and Interventions, Society of Interventional Radiology, Society of NeuroInterventional Surgery, Society for Vascular Medicine, and Society for Vascular Surgery. Circulation 2011;124:489–532.

24. Brott TG, Halperin JL, Abbara S, et al. 2011 ASA/ACCF/AHA/AANN/AANS/ACR/ASNR/ CNS/SAIP/SCAI/SIR/SNIS/SVM/SVS guideline on the management of patients with extracranial carotid and vertebral artery disease: a report of the American College of Cardiology Foundation/American Heart Association Task Force on Practice Guidelines, and the American Stroke Association, American Association of Neuroscience Nurses, American Association of Neurological Surgeons, American College of Radiology, American Society of Neuroradiology, Congress of Neurological Surgeons, Society of Atherosclerosis Imaging and Prevention, Society for Cardiovascular Angiography and Interventions, Society of Interventional Radiology, Society of NeuroInterventional Surgery, Society for Vascular Medicine, and Society for Vascular Surgery. Stroke 2011;42:e464–540.

25. Randomised trial of endarterectomy for recently symptomatic carotid stenosis: final results of the MRC European Carotid Surgery Trial (ECST). Lancet 1998;351:1379–87.

26. Beneficial effect of carotid endarterectomy in symptomatic patients with high-grade carotid stenosis. North American Symptomatic Carotid Endarterectomy Trial Collaborators. N Engl J Med 1991; 325:445–53.

27. Sillesen H. The natural history of patients with carotid stenosis. Pathophysiol Haemost Thromb 2002;32:378–80.

28. Gronholdt ML, Wiebe BM, Laursen H, et al. Lipid-rich carotid artery plaques appear echolucent on ultrasound B-mode images and may be associated with intraplaque haemorrhage. Eur J Vasc Endovasc Surg 1997;14:439–45.

29. Eesa M, Hill MD, Al-Khathaami A, et al. Role of CT angiographic plaque morphologic characteristics in addition to stenosis in predicting the symptomatic side in carotid artery disease. AJNR Am J Neuroradiol 2010;31:1254–60.

30. Morgenstern LB, Fox AJ, Sharpe BL, et al. The risks and benefits of carotid endarterectomy in patients with near occlusion of the carotid artery. North American Symptomatic Carotid Endarterectomy Trial (NASCET) Group. Neurology 1997;48:911–5.

31. Klijn CJ, Kappelle LJ, Tulleken CA, et al. Symptomatic carotid artery occlusion. A reappraisal of hemodynamic factors. Stroke 1997;28:2084–93.

32. Persoon S, Luitse MJ, de Borst GJ, et al. Symptomatic internal carotid artery occlusion: a long-term follow-up study. J Neurol Neurosurg Psychiatry 2011;82:521–6.

33. Ozgur Z, Govsa F, Ozgur T. Anatomic evaluation of the carotid artery bifurcation in cadavers: implications for open and endovascular therapy. Surg Radiol Anat 2008;30:475–80.

34. Hayashi N, Hori E, Ohtani Y, et al. Surgical anatomy of the cervical carotid artery for carotid endarterectomy. Neurol Med Chir (Tokyo) 2005;45:25–9 [discussion: 30].

35. Lo A, Oehley M, Bartlett A, et al. Anatomical variations of the common carotid artery bifurcation. ANZ J Surg 2006;76:970–2.

36. Zarins CK, Giddens DP, Bharadvaj BK, et al. Carotid bifurcation atherosclerosis. Quantitative correlation of plaque localization with flow velocity profiles and wall shear stress. Circ Res 1983;53:502–14.

37. Liu Y, Chen BP, Lu M, et al. Shear stress activation of SREBP1 in endothelial cells is mediated by integrins. Arterioscler Thromb Vasc Biol 2002;22: 76–81.

38. Malek AM, Alper SL, Izumo S. Hemodynamic shear stress and its role in atherosclerosis. JAMA 1999; 282:2035–42.

39. McNally JS, Davis ME, Giddens DP, et al. Role of xanthine oxidoreductase and NAD(P)H oxidase in endothelial superoxide production in response to oscillatory shear stress. Am J Physiol Heart Circ Physiol 2003;285:H2290–7.

40. Hwang J, Ing MH, Salazar A, et al. Pulsatile versus oscillatory shear stress regulates NADPH oxidase subunit expression: implication for native LDL oxidation. Circ Res 2003;93:1225–32.

41. Nagel T, Resnick N, Dewey CF Jr, et al. Vascular endothelial cells respond to spatial gradients in fluid shear stress by enhanced activation of transcription factors. Arterioscler Thromb Vasc Biol 1999;19:1825–34.

42. Orr AW, Sanders JM, Bevard M, et al. The subendothelial extracellular matrix modulates NF-kappaB activation by flow: a potential role in atherosclerosis. J Cell Biol 2005;169:191–202.

43. Chatzizis YS, Coskun AU, Jonas M, et al. Role of endothelial shear stress in the natural history of coronary atherosclerosis and vascular remodeling: molecular, cellular, and vascular behavior. J Am Coll Cardiol 2007;49:2379–93.

44. Koskinas KC, Chatzizis YS, Baker AB, et al. The role of low endothelial shear stress in the conversion of atherosclerotic lesions from stable to unstable plaque. Curr Opin Cardiol 2009;24:580–90.

45. Jaff MR, Goldmakher GV, Lev MH, et al. Imaging of the carotid arteries: the role of duplex ultrasonography, magnetic resonance arteriography, and computerized tomographic arteriography. Vasc Med 2008;13:281–92.

46. Sabeti S, Schillinger M, Mlekusch W, et al. Quantification of internal carotid artery stenosis with duplex US: comparative analysis of different flow velocity criteria. Radiology 2004;232:431–9.

47. Nederkoorn PJ, van der Graaf Y, Hunink MG. Duplex ultrasound and magnetic resonance angiography compared with digital subtraction angiography in carotid artery stenosis: a systematic review. Stroke 2003;34:1324–32.

48. Koelemay MJ, Nederkoorn PJ, Reitsma JB, et al. Systematic review of computed tomographic angiography for assessment of carotid artery disease. Stroke 2004;35:2306–12.

49. Hirai T, Korogi Y, Ono K, et al. Prospective evaluation of suspected stenoocclusive disease of the intracranial artery: combined MR angiography and CT angiography compared with digital subtraction angiography. AJNR Am J Neuroradiol 2002;23:93–101.

50. Wetzel S, Bongartz G. MR angiography: supra-aortic vessels. Eur Radiol 1999;9:1277–84.

51. Hankey GJ, Warlow CP, Sellar RJ. Cerebral angiographic risk in mild cerebrovascular disease. Stroke 1990;21:209–22.

52. Alexandrov AV. Ultrasound and angiography in the selection of patients for carotid endarterectomy. Curr Cardiol Rep 2003;5:141–7.

53. Williams MA, Nicolaides AN. Predicting the normal dimensions of the internal and external carotid arteries from the diameter of the common carotid. Eur J Vasc Surg 1987;1(2):91–6.

54. Bladin CF, Alexandrov AV, Murphy J, et al. Carotid stenosis index. A new method of measuring internal carotid artery stenosis. Stroke 1995;26:230–4.

55. Alexandrov AV, Bladin CF, Maggisano R, et al. Measuring carotid stenosis. Time for a reappraisal. Stroke 1993;24:1292–6.

56. Bousser M. Benefits from carotid surgery? Yes, but.... Cerebrovasc Dis 1992;2:122–6.

57. Fox AJ. How to measure carotid stenosis. Radiology 1993;186:316–8.

58. Rothwell PM, Gibson RJ, Slattery J, et al. Equivalence of measurements of carotid stenosis. A comparison of three methods on 1001 angiograms. European Carotid Surgery Trialists' Collaborative Group. Stroke 1994;25:2435–9.

59. Bartlett ES, Walters TD, Symons SP, et al. Carotid stenosis index revisited with direct CT angiography measurement of carotid arteries to quantify carotid stenosis. Stroke 2007;38:286–91.

60. Mantese VA, Timaran CH, Chiu D, et al. The Carotid Revascularization Endarterectomy versus Stenting Trial (CREST): stenting versus carotid endarterectomy for carotid disease. Stroke 2010;41:S31–4.

61. Barrett KM, Brott TG. Management of stenosis of the extracranial internal carotid artery: endarterectomy versus angioplasty and stenting. Curr Treat Options Neurol 2010;12:475–82.

62. Hopkins LN, Roubin GS, Chakhtoura EY, et al. The Carotid Revascularization Endarterectomy versus Stenting Trial: credentialing of interventionalists and final results of lead-in phase. J Stroke Cerebrovasc Dis 2010;19:153–62.

63. Coggia M, Goeau-Brissonniere O, Duval JL, et al. Embolic risk of the different stages of carotid bifurcation balloon angioplasty: an experimental study. J Vasc Surg 2000;31:550–7.

64. Rapp JH, Pan XM, Sharp FR, et al. Atheroemboli to the brain: size threshold for causing acute neuronal cell death. J Vasc Surg 2000;32:68–76.

65. Ohki T, Marin ML, Lyon RT, et al. Ex vivo human carotid artery bifurcation stenting: correlation of lesion characteristics with embolic potential. J Vasc Surg 1998;27:463–71.

66. Naggara O, Touze E, Beyssen B, et al. Anatomical and technical factors associated with stroke or death during carotid angioplasty and stenting: results from the endarterectomy versus angioplasty in patients with symptomatic severe carotid stenosis (EVA-3S) trial and systematic review. Stroke 2011;42:380–8.

67. Mas JL, Chatellier G, Beyssen B, et al. Endarterectomy versus stenting in patients with symptomatic severe carotid stenosis. N Engl J Med 2006;355:1660–71.

68. Carotid revascularization using endarterectomy or stenting systems (CARESS): phase I clinical trial. J Endovasc Ther 2003;10:1021–30.

69. Halliday A, Mansfield A, Marro J, et al. Prevention of disabling and fatal strokes by successful carotid endarterectomy in patients without recent neurological symptoms: randomised controlled trial. Lancet 2004;363:1491–502.

Endovascular Treatment of Intracranial Atherosclerotic Disease

Christopher J. Lenart, MD, Mandy J. Binning, MD,
Erol Veznedaroglu, MD*

KEYWORDS

• Atherosclerosis • Ischemic stroke • Risk factors • Endovascular treatment

KEY POINTS

- Intracranial atherosclerosis is an important cause of ischemic stroke.
- Modifiable and nonmodifiable risk factors exist.
- Systemic anticoagulation does not confer any significant advantage compared with antiplatelet medications.
- Surgical bypass has so far not proved to be better than medical therapy, although further trials are necessary to determine whether subgroups of patients exist who may benefit.
- Angioplasty and stenting so far has not proved to be better than maximal medical therapy, although further trials are necessary to determine whether subgroups of patients exist who may benefit.

INTRODUCTION

The estimated prevalence of strokes in 2006 was 6.4 million adults, with an incidence of about 795,000 new or recurrent strokes,[1,2] 87% of which were ischemic. Intracranial atherosclerotic disease (ICAD) is responsible for an estimated 40,000 to 60,000 ischemic strokes per year in the United States,[3] and has been identified as the sole cause of ischemic stroke in 8% to 9% of patients.[4,5] According to the US Centers for Disease Control and Prevention, the death rate in 2010 for stroke was 42 per 100,000.

Race as a nonmodifiable risk factor has been well characterized.[6] African American, Asian,[7] and Hispanic[4] populations have a higher incidence of intracranial disease compared with white people, who suffer more frequently from extracranial disease.[7] However, men have a tendency toward extracranial atherosclerosis,[5,7] and develop intracranial disease at an earlier age than women.

The rate of disease progression in women is more rapid than in men.[8] Thus, the male/female incidence rate changes with age: 1.25 at ages 55 to 64 years; 0.76 at 85 years and older.[1] In an asymptomatic Japanese population, age, hypertension, and diabetes mellitus were identified as risk factors for intracranial stenosis.[9] Because reports of ICAD prevalence are based on different methodologies (g, population, screening, autopsy) and imaging modalities (g, computed tomography angiography, transcranial Doppler, magnetic resonance (MR) angiography, digitally subtracted angiography (DSA)), it is likely that the prevalence exceeds stated values.

The precise role of smoking has been difficult to characterize. Although smoking is a demonstrable risk factor for extracranial carotid atherosclerosis,[10] in a study of 1200 asymptomatic patients, smoking was not identified as a risk factor for ICAD.[8] Current smokers have a risk of ischemic stroke twice that of nonsmokers.[1]

Stroke and Cerebrovascular Center of New Jersey, 750 Brunswick Avenue, Trenton, NJ 08638, USA
* Corresponding author. Department of Neurosurgery, Capital Institute for Neurosciences, Trenton, NJ 609-537-7300.
E-mail address: veznedaroglu@yahoo.com

Neuroimag Clin N Am 23 (2013) 653–659
http://dx.doi.org/10.1016/j.nic.2013.03.012
1052-5149/13/$ – see front matter © 2013 Elsevier Inc. All rights reserved.

Metabolic syndrome, a constellation of atherosclerosis risk factors linked to insulin resistance, has been associated with intracranial stenosis.[11] Diabetes mellitus, hypertension, and dyslipidemia contribute to intimal medial thickness, which in turn is an early marker of atherosclerosis. The odds ratio of developing intracranial atherosclerosis increased with each additional component of metabolic syndrome.[12]

NATURAL HISTORY

The rate of radiographic disease progression is variable. In a retrospective review of 23 patients who underwent serial angiography with moderate or severe atherosclerosis (average follow-up time 26.7 months), those without carotid bifurcation disease were more likely to have intracranial disease progression; overall, 40% of intracranial stenoses progressed, 20% regressed, and 40% were unchanged.[13] This finding is similar to that seen in patients assessed using transcranial Doppler (average follow-up time 21 months): 35% disease progression, 7% regression, 45% unchanged (inconclusive in 14%).[14]

The severity of ischemic injury is variable. Intracranial large-artery atherosclerotic stroke shows higher MR angiography–diffusion weighted imaging mismatch and lower hypoperfusion than other stroke subtypes, although the penumbra volume was similar among all stroke subtypes.[15] This finding is hypothesized to be caused by the presence of better collaterals in intracranial large-artery atherosclerotic–related strokes.

The Groupe dEtude des Stenoses Intra-Craniennes (GESICA) study examined patients symptomatic from greater than 50% stenosis of intracranial vessels and found an annual risk of transient ischemic attack (TIA) or stroke in the affected area of 19.2% (annual risk of TIA 12.6%; stroke 7%).[16] A 2-year event rate of 60.7% was seen in patients with more severe lesions.

Mortality seems to vary based on which vessel is affected: annual mortality of 6.8% for middle cerebral artery (MCA) stenosis; 11.6% for vertebrobasilar stenosis; 12.4% for intracranial internal carotid artery (ICA) stenosis.[17]

MEDICAL THERAPY

The Warfarin-Aspirin Symptomatic Intracranial Disease (WASID) trial was a retrospective study of symptomatic patients with greater than 50% stenosis of a major intracranial artery, comparing the efficacy of warfarin with aspirin for the prevention of major vascular events. The initial analysis revealed a stroke rate of 10.4 per 100 patient years in those taking aspirin, compared with 3.6 per 100 patient years in those taking warfarin.[18] However, when similar patients were assessed in a randomized, prospective study (the comparison of warfarin and aspirin for symptomatic intracranial arterial stenosis), the rate of death from nonvascular causes, major hemorrhage (ie, brain, gastrointestinal, and so forth) and myocardial infarction was significantly higher in those receiving warfarin, without conferring a therapeutic advantage in stroke prevention compared with aspirin, causing the trial to be stopped prematurely.[19] Over 2 years, the rate of ischemic stroke in patients with greater than 50% stenosis of intracranial vessels was 17.2% to 19.7%, higher than that observed in other trials (8% to 14%) assessing other causes of stroke.[19] In the 2006 subgroup analysis, patients thought to be at exceptionally high risk for ischemic events were studied separately to establish whether certain groups of patients may benefit from systemic anticoagulation. These subgroups included vertebral artery stenosis, basilar artery stenosis, and failed thrombotic therapy. The investigators concluded at the end of this analysis that, even in patients in potentially high-risk subgroups, warfarin did not provide significant benefit.[20]

In a post hoc analysis of 287 patients from the WASID trial, the degree of collateral circulation predicted risk of stroke.[21] There was a statistically significant difference in the presence of collaterals in those with moderate stenosis: 23% of women and 8% of men. However, the rate of disabling or fatal strokes was equivalent in patients with either moderate or severe stenoses. Although any collaterals in the setting of moderate stenosis was a significant predictor of stroke, there was a protective effect in patients with both severe stenosis and extensive collaterals.

MEDICAL THERAPY VERSUS SURGICAL BYPASS

In 1985, the initial results of the Extracranial-Intracranial (EC-IC) Arterial Bypass Trial were published, in which 1377 patients with symptomatic severe stenosis or occlusion of the internal carotid and middle cerebral arteries were randomized to best medical treatment (714 patients) or surgical bypass (663 patients) (Table 1). In the medically treated arm, 36% of those with distal ICA stenosis and 24% of those with MCA stenoses suffered a stroke despite receiving aspirin.[22] Despite these findings, the study failed to prove that surgery decreased the number of strokes. Eighteen percent of the medical patients and 20% of the surgical patients went on to have a single stroke, whereas 10% and 11% respectively

Table 1
Summary of surgical bypass results for intracranial stenosis

	Type of Study	Number of Patients	Outcome
EC-IC Arterial Bypass Trial[22]	Prospective randomized	714 medical 663 surgery	EC-IC bypass not effective in preventing cerebral ischemia in patients with atherosclerotic disease in the carotid and middle cerebral arteries
COSS[23]	Prospective randomized	98 medical 97 surgery	EC-IC bypass surgery plus medical therapy compared with medical therapy alone did not reduce the risk of recurrent ipsilateral ischemic stroke at 2 y

of patients had a second stroke.[22] A common criticism of this trial is that it failed to identify the subgroup of patients for whom bypass was thought to be the most effective: patients with poor collateral circulation. As neuroimaging has improved, identification of these patients has become possible.

More recently, the Carotid Occlusion Surgery Study (COSS) was designed to evaluate these patients with hemodynamic cerebral ischemia based on positron emission tomography measurements of oxygen extraction fraction.[23] One-hundred and ninety-five patients were randomized, 97 to surgery and 98 to the medical arm. The trial was terminated early because it failed to show benefit against medical therapy in this subgroup of patients with symptomatic carotid occlusions.[23,24] Further investigation has been suggested to evaluate cognitive and functional benefits in patients who have undergone surgical revascularization, rather than stroke risk reduction alone.

MEDICAL THERAPY VERSUS INTRACRANIAL ANGIOPLASTY AND STENTING

Intracranial atherosclerosis is a heterogeneous disease, as shown by outcomes analysis of percutaneous transluminal angioplasty, which differentiated angiographic characteristics.[25] Type A is less than 5 mm, concentric or moderately eccentric; type B is 5 to 10 mm, tubular, extremely eccentric of totally occluded lesions less than 3 months old; type C is greater than 10 mm, diffuse, angulated more than 90° with tortuosity or complete occlusion more than 3 months old. The risk of restenosis at 3 months was 0%, 30%, and 66%, and the risk of stroke was 8%, 26%, and 87% in types A, B, and C respectively (**Table 2**).

The mainstay of ICAD treatment has traditionally been aggressive management of modifiable risk factors. Smoking cessation, normalization of hyperlipidemia, treatment of hypertension, and management of diabetes mellitus can be

Table 2
Summary of major intracranial stent articles

Author	Type of Study	Number of Patients	Type of Stent	30-d Outcome
SSYLVIA,[27] 2004	Prospective, nonrandomized	61	Neurolink	4% stroke
Fiorella et al,[28] 2007	Prospective nonrandomized	78	Wingspan	6% stroke/death
Bose et al,[29] 2007	Prospective nonrandomized	45	Wingspan	5% stroke/death
Costalat et al,[30] 2010	Prospective nonrandomized	42	Wingspan, coronary, none	7% stroke/death
SAMMPRIS,[36] 2011	Prospective randomized	451	Wingspan	14.7% stroke/death

Abbreviations: SAMMPRIS, Stenting versus Aggressive Medical Management for Preventing Recurrent Stroke in Intracranial Stenosis; SSYLVIA, Stenting of Symptomatic Atherosclerotic Lesions in the Vertebral or Intracranial Arteries.

combined with antiplatelet therapy. However, percutaneous transluminal angioplasty and stenting for intracranial stenosis have recently undergone an evolution in techniques in response to suboptimal outcomes with medical therapy alone and with treatment using technology borrowed from cardiology.[26]

The Stenting of Symptomatic Atherosclerotic Lesions in the Vertebral or Intracranial Arteries (SSYLVIA) trial was the first to assess a dedicated intracranial balloon-expanded stent, the Neurolink System.[27] This prospective, nonrandomized feasibility study enrolled 43 patients with symptomatic intracranial stenosis and 18 patients with extracranial vertebral artery stenosis. The mean duration between TIA/stroke and procedure was 72.8 days. Stent deployment was successful in 95% of cases. Intraprocedural complications included stroke, dissection, carotid-cavernous fistula, and acute stent occlusion. At 30 days after the procedure, 4 (6.6%) strokes were observed; at 1 year, an additional 4 (7.3%) strokes occurred. Stenosis of greater than 50% at 6 months was observed in 32.4% of intracranial and 42.9% extracranial vertebral stents. Of these 18 patients, 39% were symptomatic with TIA or stroke. Risk factors associated with restenosis were diabetes, greater postprocedure stenosis, and smaller vessel size, consistent with findings in the cardiac literature. Based on these results, the Neurolink System (Guidant Corporation, Santa Clara, CA) received the US Food and Drug Administration designation of Humanitarian Device Exemption for use in patients with TIA or stroke despite medical therapy.

The balloon-expanded Neurolink System has been superseded by the self-expanding Wingspan System (Stryker Neurovascular, Fremont, CA). The Wingspan System differs significantly from the cardiac devices that have been used off label for intracranial applications, most notably in its flexibility and self-expansion. Tortuous intracranial vasculature requires more flexibility than is typically required by cardiac disorders. Because the stent is self-expanding, and the Gateway balloon for angioplasty can be undersized this avoids parent vessel barotrauma. The self-expanding design also allows it to conform to tapered or curving vessels.

Fiorello and colleagues[28] presented their periprocedural outcomes of a prospective, nonrandomized study of patients with symptomatic stenosis. Seventy-eight patients with greater than 50% stenosis of intracranial vessels 2.5 to 4.5 mm in diameter underwent angioplasty and stenting with the Gateway balloon–Wingspan stent system. Eighty-one of 82 lesions (98.8%) were successfully treated, with a 6.1% major periprocedural complication rate (4 mortalities, 1 reperfusion hemorrhage with aphasia and hemiparesis).

Bose and colleagues[29] presented their prospective, nonrandomized results of similar patients treated with the Wingspan System. Forty-five patients were treated, with stenosis reduced from a presentation of 74.9% to 50% after angioplasty, and further reduction to 31.9% after stenting. Two of 44 patients (4.5%) expired in the first month after the procedure. At the 6-month follow-up, an ipsilateral stroke rate of 7.1% (3/43) and total stroke rate of 9.7% (4/43) was observed. There was no observed symptomatic restenosis in Wingspan-treated lesions, although 3 (6.8%) showed restenosis greater than 50%.

A multicenter report from France describes the Wingspan stent in 60 symptomatic patients refractory to medical treatment with a mean of 80% stenosis: procedural complications occurred in 20%, with 4.8% permanent morbidity and death, and in-stent restenosis (ISR) was observed in 17%.[30]

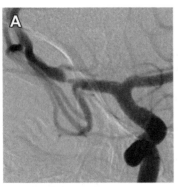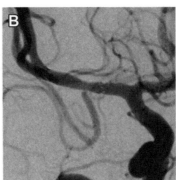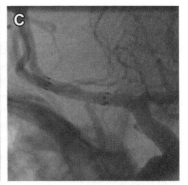

Fig. 1. A 57-year-old man on dual antiplatelet therapy with recurrent symptoms referable to right MCA stenosis. (A) Anteroposterior (AP) frontal angiogram shows a severe stenosis of the right MCA. (B) Repeat frontal angiogram after balloon angioplasty and stent placement shows a widely patent right MCA with minimal residual stenosis. (C) Unsubtracted spot fluoroscopic image shows the stent.

The National Institutes of Health registry on the use of the Wingspan stent compiled results from 16 medical centers that treated 129 patients with symptomatic stenosis greater than 70%.[31] There was an observed frequency of primary end points at 6-month follow-up of 14% and restenosis of at least 50% observed in 25%. There was an observed difference in the number of patients who experienced stroke or death between low-enrolling and high-enrolling centers (1–8 vs 14–19 patients), although statistical significance was not reported (Fig. 1).

Acute intraprocedural thrombus formation has been reported.[32] Six of 41 (14.6%) patients treated with the Wingspan system developed in-stent thrombosis within 30 minutes of stent deployment. All 6 were successfully recanalized with abciximab alone or in combination with tissue plasminogen activator (tPA) and/or angioplasty.

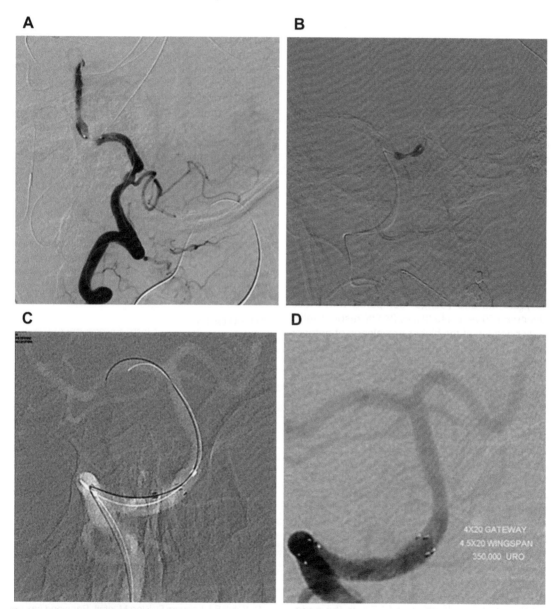

Fig. 2. A 63-year-old woman on dual antiplatelet therapy with recurrent complaints caused by right vertebral artery (VA) stenosis. (A) Lateral right vertebral arteriogram shows a severe focal stenosis within the V4 segment. (B) AP roadmap image shows balloon during midinflation across the stenosis. (C) AP roadmap image shows the stent being deployed across the lesion. (D) After balloon angioplasty and stent placement, repeat AP right VA arteriogram shows a widely patent VA.

Delayed restenosis following Wingspan percutaneous transluminal angioplasty (PTAS) has been observed in a third of treated patients, compared with 7.5% of patients in the initial Eurasian Humanitarian Device Exemption study.[33] Anterior circulation lesions are more prone to restenosis, with a more focal lesion predominating. When restenosis was diffuse or more severe than the initial lesion, patients were more likely to be symptomatic. ISR has been categorized using a modified Mehran system, originally developed to describe ISR following coronary PTAS.[34] Class I represents focal restenosis, with subtypes included; class II, diffuse; class III, proliferative; class IV, complete stent occlusion. One-hundred and twenty-seven intracranial stenotic lesions treated with the Wingspan PTAS with 3-month to 15-month follow-up were assessed for ISR, with a mean interval between treatment and follow-up of 8.5 months. Thirty-six (28.3%) lesions developed ISR and 5 (3.9%) progressed to complete occlusion. Twenty-five of 41 (61%) were focal lesions of less than 50% stent length. Sixteen of 36 ISR were described as being no worse than the originally treated lesion, whereas 20 of 36 were more severe. Nine of 10 (90%) supraclinoid ICA and 9 of 13 (69.2%) MCA lesions treated showed more ISR of greater severity than the initial lesion. Restenosis was symptomatic in 13 of 36 ISR and 2 of 5 with complete occlusion.

ISR was observed more commonly in patients 55 years old and younger compared with those older than 55 years (45.2% vs 24.2% respectively), likely because of the higher prevalence of anterior circulation lesions in the younger cohort.[35] The supraclinoid segment of the ICA had higher rates of restenosis (66.6% vs 24.4%) and symptomatic ISR (40% vs 3.9%) compared with all other lesion locations.

The Stenting versus Aggressive Medical Management for Preventing Recurrent Stroke in Intracranial Stenosis (SAMMPRIS) trial is a trial in which patients with TIA or stroke within 30 days of enrollment, secondary to 70% to 99% major intracranial artery stenosis, were randomized to maximal medical therapy alone or in conjunction with Gateway balloon angioplasty and Wingspan stent placement.[36] Patients were not required to fail medical therapy or undergo significant risk modification before being enrolled in the trial. Enrollment was stopped after randomization of 451 patients because the primary end point (30-day stroke or death) was 14.7% in the endovascular group, versus 5.8% in the medical arm (**Fig. 2**). Further trials are necessary to identify patients who will benefit from intracranial arterial angioplasty and stenting. Patients who are medically refractory with high-grade stenoses could be an important subgroup to follow.

SUMMARY

Cerebrovascular accidents are a significant source of morbidity and mortality, both for the individual, for families, and for society. Intracranial atherosclerosis has a demonstrable effect on the incidence of stroke. Maximum medical intervention is an appropriate first line of prevention and treatment, including modification of risk factors and antiplatelet therapy. However, in highly selected patients who have progression of symptomatic disease with high-grade intracranial stenosis, stenting may be an option. As with any new device, proper patient selection and vessel selection are essential; the addition of a new hammer to the interventionalist's armamentarium should not lead to an indiscriminate search for nails. The learning curve associated with novel interventions and the potential for catastrophic complications (eg, thromboembolic events, vessel dissection, perforation, or rupture) should not be underestimated. The risk of ISR, as with that seen in stents placed elsewhere in the body, requires surveillance. Given these caveats, the addition of stenting to the treatment options for symptomatic intracranial atherosclerosis is a significant event: the natural history of potentially devastating disease can be positively altered.

REFERENCES

1. Lloyd-Jones D, Adams RJ, Brown TM, et al. Heart disease and stroke statistics–2010 update: a report from the American Heart Association. Circulation 2010;121(7):e46–215.
2. Writing Group Members. Heart disease and stroke statistics-2012 update: a report from the American Heart Association. Circulation 2012;125:e2–e220.
3. Higashida RT, Meyers PM, Connors JJ 3rd, et al. Intracranial angioplasty & stenting for cerebral atherosclerosis: a position statement of the American Society of Interventional and Therapeutic Neuroradiology, Society of Interventional Radiology, and the American Society of Neuroradiology. AJNR Am J Neuroradiol 2005;26(9):2323–7.
4. Sacco RL, Roberts JK, Boden-Albala B, et al. Race-ethnicity and determinants of intracranial atherosclerotic cerebral infarction. The Northern Manhattan Stroke Study. Stroke 1995;26(1):14–20.
5. Wityk RJ, Lehman D, Klag M, et al. Race and sex differences in the distribution of cerebral atherosclerosis. Stroke 1996;27(11):1974–80.
6. Suri MF, Johnston SC. Epidemiology of intracranial stenosis. J Neuroimaging 2009;19(Suppl 1):11S–6S.

7. Caplan LR, Gorelick PB, Hier DB. Race, sex and occlusive cerebrovascular disease: a review. Stroke 1986;17(4):648–55.

8. Bae HJ, Lee J, Park JM, et al. Risk factors of intracranial cerebral atherosclerosis among asymptomatics. Cerebrovasc Dis 2007;24(4):355–60.

9. Uehara T, Tabuchi M, Mori E. Risk factors for occlusive lesions of intracranial arteries in stroke-free Japanese. Eur J Neurol 2005;12(3):218–22.

10. Fine-Edelstein JS, Wolf PA, O'Leary DH, et al. Precursors of extracranial carotid atherosclerosis in the Framingham Study. Neurology 1994;44(6):1046–50.

11. Park JH, Kwon HM, Roh JK. Metabolic syndrome is more associated with intracranial atherosclerosis than extracranial atherosclerosis. Eur J Neurol 2007;14(4):379–86.

12. Bang OY, Kim JW, Lee JH, et al. Association of the metabolic syndrome with intracranial atherosclerotic stroke. Neurology 2005;65(2):296–8.

13. Akins PT, Pilgram TK, Cross DT 3rd, et al. Natural history of stenosis from intracranial atherosclerosis by serial angiography. Stroke 1998;29(2):433–8.

14. Schwarze JJ, Babikian V, DeWitt LD, et al. Longitudinal monitoring of intracranial arterial stenoses with transcranial Doppler ultrasonography. J Neuroimaging 1994;4(4):182–7.

15. Kim SJ, Seok JM, Bang OY, et al. MR mismatch profiles in patients with intracranial atherosclerotic stroke: a comprehensive approach comparing stroke subtypes. J Cereb Blood Flow Metab 2009; 29(6):1138–45.

16. Mazighi M, Tanasescu R, Ducrocq X, et al. Prospective study of symptomatic atherothrombotic intracranial stenoses: the GESICA study. Neurology 2006; 66(8):1187–91.

17. Komotar RJ, Wilson DA, Mocco J, et al. Natural history of intracranial atherosclerosis: a critical review. Neurosurgery 2006;58(4):595–601 [discussion: 595–601].

18. Chimowitz MI, Kokkinos J, Strong J, et al. The Warfarin-Aspirin Symptomatic Intracranial Disease Study. Neurology 1995;45(8):1488–93.

19. Chimowitz MI, Lynn MJ, Howlett-Smith H, et al. Comparison of warfarin and aspirin for symptomatic intracranial arterial stenosis. N Engl J Med 2005; 352(13):1305–16.

20. Kasner SE, Lynn MJ, Chimowitz MI, et al. Warfarin vs aspirin for symptomatic intracranial stenosis: subgroup analyses from WASID. Neurology 2006;67: 1275–8.

21. Liebeskind DS, Fukuoka M, Kazita K, et al. Collaterals dramatically alter stroke risk in intracranial atherosclerosis. Ann Neurol 2010;69(9):963–74.

22. The EC/IC Bypass Study Group. Failure of extracranial-intracranial arterial bypass to reduce the risk of ischemic stroke. Results of an international randomized trial. The EC/IC Bypass Study Group. N Engl J Med 1985;313(19):1191–200.

23. Powers WJ, Clarke WR, Grubb RL, et al. Extracranial-intracranial bypass surgery for stroke prevention in hemodynamic cerebral ischemia. The Carotid Occlusion Surgery Study Randomized Trial. JAMA 2011;306(18):1983–92.

24. Amin-Hanjani S, Barker FG, Charbel FT, et al. EC-IC bypass for stroke—is this the end of the line or a bump in the road? Neurosurgery 2012;71(3):557–61.

25. Mori T, Fukuoka M, Kazita K, et al. Follow-up study after intracranial percutaneous transluminal cerebral balloon angioplasty. AJNR Am J Neuroradiol 1998; 19(8):1525–33.

26. Connors JJ, Wojak JC. Percutaneous transluminal angioplasty for intracranial atherosclerotic lesions: evolution of technique and short-term results. J Neurosurg 1999;91(3):415–23.

27. SSYLVIA Study Investigators. Stenting of Symptomatic Atherosclerotic Lesions in the Vertebral or Intracranial Arteries (SSYLVIA): study results. Stroke 2004;35(6):1388–92.

28. Fiorella D, Levy EI, Turk AS, et al. US multicenter experience with the wingspan stent system for the treatment of intracranial atheromatous disease: periprocedural results. Stroke 2007;38(3):881–7.

29. Bose A, Hartmann M, Henkes H, et al. A novel, self-expanding, nitinol stent in medically refractory intracranial atherosclerotic stenoses: the Wingspan study. Stroke 2007;38(5):1531–7.

30. Costalat V, Maldonado IL, Zerlauth JB, et al. Endovascular treatment of symptomatic intracranial arterial stenosis: six-year experience in a single-center series of 42 consecutive patients with acute and mid-term results. Neurosurgery 2010;67(6):1505–13 [discussion: 1513–4].

31. Zaidat OO, Klucznik R, Alexander MJ, et al. The NIH Registry on use of the Wingspan stent for symptomatic 70–99% intracranial arterial stenosis. Neurology 2008;70(17):1518–24.

32. Vajda Z, Schmid E, Güthe T, et al. The modified Bose-method for the endovascular treatment of intracranial atherosclerotic arterial stenoses using the Enterprise stent. Neurosurgery 2012;70(1): 91–101.

33. Levy EI, Turk AS, Albuquerque FC, et al. Wingspan in-stent restenosis and thrombosis: incidence, clinical presentation, and management. Neurosurgery 2007;61(3):644–50 [discussion: 650–1].

34. Albuquerque FC, Levy EI, Turk AS, et al. Angiographic patterns of Wingspan in-stent restenosis. Neurosurgery 2008;63(1):23–7 [discussion: 27–8].

35. Turk AS, Levy EI, Albuquerque FC, et al. Influence of patient age and stenosis location on wingspan in-stent restenosis. AJNR Am J Neuroradiol 2008; 29(1):23–7.

36. Chimowitz MI, Lynn MJ, Deredyn CP. Stenting vs aggressive medical therapy for intracranial arterial stenosis. N Engl J Med 2011;365:993–1003.

Spontaneous Cervical and Cerebral Arterial Dissections
Diagnosis and Management

Rudy J. Rahme, MD, Salah G. Aoun, MD,
Jamal McClendon Jr, MD, Tarek Y. El Ahmadieh, MD,
Bernard R. Bendok, MD*

KEYWORDS

- Stroke • Cervical artery dissection • Cerebral artery dissection • Transient ischemic attack
- Balloon angioplasty • Stent placement

KEY POINTS

- Cervicocranial dissections are thought to be spontaneous if no evidence of preceding trauma is found.
- They occur primarily in middle-aged men with a yearly incidence of 2.6 per 100,000 for carotid artery dissection and 1 to 1.5 per 100,000 for vertebral artery dissections.
- Ischemic symptoms are often delayed in onset compared with the dissection event.
- Arterial dissection often heal with medical management within 3 to 6 months, and associated aneurysms tend to stabilize or even decrease in size and completely resolve in some cases.
- The risk of recurrent spontaneous dissection is 2% within the first month and decreases to 1% 1 year thereafter.
- No level I evidence is available to guide the treatment of this disease.
- Antithrombotic therapy is typically started in the acute phase of a cervicocerebral arterial dissection unless specific contraindications are present.
- For extracranial arterial dissections, endovascular management is usually reserved for cases in which medical therapy fails.
- For intracranial arterial dissections, cases with hemorrhagic presentation are best treated with trapping of the dissected segment either endovascularly or surgically with or without a bypass. This approach offers the lowest risk for recurrent hemorrhage. For nonhemorrhagic presentation, surgical and/or endovascular approaches are typically reserved for failed medical therapy.

INTRODUCTION

Arterial dissections of head and neck arteries were first identified pathologically in the 1950s,[1] but not until the 1970s and the 1980s did they begin to be widely recognized as a clinical entity.[2–4] Carotid and vertebral artery dissections account for only 2% of all ischemic strokes, but they account for approximately 20% of thromboembolic strokes in patients younger than 45 years.[5–9] The cause of supra-aortic dissections can be either spontaneous or traumatic. A dissection is deemed spontaneous if no evidence of preceding trauma is found. In some cases, the preceding traumatic event might be missed because of its benign nature (eg, violent coughing or simple neck manipulations).[10] Therefore, these cases might be

Department of Neurological Surgery, Northwestern University Feinberg School of Medicine, 676 North Saint Clair Street, Suite 2210, Chicago, IL 60611, USA
* Corresponding author.
E-mail address: bbendok@nmff.org

Neuroimag Clin N Am 23 (2013) 661–671
http://dx.doi.org/10.1016/j.nic.2013.03.013
1052-5149/13/$ – see front matter © 2013 Elsevier Inc. All rights reserved.

misdiagnosed as spontaneous dissections. This article addresses spontaneous cervical and cerebral artery dissections.

Because of the inconsistent use of terminology throughout the literature and to avoid any confusion, this article uses the following definitions:

- Dissection: a tear alongside the internal wall of an artery with extravasation of blood between the intima and media, with potential luminal narrowing.
- Dissecting aneurysm: aneurysmal dilatation caused by dissection of blood between the media and the adventitia.
- Pseudoaneurysm: leaking of blood outside of the artery with subsequent confinement of the extravascular hematoma; may or may not produce narrowing of the lumen.

EPIDEMIOLOGY

Spontaneous cerebral artery dissections occur primarily in middle-aged patients with a higher frequency in men, whereas traumatic dissections tend to occur at a slightly younger age.[11] Women on average are 5 years younger than men at the time of the dissection and are more likely to have dissections in multiple vessels.[10,12] The real incidence of cervicocranial dissections is hard to determine because some patients might experience minimal to no symptoms and thus remain undiagnosed.[10] Nonetheless, the yearly detected incidence of spontaneous carotid artery dissection is thought to be around 2.6 per 100,000, whereas that of vertebral artery dissection is estimated to be at 1 to 1.5 per 100,000.[7,13–16] Although spontaneous dissection is largely thought to be idiopathic, up to 15% of patients with spontaneous dissection are diagnosed with fibromuscular dysplasia.[13–15,17] Other connective tissue diseases, such as Marfan syndrome, Ehlers-Danlos syndrome type IV, autosomal polycystic kidney disease, and osteogenesis imperfecta are also thought to be involved to a lesser extent.[18,19]

PATHOPHYSIOLOGY

The common pathologic finding in all dissections is a longitudinal tear within the arterial wall in the tunica media.[11,20] The nature of the inciting event is debatable. The dissection is thought to be caused by a tear in the intima leading to a direct connection between intraluminal blood and the tunica media.[5,11,20] Another hypothesis is direct extravasation of blood from the vasa vasorum into the media with subsequent proximal and distal extension of the hematoma along the vessel wall.[11,20] Regardless of the inciting event, the hematoma formation may be associated with narrowing or occlusion of the arterial lumen. In addition, the dissection can potentially expose the blood stream to the prothrombotic components of the subendothelial layer, potentially leading to thrombus and distal embolic complications.[21]

The extracranial segments of the vertebral and carotid arteries are more prone to dissections than their intracranial counterparts. The extracranial segments have greater mobility and thus have a greater risk of injury through contact with bony structures, such as the vertebral bodies for the vertebral arteries and the styloid process for the carotid arteries.[3,22,23]

NATURAL HISTORY

The true natural history of cervicocranial arterial dissection is not entirely clear, but the risk of stroke would make any prospective natural history study without treatment difficult to justify. The reported mortality rate from carotid and vertebral artery dissection is approximately 5%.[3,12,22,24] Although stroke might be the presenting symptom occurring at the time of dissection, it is often delayed and its onset can occur as late as 31 days after the initial injury.[24,25] Ischemic manifestations typically occur within the few days after the dissection.[24,25] Most dissections heal spontaneously within 3 to 6 months with medical treatment, as revealed by serial imaging.[24–29] The likelihood of a dissection healing after 6 months decreases significantly.[5,24] In a prospective study, however, Kremer and colleagues[28] showed that the long-term outcome of internal carotid artery stenosis is benign, with the rate of stroke not related to the persistence of stenosis or occlusion. Nedeltchev and colleagues[29] prospectively followed 249 consecutive patients with 268 spontaneous carotid artery dissections using ultrasound imaging at 1, 3, 6, and 12 months. Of 268 cases, 20 presented with 50% or less stenosis, 30 with 51% to 80% stenosis, 92 with 81% to 99% stenosis, and 125 with complete occlusion. The rate of complete recanalization after medical treatment was 12% at 1 month, 50% at 3 months, and 60% at 6 and 12 months. Dissecting aneurysms tend to stabilize, and they rarely grow.[26,27] They can in some cases either decrease in size or even completely resolve.[26,27] The risk of recurrence of spontaneous dissection within the first month is 2%, and thereafter decreases to 1% a year.[12,30]

CLINICAL PRESENTATION

Craniocervical dissections can in some cases remain asymptomatic and undiagnosed.[5] However, they can cause symptoms typically through 2 mechanisms:

- Thromboembolic: exposure of subendothelial prothrombotic components leading to platelet aggregation,[21] with subsequent dislodgment of the thrombus and release of distal emboli.
- Hemodynamic: stenosis or occlusion of the true arterial lumen secondary to the expansion of the mural hematoma and to the potential formation of intraluminal thrombus, causing a decrease in distal blood flow.

In addition to these 2 mechanisms, dissections might also cause symptoms associated with subarachnoid hemorrhage (SAH) from intracranial extension of the dissection, more frequently seen with dissection in the vertebrobasilar circulation.[31–33]

Dissection of the Internal Carotid Artery

The typical presentation of internal carotid artery dissection includes the triad of ipsilateral facial pain, partial Horner syndrome (oculosympathetic palsy) and subsequent ischemia.[5,10,34] Although this presentation is encountered in fewer than a third of the cases,[5,34] a high index of suspicion should be maintained in patients who present with at least 2 of these symptoms or with nonspecific focal neurologic complaints, particularly if a history of trauma can be found.

In spontaneous dissections, pain is most frequently the initial symptom.[5,34] Most often it is characterized as a unilateral headache affecting the frontotemporal area, nonthrobbing in nature, with gradual onset, although it can also present as an acute-onset severe "thunderclap" headache.[5,34–37] Orbital pain may also be present in half of the patients.[36] In fewer than 10% of cases, pain is the only presenting symptom.[36,38]

Oculosympathetic palsy is defined as ptosis with meiosis without anhidrosis. It is recognized as a typical finding of internal carotid artery dissection because the sympathetic fibers innervating the facial sweat glands follow the external carotid artery and are thus spared.[5,34,36,37] Found in up to 50% of cases,[3,22,36,37] any patient with a partial Horner syndrome should be considered to have an internal carotid artery dissection until proven otherwise.[5,34]

In addition to pain and an incomplete Horner syndrome, an internal carotid artery dissection might also cause cranial nerve palsies in approximately 12% of patients, with a predilection for lower cranial nerves.[39,40] The most commonly affected nerve is the hypoglossal (XII) because of its location in proximity to the carotid sheath.[40] Other nerves that might be injured are the oculomotor (III), trigeminal (V), and facial nerves (VII).[39,40] The clinical presentation of lower cranial nerve palsy associated with oculosympathetic impairment might therefore mimic a brain stem infarct.

Because of the potential narrowed lumen, an audible pulsatile tinnitus has been reported in up to one-fourth of cases.[3,22,34,36] The bruit can be heard by the patients, and sometimes objectively presents on auscultation.[3,22,34,36]

Ischemic manifestations are common in patients with carotid artery dissection, with a reported frequency of 50% to 95%.[5,34] The most common mechanism of ischemia is thromboembolism. In certain cases, however, when dissection results in acute severe stenosis or occlusion, ischemic symptoms can be from hemodynamic insufficiency.[20,34] Because of increased early recognition of arterial dissections as a clinical entity, added to the fact that ischemic symptoms often are a delayed manifestation of dissections, the frequency of ischemic presentations has declined over the years.[24,36,39,40] Usually, ischemic stroke is preceded by warning signs, such as transient ischemic attacks and amaurosis fugax[24,36,37]; however, approximately 20% of patients present with an ischemic stroke without any warning signs.[24]

Dissection of the Vertebral Artery

Patients with vertebral artery dissections typically present with pain in the posterior half of the neck, followed by ischemic manifestations in the posterior circulation.[5,36] In addition to neck pain, patients often complain of headache most commonly localized in the occipital area but sometimes extending to the entire cranium or the frontal area.[5,36] Patients with vertebral artery dissections also rarely present with upper extremity weakness from involvement of the C5–C6 nerve roots.[5,41]

In patients with vertebral artery dissections, ischemic manifestations are very common and may present as a lateral medullary syndrome (Wallenberg syndrome), specifically if the dissection is localized in the third or fourth segment of the vertebral artery.[2,3,5,22,36] The transient ischemic attacks or stroke may also involve other areas of the brain stem, the thalamus, the cerebral and cerebellar hemispheres,[3,5,22,36] and, rarely, the spinal cord in isolation.[42,43]

DIAGNOSTIC IMAGING

The conventional gold standard for diagnosing arterial dissection is cerebral angiography.[5,20,34]

However, with the vast improvements in magnetic resonance imaging (MRI) technology in the past decade, the use of MRI and magnetic resonance angiography (MRA) for diagnostic purposes and, more commonly, for follow-up of patients has increased significantly.[5,20,34,41,44,45] The major disadvantage of magnetic resonance technology is acquisition time, which limits its use in emergency situations. Computed tomography (CT) scans, however, can be obtained quickly, can assess with high accuracy the presence of subarachnoid hemorrhage and stroke or other signs of hypoperfusion, and are widely available in most centers.[5,20,34]

Cerebral Angiography

The most common finding on conventional angiography is segmental arterial stenosis or "string sign."[20,34,46] A "string sign" is caused by the narrowing of the vessel lumen and is not specific to dissection. It can also be seen in other conditions, such as atherosclerotic stenosis.[46–48] Other findings include fusiform dilation with proximal or distal narrowing, termed the "string and pearl sign"; an intimal flap; occlusion of the vessel usually tapered to a point; and a double lumen with retention of the contrast in the false lumen well into the venous phase.[5,20,34,47,48] The pathognomonic signs of dissection such as the double lumen and the intimal flap are seen in fewer than 10% of cases.[47,49]

A typical carotid artery dissection presents with an irregular stenosis starting 2 to 3 cm above the carotid bulb and extends distally without reaching past the petrous segment where the lumen reconstitutes precipitously.[3,22,49] Aneurysmal dilation typically occurs in the cervical portion of the artery, although these dissections can occur intracranially.[3,22,49,50] Carotid arterial dissections are fusiform in nature and occur in a third of the patients.[49–51]

As for vertebral artery dissections, they most commonly occur at the level of the first and second vertebrae and can extend intracranially in approximately 10% of cases.[3,12,22,49] This finding occurs because, unlike the carotid artery, the vertebral artery enters the cranium through a wide foramen. The angiographic appearance is less specific than that of a carotid artery dissection.

Regardless of its location, a risk of misdiagnosis exists because the dissection could be misinterpreted on the images as either a saccular aneurysm, an atherosclerotic lesion, or a vasospasm after an SAH. With regard to atherosclerotic lesions, patients with dissection are usually younger, their lesions are typically isolated, and the stenosis is smooth. As for vasospasm, the timing of events should help clarify the diagnosis in most cases; as with dissection, the stenotic appearance is present from the start. The confusion might occur in patients who present to the emergency room in delayed fashion.

MRI

Because of its invasive nature, conventional angiography is being replaced as the standard diagnostic procedure for dissection by other noninvasive tests, such as MRI and MRA.[5,48,52] Different magnetic resonance sequences allow for various visualizations of the arterial dissection. Although MRA would help detect any potential luminal stenosis or occlusion, T1-weighted, T2-weighted, and proton density images allow direct evaluation of the vessel wall.[47,48,53,54] Although the manifestations of dissection described on conventional angiography can be seen on an MRI,[52,53] the most common finding is the intramural hematoma.[53] The hematoma appearance follows a typical pattern of blood signal change on an MRI over time caused by hemoglobin breakdown, and goes from hypointense on T1- and T2-weighted images in the hyperacute phase to a characteristic hyperintense crescent shape around a flow void on T1-weighted images in the subacute phase.[48,53] Fat-saturation sequences might help differentiate small hematomas from surrounding soft tissue.[5] Another typical finding of arterial dissection on an MRI is an increased external diameter of the vessel, with a decreased luminal diameter resulting from the stenosis.

CT

CT angiography (CTA) has been reported to show similar results to magnetic resonance techniques, with CT the preferred modality in emergency situations and trauma cases.[5,20,34,55,56] CTA can typically show luminal stenosis and occlusion, a crescent-shaped mural thickening representing the hematoma, the intimal flap, and a dissecting aneurysm.[47,56]

Ultrasound with gray-scale and Doppler color is another noninvasive imaging technique, although it should not be considered a diagnostic tool but more a screening tool because it is highly operator-dependent and has a low diagnostic performance with dissections close to the skull base.[53] The gray-scale ultrasound might show the intimal flap, an intramural hematoma, and, in some cases, a luminal narrowing.[47,57] The color Doppler typically shows a high-resistance flow.[58]

TREATMENT

The major treatment objective of cervical cerebral arterial dissections is to avoid or limit neurologic deficits.[5,20,34,41] Because ischemic manifestations are often delayed in their presentation,[5,24] the priority in managing these patients is determining whether they can be managed medically or whether surgical or endovascular intervention is needed. In addition, although it is widely accepted that the most likely pathophysiologic mechanism of ischemic complications is embolic,[20,21,59] hemodynamic compromise can play a role in certain cases, particularly in patients with acute arterial occlusion.[20] These patients might benefit from more-aggressive approaches. Treatment options include thrombolysis, anticoagulation, endovascular interventions, and surgical intervention. Unfortunately, no randomized trial has compared the various treatment options and their efficacy.

Medical Management

Thrombolysis

Little evidence in the literature shows thrombolysis in the setting of cervical cerebral arterial dissection.[34] However, the use of intravenous or intra-arterial recombinant tissue plasminogen activator or urokinase could be warranted in patients in whom ischemic symptoms stem from an acute blockage of blood flow.[30] Potential complications of thrombolysis include an increase in size of mural thrombus with worsening of the luminal stenosis, or even mobilization of the mural thrombus with distal embolization. In addition, thrombolysis could cause an SAH because of leakage, with the potential subsequent development of a pseudoaneurysm. The risk of developing these complications is difficult to assess because of the lack of data in the literature. Georgiadis and colleagues[60] reviewed 33 patients treated with intravenous thrombolysis for acute stroke because of spontaneous cervical carotid artery dissection and found no new or worsening of local signs, SAH, or pseudoaneurysms. In addition, a meta-analysis of individual patient data of 180 patients from 14 retrospective series and 22 case reports showed that thrombolysis had a similar safety and outcome profile in patients with stroke caused by cervical artery dissections and those with all causes of stroke.[61] Thrombolysis seems to be a safe treatment modality, but further studies are warranted to evaluate its efficacy.

Antithrombotic therapy

In 2007, the Cervical Artery Dissection in Ischemic Stroke Patients (CADISP) study group published a summary of the pathophysiologic and clinical considerations regarding the use of antithrombotic agents in arterial dissection, and performed a systematic meta-analysis of the published data comparing their efficacy.[21]

Several arguments support the hypothesis of an embolic mechanism behind the ischemic manifestations of dissections, and thus are in favor of antithrombotic therapy. The infarct pattern on brain imaging,[59] the presence of distal branch occlusion, and the observation of microemboli[21] all favor a thromboembolic mechanism. Transcranial Doppler studies in extracranial vertebral and carotid artery dissections revealed findings suggesting emboli in the posterior and middle cerebral artery, respectively.[62–65] Also, theoretically, because most dissections heal and recanalize spontaneously, the intramural thrombus might be mobilized and throw clots into the bloodstream, thereby causing infarctions.[21]

However, the same arguments that could potentially complicate the use of thrombolytics in arterial dissection patients apply to anticoagulation, including increase of intramural thrombus with local compression symptoms (cranial nerve palsies, Horner syndrome), and hemodynamic-induced infarcts.[21] Unlike with thrombolytics, delayed occlusion of the internal carotid artery has been reported with the use of heparin.[21,66] Finally, the risk of hemorrhagic transformation in patients with severe ischemic strokes should always be considered before an anticoagulation therapy is administered.

Because no randomized trials have been performed, no high-level recommendation can be produced. Nonetheless, it is widely thought that, unless specific contraindications are present, antithrombotic therapy should be started in the acute phase of a cervical cerebral arterial dissection.[10,20,34,41]

Antithrombotic treatment consists of either anticoagulation with intravenous heparin followed by warfarin, or antiplatelet therapy with aspirin.[34] Currently no clear evidence supports the use of one treatment over the other, although anticoagulation is typically preferred and more widely used.[34,41] Anticoagulation might be preferred in patients with severe stenosis, occlusion, or pseudoaneurysm, based on the hypothesis that it is more effective in preventing a thromboembolic complication.[34,41] Applying the superiority of anticoagulation to antiplatelet therapy in preventing secondary stroke in cases involving cardioembolic causes[67] as an argument in favor of anticoagulation in preventing cervical artery dissection is questionable.[21] Antiplatelet use might be preferable for patients with a poor prognosis or those with large infarcts.[21,41,68] The CADISP study group performed a meta-analysis comparing the 2 treatment modalities.[21] Their analysis included 26 studies and 327 patients, and showed no significant differences between the treatment modalities in terms of "death from all causes" and "death and disability."[21] A Cochrane systematic meta-analysis of nonrandomized studies showed similar results.[68] However, both analyses cite a lack of data from randomized trials, which therefore limits the potential for a real evaluation of their efficacy, let alone a true comparison between anticoagulation and antiplatelet therapies in cervical cerebral dissections.

Duration of treatment is open to debate. Typically, because dissections heal within 6 months of onset and rarely recur after,[5] treatment should be continued for 3 to 6 months.[41] Imaging findings have been suggested as potential guidelines for continued anticoagulation of lack thereof, but this method has not been proven.

Endovascular Management

Indications

Endovascular interventions should not typically be considered as first-line treatment for spontaneous cervical cerebral dissections because of the low recurrence rate of dissections combined with the risk of iatrogenic complications of invasive interventions.[10,34] However, certain clinical scenarios exist in which an endovascular or a surgical intervention is warranted. First and foremost, patients presenting with an SAH should be considered surgical or endovascular emergencies, particularly those with intracranial dissections in the posterior circulation.[20,45,69] These patients should first undergo a diagnostic angiogram to assess for a direct cause of the hemorrhage, such as a pseudoaneurysm. The diagnostic angiogram would also study the collateral circulation, the length of the dissected segment, and vertebral dominance.[20] Intracranial pseudoaneurysms have a reported mortality rate as high as 83% and a rerupture rate of approximately 70% within the first 24 hours of presentation.[20,45,70,71] Occlusion of the entire dissected segment with or without flow replacement is the treatment option associated with the lowest risk of rehemorrhage.[20,45,72] Although this could be achieved through proximal occlusion, trapping of the dissected segment might be a better option to avoid filling of the occluded segment through a retrograde flow from the contralateral vertebral artery. The procedure can be performed endovascularly, although in certain cases an open surgical approach might be preferable to visualize and preserve the

posteroinferior cerebellar artery (PICA) and brainstem perforators.[20,45,72] In cases of ruptured vertebral artery dissection that extends to the basilar artery, treatment options are limited. These lesions are notoriously difficult to treat. If the patient passes the balloon test, occlusion and then a proximal occlusion of the basilar artery or bilateral occlusion of the vertebral arteries might be the best option. Otherwise, a stent-in-stent technique can be attempted with potential stent coiling of the pseudoaneurysm.[20,45,72]

Another clinical vignette in which endovascular treatment is indicated in the acute setting is when dissection results in acute arterial occlusion. In these cases, hemodynamic compromise, and not thromboembolism, is the mechanism behind ischemia of cerebral tissue.[20] In these patients, attempts can be consistent to restore flow. First, high-volume fluid resuscitation should be started to reach a normotensive state with a likely benefit of a slight hypertensive state. An arterial line and a Foley catheter could also help strictly monitor the patient's volemic state, the objective being a euvolemic or a slightly hypervolemic state.[20] Once the patient is stabilized, an intervention to restore normal flow should be considered.[20]

Other than these 2 indications, endovascular therapy should be considered if medical management fails or the patient has a contraindication to antithrombotic agents.[8,73–76] Although no textbook definition of failure of medical therapy exists, it is generally agreed that progression of neurologic symptoms and new ischemic events despite adequate antithrombotic therapy define failure of medical therapy.[8] Whether pseudoaneurysm enlargement can be considered failure of medical therapy is controversial.[8]

Technical nuances

Preoperative assessment of images is critical. Length of the dissected segment, associated pseudoaneurysm, and location of important arteries and perforators should be assessed before the patient is taken to the interventional suite. Furthermore, understanding of the clinical presentation is important and might help determine the antithrombotic strategy after intervention. Because guidewires and catheters are thrombogenic, efforts should be made to perform the procedure as efficiently and quickly as possible without compromising patient safety. To avoid iatrogenic complications, including thromboemboli, every effort should be made to minimize intravascular manipulation. A microcatheter should be passed atraumatically over the dissection. At that point, contrast material should be injected to ensure that the catheter is actually in the true

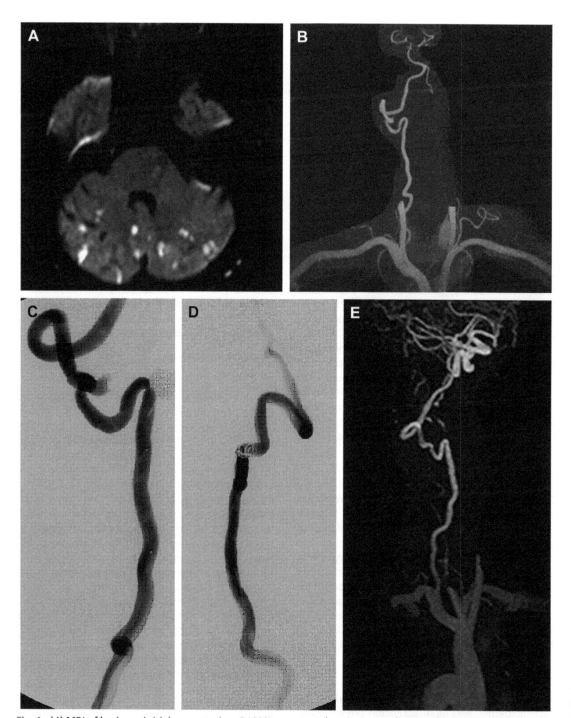

Fig. 1. (A) MRI of brain on initial presentation, B1000 sequence, showing several areas of cerebellar infarction. (B) MRA head on initial presentation, 3-dimensional reconstruction, showing left vertebral artery occlusion and right vertebral artery pseudoaneurysm. (C) Cerebral angiogram, right vertebral artery injection, oblique view showing a 7-mm, broad-based, irregular right vertebral artery pseudoaneurysm. (D) Cerebral angiogram, right vertebral artery injection, oblique view poststent placement and coil embolization of pseudoaneurysm showing decreased filling of pseudoaneurysm. (E) MRA neck, 3-dimensional reconstruction, 14 months poststent placement showing resolution of right vertebral artery pseudoaneurysm.

lumen. Once confirmed, an exchange wire should be left beyond the dissected segment. Ideally, wire access should not be lost until stenting is completed. Different types of stents can be used. Balloon-expandable stents exert a high radial force on the vessel wall and have an increased metal-to-artery wall surface. They can therefore be used to great advantage in patients with extracranial artery dissections.[77–80] Their high radial force reapposes the intimal flap and attaches the thrombus on the vessel wall. Their limitation is that they are rigid and cannot be guided into the smaller, more tortuous intracranial vasculature. Furthermore, their lack of flexibility limits their use in the skull base, where flexion and extension of the neck might kink and thus occlude the stent.[20] Self-expandable stents offer more flexibility and a lower radial force, and are thus better suited for intracranial placement. They can be more easily guided into the intracranial vessels and resist compression after placement.[8,20,81]

Finally, unlike stenting for carotid artery stenosis, it is generally agreed that the risk of worsening the dissection with the use of distal embolic protection devices outweighs any benefits that might stem from their deployment.[8,81,82] Investigators have hypothesized that perhaps proximal protection devices might prove beneficial in this patient population.[83]

Surgical Management

Endovascular management has largely replaced surgical treatment of arterial dissections. It is still useful in patients who present with SAH and in whom proximal occlusion or trapping of the dissected segment is indicated. Surgery offers the benefit of better visualization of the perforators and PICA. Other surgical procedures indicated for managing dissection include extracranial-intracranial bypass as flow replacement for cases treated with trapping, and thromboendarterectomy for carotid dissections.[5,9,30,68,84–86]

CASE ILLUSTRATION

A 61-year-old man with a history of hypertension, hyperlipidemia, and atrial fibrillation presented to the emergency department with nausea and gait imbalance. He reported that after turning his head to the right, he suddenly felt nauseous, vomited, and had difficulty walking. An MRA showed several cerebellar infarcts associated with a completely occluded left vertebral artery and a 7-mm right vertebral artery pseudoaneurysm (Fig. 1A, B). A diagnosis of vertebral artery dissection was made. He was initially managed medically with

warfarin and clopidogrel, but he reported continued nausea and vomiting during a follow-up clinical visit 1 month later. A repeat CTA at that time showed progression of the pseudoaneurysm to 9 mm. Because of the new symptoms and lesion progression despite medical therapy, endovascular therapy was recommended. Cerebral angiography showed a broad-based, irregular, 7-mm pseudoaneurysm of the distal V2 segment of the right vertebral artery (see Fig. 1C). One self-expanding Enterprise VRD stent (Codman Neurovascular, Raynham, MA) was placed, followed by deployment of platinum coils into the pseudoaneurysm. No complications occurred and filling of the pseudoaneurysm immediately decreased (see Fig. 1D). He was discharged in stable condition with instructions to continue his warfarin and antiplatelet therapy indefinitely. Clinical follow-up over 12 months showed complete resolution of symptoms with no further neurologic events. Imaging follow-up over 14 months showed complete resolution of the pseudoaneurysm (see Fig. 1E).

SUMMARY

Cervical cerebral dissections are an important cause of stroke in the young population. Conservative management with antithrombotic therapy is the most widely accepted first line of treatment in most cases. Endovascular management in patients with cervical dissections is most often a "back-up" option in case of failure of medical treatment. Patients with intracranial extension of the dissection and SAH presentation should be considered for endovascular or surgical management. Many unanswered questions remain with regard to this disease: Is thrombolysis warranted? Should antiplatelet therapy or anticoagulant therapy be used? What is the optimal duration of antithrombotic treatment? Unfortunately, no level I evidence is available to guide treatment of this disease. Randomized trials are needed to really understand this disease and to validate the established treatment modalities.

REFERENCES

1. Wolman L. Cerebral dissecting aneurysms. Brain 1959;82:276–91.
2. Caplan LR, Zarins CK, Hemmati M. Spontaneous dissection of the extracranial vertebral arteries. Stroke 1985;16(6):1030–8.
3. Fisher CM, Ojemann RG, Roberson GH. Spontaneous dissection of cervico-cerebral arteries. Can J Neurol Sci 1978;5(1):9–19.

4. Ojemann RG, Fisher CM, Rich JC. Spontaneous dissecting aneurysm of the internal carotid artery. Stroke 1972;3(4):434–40.

5. Schievink WI. Spontaneous dissection of the carotid and vertebral arteries. N Engl J Med 2001; 344(12):898–906.

6. Chandra A, Suliman A, Angle N. Spontaneous dissection of the carotid and vertebral arteries: the 10-year UCSD experience. Ann Vasc Surg 2007;21(2):178–85.

7. Bogousslavsky J, Regli F. Ischemic stroke in adults younger than 30 years of age. Cause and prognosis. Arch Neurol 1987;44(5):479–82.

8. Pham MH, Rahme RJ, Arnaout O, et al. Endovascular stenting of extracranial carotid and vertebral artery dissections: a systematic review of the literature. Neurosurgery 2011;68(4):856–66 [discussion: 866].

9. Bassetti C, Carruzzo A, Sturzenegger M, et al. Recurrence of cervical artery dissection. A prospective study of 81 patients. Stroke 1996;27(10): 1804–7.

10. Shah Q, Messe SR. Cervicocranial arterial dissection. Curr Treat Options Neurol 2007;9(1):55–62.

11. Anson J, Crowell RM. Cervicocranial arterial dissection. Neurosurgery 1991;29(1):89–96.

12. Schievink WI, Mokri B, O'Fallon WM. Recurrent spontaneous cervical-artery dissection. N Engl J Med 1994;330(6):393–7.

13. Schievink WI, Mokri B, Whisnant JP. Internal carotid artery dissection in a community. Rochester, Minnesota, 1987-1992. Stroke 1993;24(11):1678–80.

14. Muller BT, Luther B, Hort W, et al. Surgical treatment of 50 carotid dissections: indications and results. J Vasc Surg 2000;31(5):980–8.

15. Schievink WI. The treatment of spontaneous carotid and vertebral artery dissections. Curr Opin Cardiol 2000;15(5):316–21.

16. Davis JW, Holbrook TL, Hoyt DB, et al. Blunt carotid artery dissection: incidence, associated injuries, screening, and treatment. J Trauma 1990;30(12): 1514–7.

17. Mas JL, Bousser MG, Hasboun D, et al. Extracranial vertebral artery dissections: a review of 13 cases. Stroke 1987;18(6):1037–47.

18. Schievink WI, Michels VV, Piepgras DG. Neurovascular manifestations of heritable connective tissue disorders. A review. Stroke 1994;25(4):889–903.

19. Schievink WI, Bjornsson J, Piepgras DG. Coexistence of fibromuscular dysplasia and cystic medial necrosis in a patient with Marfan's syndrome and bilateral carotid artery dissections. Stroke 1994; 25(12):2492–6.

20. Amenta PS, Jabbour PM, Rosenwasser RH. Approaches to extracranial and intracranial dissection. In: Bendok BR, Naidech AM, Walker MT, et al, editors. Hemorrhagic and ischemic stroke: medical, imaging, surgical, and interventional approaches. New York: Thieme; 2011. p. 461–72.

21. Engelter ST, Brandt T, Debette S, et al. Antiplatelets versus anticoagulation in cervical artery dissection. Stroke 2007;38(9):2605–11.

22. Hart RG, Easton JD. Dissections of cervical and cerebral arteries. Neurol Clin 1983;1(1):155–82.

23. Sundt TM Jr, Pearson BW, Piepgras DG, et al. Surgical management of aneurysms of the distal extracranial internal carotid artery. J Neurosurg 1986; 64(2):169–82.

24. Biousse V, D'Anglejan-Chatillon J, Touboul PJ, et al. Time course of symptoms in extracranial carotid artery dissections. A series of 80 patients. Stroke 1995;26(2):235–9.

25. Rao AS, Makaroun MS, Marone LK, et al. Long-term outcomes of internal carotid artery dissection. J Vasc Surg 2011;54(2):370–4 [discussion: 375].

26. Benninger DH, Gandjour J, Georgiadis D, et al. Benign long-term outcome of conservatively treated cervical aneurysms due to carotid dissection. Neurology 2007;69(5):486–7.

27. Guillon B, Brunereau L, Biousse V, et al. Long-term follow-up of aneurysms developed during extracranial internal carotid artery dissection. Neurology 1999;53(1):117–22.

28. Kremer C, Mosso M, Georgiadis D, et al. Carotid dissection with permanent and transient occlusion or severe stenosis: long-term outcome. Neurology 2003;60(2):271–5.

29. Nedeltchev K, Bickel S, Arnold M, et al. R2-recanalization of spontaneous carotid artery dissection. Stroke 2009;40(2):499–504.

30. Kim YK, Schulman S. Cervical artery dissection: pathology, epidemiology and management. Thromb Res 2009;123(6):810–21.

31. Sakamoto S, Ohba S, Eguchi K, et al. Churg-Strauss syndrome presenting with subarachnoid hemorrhage from ruptured dissecting aneurysm of the intracranial vertebral artery. Clin Neurol Neurosurg 2005;107(5):428–31.

32. Friedman AH, Drake CG. Subarachnoid hemorrhage from intracranial dissecting aneurysm. J Neurosurg 1984;60(2):325–34.

33. Lanzino G, Kaptain G, Kallmes DF, et al. Intracranial dissecting aneurysm causing subarachnoid hemorrhage: the role of computerized tomographic angiography and magnetic resonance angiography. Surg Neurol 1997;48(5):477–81.

34. Patel RR, Adam R, Maldjian C, et al. Cervical carotid artery dissection: current review of diagnosis and treatment. Cardiol Rev 2012;20(3):145–52.

35. Bogousslavsky J, Despland PA, Regli F. Spontaneous carotid dissection with acute stroke. Arch Neurol 1987;44(2):137–40.

36. Silbert PL, Mokri B, Schievink WI. Headache and neck pain in spontaneous internal carotid and

vertebral artery dissections. Neurology 1995;45(8):
1517–22.

37. Dziewas R, Konrad C, Drager B, et al. Cervical artery dissection–clinical features, risk factors, therapy and outcome in 126 patients. J Neurol 2003;250(10):1179–84.

38. Arnold M, Cumurciuc R, Stapf C, et al. Pain as the only symptom of cervical artery dissection. J Neurol Neurosurg Psychiatry 2006;77(9):1021–4.

39. Gout O, Bonnaud I, Weill A, et al. Facial diplegia complicating a bilateral internal carotid artery dissection. Stroke 1999;30(3):681–6.

40. Mokri B, Silbert PL, Schievink WI, et al. Cranial nerve palsy in spontaneous dissection of the extracranial internal carotid artery. Neurology 1996;46(2):356–9.

41. Debette S, Leys D. Cervical-artery dissections: predisposing factors, diagnosis, and outcome. Lancet Neurol 2009;8(7):668–78.

42. Crum B, Mokri B, Fulgham J. Spinal manifestations of vertebral artery dissection. Neurology 2000;55(2):304–6.

43. Weidauer S, Claus D, Gartenschlager M. Spinal sulcal artery syndrome due to spontaneous bilateral vertebral artery dissection. J Neurol Neurosurg Psychiatry 1999;67(4):550–1.

44. Provenzale JM, Barboriak DP, Taveras JM. Exercise-related dissection of craniocervical arteries: CT, MR, and angiographic findings. J Comput Assist Tomogr 1995;19(2):268–76.

45. Boet R, Wong HT, Yu SC, et al. Vertebrobasilar artery dissections: current practice. Hong Kong Med J 2002;8(1):33–8.

46. Pappas JN. The angiographic string sign. Radiology 2002;222(1):237–8.

47. Flis CM, Jager HR, Sidhu PS. Carotid and vertebral artery dissections: clinical aspects, imaging features and endovascular treatment. Eur Radiol 2007;17(3):820–34.

48. Rodallec MH, Marteau V, Gerber S, et al. Craniocervical arterial dissection: spectrum of imaging findings and differential diagnosis. Radiographics 2008;28(6):1711–28.

49. Houser OW, Mokri B, Sundt TM Jr, et al. Spontaneous cervical cephalic arterial dissection and its residuum: angiographic spectrum. AJNR Am J Neuroradiol 1984;5(1):27–34.

50. Djouhri H, Guillon B, Brunereau L, et al. MR angiography for the long-term follow-up of dissecting aneurysms of the extracranial internal carotid artery. AJR Am J Roentgenol 2000;174(4):1137–40.

51. Schievink WI, Piepgras DG, McCaffrey TV, et al. Surgical treatment of extracranial internal carotid artery dissecting aneurysms. Neurosurgery 1994;35(5):809–15 [discussion: 815–6].

52. Levy C, Laissy JP, Raveau V, et al. Carotid and vertebral artery dissections: three-dimensional time-of-flight MR angiography and MR imaging versus conventional angiography. Radiology 1994;190(1):97–103.

53. Provenzale JM. MRI and MRA for evaluation of dissection of craniocerebral arteries: lessons from the medical literature. Emerg Radiol 2009;16(3):185–93.

54. Aggarwal S, Kucharczyk W, Keller MA. Asymptomatic postendarterectomy dissection of the internal carotid artery detected incidentally on MRI. Neuroradiology 1993;35(8):586–7.

55. Provenzale JM, Sarikaya B. Comparison of test performance characteristics of MRI, MR angiography, and CT angiography in the diagnosis of carotid and vertebral artery dissection: a review of the medical literature. AJR Am J Roentgenol 2009;193(4):1167–74.

56. Leclerc X, Godefroy O, Salhi A, et al. Helical CT for the diagnosis of extracranial internal carotid artery dissection. Stroke 1996;27(3):461–6.

57. Sturzenegger M, Mattle HP, Rivoir A, et al. Ultrasound findings in carotid artery dissection: analysis of 43 patients. Neurology 1995;45(4):691–8.

58. Steinke W, Rautenberg W, Schwartz A, et al. Noninvasive monitoring of internal carotid artery dissection. Stroke 1994;25(5):998–1005.

59. Benninger DH, Georgiadis D, Kremer C, et al. Mechanism of ischemic infarct in spontaneous carotid dissection. Stroke 2004;35(2):482–5.

60. Georgiadis D, Lanczik O, Schwab S, et al. IV thrombolysis in patients with acute stroke due to spontaneous carotid dissection. Neurology 2005;64(9):1612–4.

61. Zinkstok SM, Vergouwen MD, Engelter ST, et al. Safety and functional outcome of thrombolysis in dissection-related ischemic stroke: a meta-analysis of individual patient data. Stroke 2011;42(9):2515–20.

62. Droste DW, Junker K, Stogbauer F, et al. Clinically silent circulating microemboli in 20 patients with carotid or vertebral artery dissection. Cerebrovasc Dis 2001;12(3):181–5.

63. Srinivasan J, Newell DW, Sturzenegger M, et al. Transcranial Doppler in the evaluation of internal carotid artery dissection. Stroke 1996;27(7):1226–30.

64. Koennecke HC, Trocio SH Jr, Mast H, et al. Microemboli on transcranial Doppler in patients with spontaneous carotid artery dissection. J Neuroimaging 1997;7(4):217–20.

65. Molina CA, Alvarez-Sabin J, Schonewille W, et al. Cerebral microembolism in acute spontaneous internal carotid artery dissection. Neurology 2000;55(11):1738–40.

66. Dreier JP, Lurtzing F, Kappmeier M, et al. Delayed occlusion after internal carotid artery dissection under heparin. Cerebrovasc Dis 2004;18(4):296–303.

67. Hart RG, Benavente O, McBride R, et al. Antithrombotic therapy to prevent stroke in patients with atrial fibrillation: a meta-analysis. Ann Intern Med 1999;131(7):492–501.

68. Lyrer P, Engelter S. Antithrombotic drugs for carotid artery dissection. Cochrane Database Syst Rev 2010;(10):CD000255.

69. Uhl E, Schmid-Elsaesser R, Steiger HJ. Ruptured intracranial dissecting aneurysms: management considerations with a focus on surgical and endovascular techniques to preserve arterial continuity. Acta Neurochir 2003;145(12):1073–83 [discussion: 1083–4].

70. Kitanaka C, Sasaki T, Eguchi T, et al. Intracranial vertebral artery dissections: clinical, radiological features, and surgical considerations. Neurosurgery 1994;34(4):620–6 [discussion: 626–7].

71. Mizutani T, Aruga T, Kirino T, et al. Recurrent subarachnoid hemorrhage from untreated ruptured vertebrobasilar dissecting aneurysms. Neurosurgery 1995;36(5):905–11 [discussion: 912–3].

72. Taha MM, Sakaida H, Asakura F, et al. Endovascular management of vertebral artery dissecting aneurysms: review of 25 patients. Turk Neurosurg 2010;20(2):126–35.

73. Malek AM, Higashida RT, Phatouros CC, et al. Endovascular management of extracranial carotid artery dissection achieved using stent angioplasty. AJNR Am J Neuroradiol 2000;21(7):1280–92.

74. Cohen JE, Leker RR, Gotkine M, et al. Emergent stenting to treat patients with carotid artery dissection: clinically and radiologically directed therapeutic decision making. Stroke 2003;34(12):e254–7.

75. Liu AY, Paulsen RD, Marcellus ML, et al. Long-term outcomes after carotid stent placement treatment of carotid artery dissection. Neurosurgery 1999; 45(6):1368–73 [discussion: 1373–4].

76. Albuquerque FC, Han PP, Spetzler RF, et al. Carotid dissection: technical factors affecting endovascular therapy. Can J Neurol Sci 2002;29(1):54–60.

77. Ansari SA, Thompson BG, Gemmete JJ, et al. Endovascular treatment of distal cervical and intracranial dissections with the neuroform stent. Neurosurgery 2008;62(3):636–46 [discussion: 636–46].

78. Benndorf G, Herbon U, Sollmann WP, et al. Treatment of a ruptured dissecting vertebral artery aneurysm with double stent placement: case report. AJNR Am J Neuroradiol 2001;22(10): 1844–8.

79. Brassel F, Rademaker J, Haupt C, et al. Intravascular stent placement for a fusiform aneurysm of the posterior cerebral artery: case report. Eur Radiol 2001;11(7):1250–3.

80. Doerfler A, Wanke I, Egelhof T, et al. Double-stent method: therapeutic alternative for small wide-necked aneurysms. Technical note. J Neurosurg 2004;100(1):150–4.

81. Schulte S, Donas KP, Pitoulias GA, et al. Endovascular treatment of iatrogenic and traumatic carotid artery dissection. Cardiovasc Intervent Radiol 2008;31(5):870–4.

82. Edgell RC, Abou-Chebl A, Yadav JS. Endovascular management of spontaneous carotid artery dissection. J Vasc Surg 2005;42(5):854–60 [discussion: 860].

83. Fanelli F, Bezzi M, Boatta E, et al. Techniques in cerebral protection. Eur J Radiol 2006;60(1):26–36.

84. Ansari SA, Parmar H, Ibrahim M, et al. Cervical dissections: diagnosis, management, and endovascular treatment. Neuroimaging Clin N Am 2009; 19(2):257–70 [table of contents].

85. Ali MJ, Bendok BR, Tawk RG, et al. Trapping and revascularization for a dissecting aneurysm of the proximal posteroinferior cerebellar artery: technical case report and review of the literature. Neurosurgery 2002;51(1):258–62 [discussion: 262–3].

86. Redekop GJ. Extracranial carotid and vertebral artery dissection: a review. Can J Neurol Sci 2008; 35(2):146–52.

Endovascular Treatment of Acute Ischemic Stroke

Sabareesh K. Natarajan, MD, MS[a,b], Jorge L. Eller, MD[a,b],
Kenneth V. Snyder, MD, PhD[b,c],
L. Nelson Hopkins, MD[b,c,d,e], Elad I. Levy, MD[b,c,d],
Adnan H. Siddiqui, MD, PhD[b,c,d],*

KEYWORDS

• Endovascular treatment • Stroke • Ischemia • Imaging

KEY POINTS

- Less than 1% of patients with acute ischemic stroke in the United States receive intravenous (IV) tissue plasminogen activator (t-PA); recanalization rates associated with IV t-PA for proximal, large vessel arterial occlusions remain poor.
- At present, patients who do not meet the eligibility criteria for thrombolytic therapy, who fail to improve neurologically after thrombolytic therapy, or who improve and then worsen (patients with reocclusion) are candidates for endovascular revascularization therapies.
- Advanced brain perfusion imaging is increasing the ability to better assess the therapeutic target (the ischemic penumbra) and better select patients who may benefit from revascularization.
- Higher rates of recanalization have been shown with endovascular methods, particularly mechanical therapies, and this has been correlated with better outcomes.
- Stent-assisted and stent platform–based thrombectomy devices have increased the ability to achieve high recanalization rates in large vessel occlusions.
- The rapidity of advances in endovascular stroke therapy has made assessment through large-scale randomized controlled trials difficult and, for many interventionists who see surprising recoveries following endovascular therapy, unethical because of a lack of clinical equipoise.

INTRODUCTION

Endovascular stroke therapy has revolutionized the management of patients with acute ischemic stroke in the last decade and has facilitated the development of sophisticated stroke imaging techniques and a multitude of thrombectomy devices. Moreover, it has changed the way in which stroke therapists have used intravenous (IV) tissue plasminogen activator (t-PA), which is the only medical therapy approved by the US Food and Drug Administration (FDA) for acute stroke treatment at present.

IV THROMBOLYSIS IS NOT A PANACEA FOR ALL PATIENTS

Less than 1% of acute patients with ischemic stroke in the United States receive t-PA, primarily because of a delay in presentation for treatment,[1] although this number may increase with the extended time window of 4.5 hours.[2] There is also reluctance in

[a] Department of Neurosurgery, School of Medicine and Biomedical Sciences, University at Buffalo, State University of New York, 100 High Street, Suite B4, Buffalo, NY 14203, USA; [b] Department of Neurosurgery, Kaleida Health, 100 High Street, Suite B4, Buffalo, NY 14203, USA; [c] Department of Neurosurgery, Toshiba Stroke Research Center, School of Medicine and Biomedical Sciences, University at Buffalo, State University of New York, 100 High Street, Suite B4, Buffalo, NY 14203, USA; [d] Department of Radiology, Toshiba Stroke Research Center, School of Medicine and Biomedical Sciences, University at Buffalo, State University of New York, 100 High Street, Suite B4, Buffalo, NY 14203, USA; [e] Jacobs Institute, 875 Ellicott Street, Buffalo, New York 14203, USA

* Corresponding author. University at Buffalo Neurosurgery, 100 High Street, Suite B4, Buffalo, NY 14203.
E-mail address: asiddiqui@ubns.com

Neuroimag Clin N Am 23 (2013) 673–694
http://dx.doi.org/10.1016/j.nic.2013.03.014

emergency physician participation because of perceived risks, particularly intracranial hemorrhage (ICH), and lack of supporting critical care and specialty neurologic services. Even when delivered early, reocclusion after thrombolysis has been shown by transcranial Doppler imaging to occur in 34% of patients receiving IV t-PA and may result in neurologic worsening in many of these patients.[2–5]

PATIENTS WHO FAIL OR ARE NOT CANDIDATES FOR IV THROMBOLYSIS

Patients who do not meet the eligibility criteria for thrombolytic therapy, fail to improve neurologically after thrombolytic therapy, or who improve and then worsen (patients with reocclusion) are currently considered candidates for endovascular revascularization therapies. At our center, 94 patients with a mean National Institutes of Health Stroke Scale (NIHSS) score of 14.7 at presentation were treated by endovascular interventions within 3 hours of stroke symptom onset.[6] In these patients, t-PA IV thrombolysis (IVT) was contraindicated or had failed. Partial to complete recanalization (Thrombolysis in Myocardial Infarction [TIMI] score of 2 or 3) was achieved in 62 of 89 (70%) patients presenting with significant occlusion (TIMI 0 or 1). Postprocedure symptomatic intracranial hemorrhage (SICH) occurred in 5 patients (5.3%), which was subarachnoid hemorrhage in 3 of these patients. The total mortality, including procedural mortality, progression of disease, or other comorbidities, was 26.6%. Overall, 36.7% of patients had a modified Rankin scale (mRS) score of less than or equal to 2 at discharge. Mean NIHSS at discharge was 6.5, representing an overall 8-point improvement in NIHSS score.

Atrial fibrillation is a surrogate parameter of cardioembolic stroke with well-known higher bleeding rates in patients who receive IVT.[7–9] The Interventional Management of Stroke (IMS) I study showed a significant increased risk of SICH in patients with atrial fibrillation.[7] At our center, patients with strokes with atrial fibrillation had high rates (14.3%) of SICH after endovascular therapy that could not be explained by their anticoagulation status.[6] It is important to identify these patients as a separate entity to weigh the risks and benefits associated with treatment.

THE CONCEPT OF CLOT BURDEN AND LOCATION

Clot extent and location are important determinants of outcomes in acute stroke and determine the ability to achieve recanalization. The recanalization rates associated with IV t-PA for proximal, large vessel arterial occlusions are poor and range from only 10% for internal carotid artery (ICA) occlusion to 30% for middle cerebral artery (MCA) occlusion.[10] IVT is not as effective in thromboembolic obstruction of these large, proximal vessels as in more distal smaller vessels.[11] The outcome of IVT after large intracranial vessel thromboembolic occlusion currently remains dismal and is associated with high morbidity and mortality.[12–15] Clinical response to thrombolysis was influenced by the site of occlusion in a multicenter cohort of patients with strokes.[11] Odds ratios (ORs) for complete recanalization (TIMI 3) of vessel occlusions were as follows: distal MCA, 2; proximal MCA, 0.7; ICA terminus, 0.1; tandem cervical ICA/MCA, 0.7; and basilar artery, 0.96. A long, proximal clot is harder to treat, leading to a worse outcome compared with a shorter distal clot.[16–21]

NIHSS IS NOT A RELIABLE ASSESSMENT OF CLOT LOCATION OR BURDEN

Previously, an NIHSS score of greater than 12 was thought to suggest an occlusion of a large, proximal vessel and, therefore, a high thrombus burden.[22] In a prospective cohort study of 699 patients with 377 (54%) large vessel occlusions and 171 (24%) MCA M1 segment occlusions, the median NIHSS score for patients found to have a large vessel occlusion was higher than the overall median score for the cohort (9 vs 5, P<.0001).[23] The median NIHSS score of patients with MCA M1 segment occlusion was 14. An NIHSS score of greater than or equal to 10 had an 81% positive predictive value for large vessel occlusion but only 48% sensitivity, with most patients with proximal occlusions presenting with lower NIHSS scores. These data suggest that all patients with NIHSS scores of greater than or equal to 2 need to have imaging to detect 90% of proximal occlusions. This finding suggests a need to revisit the current practice of administering IV t-PA to patients because of NIHSS scores alone in the absence of any vascular or perfusion imaging studies. Further, many distally located clots (M2, M3, P2, P3) may cause the patient to present with a high NIHSS score; this confounding finding may be explained by intrinsic thrombolysis that results in a large proximal occlusion (the original cause of the high NIHSS score) resolving into smaller distal residual emboli.

ENDOVASCULAR THERAPY ACHIEVES HIGHER RECANALIZATION RATES AND IMPROVED OUTCOMES

In the Mechanical Embolus Removal in Cerebral Ischemia (MERCI)[24,25] and Multi-MERCI[26] studies and the combined analysis of IMS-I and IMS-II data,[27] functional outcome (measured by an mRS score of $\leq$2 at 3 months) was significantly better and 3-month mortality was significantly lower in patients who had TIMI 2 or 3 recanalization than in patients in whom vessels failed to recanalize after endovascular therapy. Rha and Saver[28] reviewed 53 studies including 2066 patients and found that good functional outcomes (mRS score $\leq$2 at 3 months) were more frequent in patients with vessel recanalization than without vessel recanalization. The 3-month mortality was reduced in patients in whom vessels were recanalized. Higher rates of recanalization were achieved with endovascular methods, particularly mechanical therapies, and consequently were associated with better outcomes.

TIME WINDOW BETWEEN SYMPTOM ONSET AND TREATMENT AFFECTS OUTCOMES

The European Cooperative Acute Stroke Study (ECASS) III trial[2] showed the value of extending the time window for IV t-PA to 4.5 hours. A meta-analysis by Lansberg and colleagues[29] included data from patients in the ECASS I, II, III, and Alteplase Thrombolysis for Acute Noninterventional Therapy in Ischemic Stroke (ATLANTIS) trials treated within the 3-hour to 4.5-hour time window, and showed at 3 months that t-PA treatment was associated with an increased probability of favorable outcome and mortality was not significantly different for IVT-treated and placebo-treated patients. A meta-analysis conducted by Wardlaw and colleagues[30] showed higher benefit (compared with risk of being dead or disabled) up to 6 hours after IVT, thus formally providing level 1 evidence, even in patients selected solely from noncontrast computed tomography (CT) imaging.

ENDOVASCULAR THERAPY CAN BE USED BEYOND THE IVT TIME WINDOW

The Prolyse in Acute Cerebral Thromboembolism (PROACT) trials[31,32] established a benefit of intra-arterial thrombolysis (IAT) up to 6 hours after stroke symptom onset with an increase in recanalization rates. Mechanical revascularization strategies reestablish flow faster than thrombolytics, and thus may increase the benefit of treatment, even when there is a delay in presentation for treatment. The MERCI,[24,25] Multi-MERCI,[26] and Penumbra[33] trials show effectiveness of mechanical revascularization therapy up to 8 hours after stroke symptom onset. There is increasing evidence that identification of potentially salvageable brain tissue with advanced magnetic resonance

(MR)–based and CT-based perfusion imaging may allow the selection of patients who can be effectively and safely treated more than 8 hours after ictus.[2,34–40] In a consecutive series of patients selected for endovascular revascularization from advanced CT perfusion imaging at our center, no difference was found in outcomes in those with known time of symptom onset of less than 8 hours and those with wake-up strokes (with unknown time of onset but suspected to be >8 hours).[6]

THE CHANGE FROM TIME IS BRAIN TO ISCHEMIC PENUMBRA BEING THE THERAPEUTIC TARGET

The concept of ischemic penumbra divides tissues in the ischemic territory supplied by the occluded vessel to be comprised of (1) ischemic core, which is tissue that is dead and cannot be salvaged; (2) ischemic penumbra, which is tissue that will rapidly convert to core if the occluded vessel is not recanalized; and (3) area of oligemia, which is the area of the brain that is underperfused but will likely survive even if the vessel is not recanalized (dependent on collateral supply). Compartmentalization of ischemic tissue is dynamic and is changing every minute from symptom onset until tissue perfusion is restored or ischemic penumbra and core are matched. The concepts of identifying the therapeutic target (the ischemic penumbra) and having an estimation of the size and location of the core are driving stroke neuroimaging research and development at a fast pace. The theoretic possibility of being able to manipulate these dynamic variables in the critical time period from patient identification to tissue reperfusion has provided a second overlay over the time of stroke onset to decide on reperfusion strategies and search for adjunctive measures to improve outcomes after stroke revascularization.

IMPORTANCE OF COLLATERALS IN STROKE OUTCOMES

Collateral supply is one of the main determinants of the dynamic balance between the relative amounts of tissue classified as ischemic penumbra and oligemia. The ability to quantify the presence and extent of collateral support to ischemic tissue and augment collateral support before recanalization may widen the time window for recanalization therapy and improve ability to prognosticate stroke outcomes. It may also further the understanding of the physiology of ischemic tissue and aid selection of patients for aggressive recanalization strategies. The extent of revascularization depends not only on recanalization of the primary arterial occlusive lesion but also on reperfusion of the distal vascular bed.[41] The degree of collateral supply through peripheral leptomeningeal sources is important and correlates with the presence of a smaller final infarct volume.[42] The evaluation of collateral supply remains challenging because of the diminutive size and complex routes of these vessels.[43,44] Collateral failure may be an important cause of delayed deterioration after successful reperfusion, and thus collateral support may need to be monitored after reperfusion to improve outcomes.[45] Several interventions that might augment collateral blood flow are being investigated.[44]

IMPORTANCE OF ASSESSING ISCHEMIC CORE BEFORE REVASCULARIZATION

The percentage and location of the ischemic core are important determinants of the risk of SICH after reperfusion. ICH occurs in the core of the infarction in most patients.[46] SICH usually occurs within 24 to 36 hours of reperfusion therapy.[46] The mortality after SICH in the National Institute of Neurologic Disorders and Stroke (NINDS) trial was 47%.[46] When dichotomized Alberta Stroke Program Early CT Scores (ASPECTS) were assessed, patients with low stroke burden (ASPECTS >7) on CT imaging had a lower occurrence of SICH after IVT and a higher chance of gaining independence (mRS score ≥2).[47] The use of CT perfusion (CTP) imaging, rather than noncontrast CT imaging, increases prognostic accuracy of the ASPECTS, with the final infarct mirroring cerebral blood volume (CBV) or cerebral blood flow (CBF) deficits when reperfusion is or is not achieved, respectively.[48] The Diffusion-weighted Imaging Evaluation for Understanding Stroke Evolution (DEFUSE) trial[49] was the first study that directly established a strong relationship between MR imaging (based on ischemic core) and tissue parameters and SICH. In this study, early reperfusion was associated with fatal ICH in patients with the malignant profile (baseline diffusion-weighted imaging volume >100 mL and/or perfusion-weighted imaging deficit >100 mL with 8 seconds or longer of T_{max} [time to peak of the deconvoluted curve]). The presence of even small ischemic cores in the basal ganglia region predicts higher rates of SICH and disability after revascularization.[50]

PERFUSION IMAGING FOR PATIENT SELECTION

Perfusion imaging for patient selection for both IVT and endovascular therapy is being investigated for its potential to identify the ischemic territory (perfusion deficit) and the location and percentage of ischemic core (perfusion mismatch). CT and MR are two perfusion imaging modalities that are being evaluated. The main limitation of both modalities is that the perfusion deficit is a sum of the therapeutic target: the real ischemic penumbra and the oligemic tissue. Any perfusion mismatch calculation is erroneous, because currently there is no definite way to differentiate between these territories. As emphasized earlier, the relative percentage of core, ischemic penumbra, and oligemic tissue is a dynamic phenomenon and has to be assessed as close to the time of the recanalization procedure as possible to achieve meaningful outcomes based on perfusion imaging findings. The assessment of collaterals through perfusion imaging and catheter-based angiography is being investigated at multiple centers.

Perfusion parameters stratify the patient's risk for hemorrhage after endovascular intervention and the potential benefit of mechanical flow restoration. In general terms, when decreased CBF and CBV (findings that suggest completed infarct) represent less than one-third of the territory exhibiting increased time to peak (TTP) (ie, putative penumbra or perfusion deficit), we have found that the patient benefits from endovascular intervention and has a lower risk of SICH. Early ischemic changes on a noncontrast CT scan that correspond with CBF and CBV deficits solidify the reliability of predicting completed infarct. Reperfusion of a larger core is ineffective and likely increases the risk of hemorrhage.[51] In contrast, patients with hyperacute presentations (ie, <2 hours) had salvageable regions after endovascular therapy, even in the face of a poor CTP profile (ie, with decreased CBV and CBF).[51] In addition, occlusion of proximal M1 perforators and attendant basal ganglionic involvement in the infarct core presage a higher risk of hemorrhage and poor clinical outcome after recanalization.[50] Recent studies suggest that clinical improvement is noted even when endovascular stroke therapy is performed more than 8 hours after ictus in patients with large penumbras identified on CTP imaging.[52,53]

There has been recent interest in estimating CTP thresholds (thresholds of CBF and CBV) and using quantitative and automated CTP maps to estimate core and penumbra to aid in choosing patients for reperfusion beyond traditional therapeutic windows or when the time of stroke onset is unknown.[54,55] Differences in CTP hardware and software can affect quantified metrics,[56,57] and clearly defined thresholds for guiding therapy have yet to be standardized.[58] Some studies suggest the use of CBF thresholds for defining areas of infarct, specifically CBF less than 25 mL/100 g/min. In an analysis of 130 patients with acute stroke, Wintermark and colleagues[59] suggested using absolute CBV less than 2 mL/100 g to define core infarct and increase in relative mean transit time by 145% of normal to define penumbra. Murphy and colleagues[60] studied 30 patients and showed CBF × CBV as the best predictor for differentiating core infarct and penumbra (better than CBF or CBV thresholds alone). CTP thresholds are also specific to the perfusion software platform being used and may not be automatically transferable to other vendors, scanners, and even software versions. Attention should be paid to technical aspects of data acquisition and postprocessing, including placement of regions of interest as well as selecting an appropriate volume of imaging commensurate with the clinical condition or symptoms.[61] Disorders such as chronic infarct, severe microvascular ischemia, and seizure can be mistaken for acute infarct. Vascular stenoses can mimic and overestimate areas of ischemic penumbra; therefore, CTP should always be performed and interpreted in conjunction with CT angiography.[51] At this time, much work remains to standardize quantitative methods of CTP interpretation, which, in the future, may be addressed by a proposed consortium for acute stroke imaging.[58]

PATIENT SELECTION FOR ENDOVASCULAR THERAPY

Because patients considered for revascularization (whether IVT or endovascular therapy) require imaging assessment of the presence of decreased tissue perfusion, location and extent of clot burden, and core location and percentage, every patient with a clinical diagnosis of ischemic stroke at our center is evaluated with stroke CT imaging. The imaging protocol includes (1) non-contrast cranial CT scan to exclude hemorrhagic conversion or other structural abnormality; (2) CTP imaging with special attention to TTP, CBF, and CBV sequences; and (3) CT angiogram from the aortic arch through the intracranial vessels. Perfusion imaging is performed on a 320-slice Aquilon scanner (Toshiba Medical Systems, Tustin, CA).

CT angiography, although not essential when proceeding directly to the performance of a catheter angiogram for diagnostic purposes, provides critical information for endovascular planning. First and foremost, the target vessel occlusion responsible for the patient's symptoms is confirmed, after clinical evaluation, with the corresponding CTP data. In addition, CT angiography allows the length of the occlusion to be determined, the presence of tandem occlusions to be identified, and access planned from the aortic arch to the lesion.

In the setting of large vessel occlusion (ICA to proximal M2) on CT angiography, the patient is always assessed for consideration of endovascular revascularization either alone or with IVT bridging therapy. We have found that patients with anterior circulation strokes with large vessel occlusions presenting more than 8 hours after symptom onset have done poorly, despite selection based on imaging findings.[6] Patients with wake-up strokes with unknown time of onset and posterior circulation strokes 24 hours, or sometimes even up to 48 hours, after stroke symptom onset are evaluated for endovascular revascularization. For patients more than 75 years of age, a more thorough risk-benefit analysis is warranted. In our series of such patients who were selected from imaging, 72% died or were disabled after endovascular treatment.[6] As mentioned earlier, patients with atrial fibrillation have a higher risk of SICH during stroke interventions, and careful selection of patients and revascularization tools is warranted in such cases.

IAT

In theory, IAT may offer a higher dose of thrombolytic drug delivery to the clot with fewer systemic complications and higher recanalization rates.[62] Intra-arterial (IA) treatment may also facilitate extension of the therapeutic window and provide an option for patients with contraindications for systemic thrombolysis (ie, postoperative stroke) or patients in whom IVT has failed. The advantages of IAT include the ability to perform angiography with gold-standard characterization of the obstructive lesion; imaging of collateral flow anatomy (to the extent possible with current technology); confirmation, exact degree, and timing of recanalization; and capability for combination with mechanical thrombectomy methods. Disadvantages of IAT include delay in treatment, risks of catheter manipulation, increased risk of SICH with pharmacologic thrombolysis, and need for skilled endovascular facilities and personnel.[62]

To perform IAT, a long 6-French (F) or 7-F sheath is placed into the femoral artery, and a 6-F or 7-F guiding catheter is advanced into the ICA or vertebral artery of the affected side. A microcatheter is then navigated to the occlusion site over a microwire, and the thrombolytic agent is injected proximal to or directly into the thrombus.

The PROACT studies evaluated IAT with recombinant prourokinase (pro-UK) in patients within

6 hours of an MCA (M1 or M2 segment) occlusion stroke.[31,32] The PROACT-II study (a phase III prospective, randomized, placebo-controlled study) enrolled 180 patients with a median NIHSS score of 17 (range, 4–30).[32] Favorable outcome (mRS score of 0–2 at 90 days) was achieved in 40% of patients treated with IA pro-UK (9 mg; plus low-dose heparin) versus only 25% of control subjects (low-dose heparin only) ($P = .04$). The recanalization rate was significantly higher in the pro-UK group (66%) than in the control group (18%) ($P<.001$). Although the rate of SICH was higher in patients given pro-UK (10%) than in control patients (2%) ($P = .06$), no difference in mortality was observed. Although only IA pro-UK was used for thrombolysis in the PROACT trials, t-PA is used for thrombolysis in the United States because of the unavailability of pro-UK here. However, the FDA has not yet approved the use of t-PA for IA thrombolysis.

Two studies in Japan evaluated IA urokinase treatment. From these IA thrombolysis studies, it is apparent that recanalization rates may differ with occlusion site and stroke cause. Lower recanalization rates were observed in patients with thromboembolic carotid terminus occlusion (30%) relative to MCA M1 segment (50%) or M2 segment (90%) occlusions.[63–65] Therefore, considerations of the nature of the occlusion may inform endovascular planning.

COMBINED IV AND IA THROMBOLYSIS

The IMS studies investigated the feasibility and safety of a combined IV and IA approach to thrombolysis. In IMS-I, 80 patients were enrolled within 3 hours of stroke onset; median baseline NIHSS score was 18.[7] The patients received 0.6 mg/kg of IV t-PA followed by 22 mg of IA t-PA via a 2-hour infusion or until thrombolysis had been achieved. The outcome of this study was compared with that for the NINDS IV t-PA stroke trial.[46] IMS subjects had a significantly better outcome at 3 months than NINDS placebo-treated subjects for all outcome measures (OR $\geq$2) but not beyond the benefit conferred to the NINDS IVT group.

IMS-II was a continuous, nonrandomized, safety and feasibility pilot study to evaluate efficacy and safety of IV t-PA (0.6 mg/kg, followed by IA t-PA [22 mg again]) coupled with low-energy sonography (via the EKOS Primo Micro-Infusion Catheter [EKOS Corporation, Bothell, WA]) to theoretically increase fluid permeation and thrombolytic infusion within the clot.[66] IMS-II subjects had significantly better outcomes at 3 months than NINDS placebo-treated subjects for all end points

(OR $\geq$2.7) and better outcomes than NINDS t-PA-treated subjects.

Pooled IMS-I and IMS-II data showed that partial or complete recanalization occurred in 74.6% of ICA terminus and MCA M1 occlusions, with good reperfusion (TIMI 2 or 3) in 61.3%.[27,28] Good reperfusion (TIMI 2 or 3) correlated strongly with good outcome ($P = .0004$). The 3-month mortality was lower (although not of statistical significance) in IMS-II patients (16%), than in placebo-treated (24%) or t-PA–treated (21%) NINDS trial patients. The rate of SICH was higher in IMS-II (9.9%) but not significantly different from that in the NINDS trial (6.6%). The definitive randomized controlled trial, IMS-III,[67] is ongoing; and the results will likely provide class I evidence for the concept of combined IV-IA therapy.

MECHANICAL THROMBECTOMY

The most common method for mechanical thrombus disruption is probing the thrombus with a microguidewire. This technique seems to be useful in facilitating pharmacologic thrombolysis.[68] Systems for mechanical recanalization can be divided into 2 major groups according to where they apply force on the thrombus. Proximal devices apply force to the proximal base of the thrombus. This group includes various aspiration catheters. Distal devices approach the thrombus proximally but then are advanced over a guide wire and microcatheter across the thrombus to be unsheathed distally, where force is applied to the distal base of the thrombus. This group includes snarelike, basketlike, or coil-like devices. In an animal model,[69] proximal devices were faster in application and were associated with a low complication rate. The distal devices were more successful at removing thrombotic material, but their method of application and attendant thrombus compaction increased the risk of thromboembolic events and vasospasm.[17,70] Advantages and disadvantages of mechanical revascularization strategies overall are summarized in Box 1. Current FDA-approved thrombectomy devices are the Merci retriever (distal device) (Concentric Medical Inc, Mountain View, CA) and the Penumbra aspiration catheter (proximal device) (Penumbra Inc, Alameda, CA).

Merci Device

The Merci retriever is a shaped wire constructed of nitinol. The flexible corkscrewlike tip can easily be delivered through a microcatheter into the vessel distal to the occlusion site. When deployed, this device returns to its preformed coiled shape to ensnare the thrombus. The thrombus is bypassed

---

Box 1
Mechanical revascularization strategies

Advantages

- Lessen, and may even preclude, the use of pharmacologic thrombolytics, and thus reduce the incidence of SICH
- May extend the treatment window beyond the limit of 6 to 8 hours
- Mechanical fragmentation of the clot increases the surface area of the clot available for endogenous and exogenous fibrinolysis
- Recanalization time may be faster
- May be effective for thrombi or other material resistant to thrombolytics that occlude the vessel
- Key option for patients who have a contraindication for pharmacologic thrombolysis, such as recent surgery or abnormal hemostasis, or have a late presentation

Disadvantages

- Technical difficulty navigating the devices through the intracranial vasculature
- Excessive trauma to the vasculature
- Distal embolization from fragmented thrombus

---

and the retriever deployed from inside the catheter distal to the thrombus. The corkscrewlike tip is pulled back slowly to ensnare the clot as a corkscrew would ensnare a cork. The retriever is then retracted into the guide catheter under proximal flow arrest. Different versions of this device are available. In the first-generation devices (X5 and X6), the nitinol wire was shaped in helical-tapering coil loops. The second-generation devices (L4, L5, and L6) differ from the X devices by the inclusion of a system of arcading filaments attached to a nontapering helical nitinol coil, which has a 90° angle in relation to the proximal wire component. The third-generation devices (V series) have variable-pitch loops in a linear configuration with attached filaments. The retriever device is deployed through a 2.4-F microcatheter (14 X or 18 L, Concentric Medical). The addition of a 4.3-F distal access catheter (DAC) has provided additional coaxial support to the system, resulting in improved delivery ability with the potential for simultaneous thromboaspiration as well. Merci devices are available in various diameters from 1.5 to 3 mm, depending on the caliber of the occluded vessel. These devices are regularly used in combination with proximal balloon occlusion in the ICA, in addition to aspiration from the guiding catheter,

to reduce the risk of distal thromboembolism. An illustrative case of Merci retrieval is provided in **Fig. 1**.

The Merci procedure is performed after femoral artery access is obtained with the Merci balloon guide, which comes in both 8-F and 9-F outer diameters. Once the balloon guide is in the conduit vessel of interest, a medium-sized catheter (available in 4.2-F and 5.3-F outer diameters), the DAC (used for triaxial support), and microcatheter of choice are advanced over the microwire to the clot under direct fluoroscopic guidance. The microwire is then exchanged for the Merci retriever system with placement distal to the clot. The balloon guide is then inflated. Using a slow, steady pulling motion, the retriever engages the clot while the DAC position is maintained. Then, as the clot moves proximally, the DAC, microcatheter, and retriever are moved toward the guide while aggressive aspiration is performed from the guide. The retriever can be resheathed and the steps repeated. The Merci device often requires 3 to 6 passes before flow is restored, which delays the time to recanalization. The aforementioned new DAC available for use with the Merci device allows placement of smaller triple coaxial guide catheter near the lesion of interest to transmit the traction force better in a straighter angle at a shorter distance.

FDA approval of the Merci device in 2004 was based on a review of data obtained in the multicenter Merci trial that involved 141 patients (mean age, 60 years; mean NIHSS score, 20) ineligible for standard thrombolytic therapy.[24,25] The Multi-MERCI trial[26] was a prospective, multicenter, single-arm registry that included 164 patients (mean age, 68 years; mean NIHSS score 19) treated with different Merci retrieval systems (X5, X6, and L5). Patients with persistent large vessel occlusion after IVT (with t-PA) were also included in the study, and adjunctive IAT (also with t-PA) was allowed. The Merci device has led to an increase in the rates of recanalization of intracranial ICA occlusions.[71] Two ongoing prospective randomized trials are using the device, namely the MR and Recanalization of Stroke Clots Using Embolectomy (MR-RESCUE) trial (NCT00389467) and the IMS-III trial.[67]

Penumbra Device

From a procedural approach, proximal devices, like the Penumbra, are comparable with IAT. The Penumbra system has 3 main components: a reperfusion catheter, separator, and a thrombus removal ring. A Penumbra procedure is performed after arterial access is obtained and usually after

A

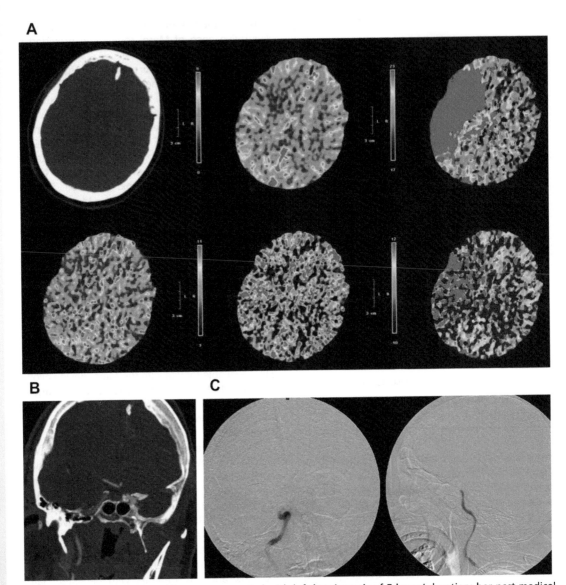

B

C

Fig. 1. Merci case: a 59-year-old woman presented with left hemiparesis of 5 hours' duration; her past medical history included hypertension, diabetes mellitus, and hypercholesterolemia. She denied use of tobacco, alcohol, or illicit drugs. Medications included antihypertensive agents and statins. Her NIHSS score on the initial examination was 16. CT perfusion imaging shows increased TTP in the right MCA territory (*A*). CT angiogram shows occlusion of the right supraclinoid ICA and the MCA (*B*). A Merci device (Concentric Medical Inc., Mountain View, CA) was used to ensnare and retrieve the clot. The first angiographic run shows no filling of the right supraclinoid ICA, anterior cerebral artery, or MCA. (*C*) Anteroposterior (AP) projection (*left*) and lateral projection (*right*). TIMI 3 flow is seen after the second pass of the Merci device.

systemic heparinization. All but the largest components of the Penumbra system are deliverable through a 6-F standard guide catheter; a 070 Neuron catheter is the guide designed for the system. The reperfusion catheter is advanced past the guide catheter over a guidewire and placed proximal to the clot. The catheters and separators are available in different sizes for various arterial diameters, including 026, 032, 041, and 057. The 057 aspiration system requires a 6-F long sheath in the access vessel for delivery (shuttle). The guidewire is then removed from the reperfusion catheter, and the penumbra separator is advanced through the reperfusion catheter. The aspiration pump is started and a continuous aspiration, clot disruption-debulking process is performed with the separator. In general, the Penumbra device works better in straight arterial segments than

D

E

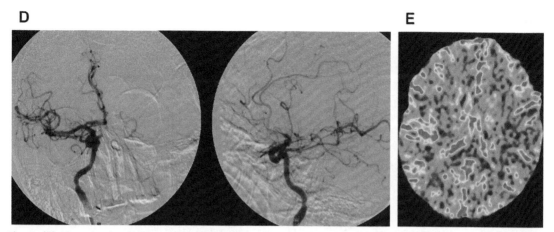

Fig. 1. (*D*) AP projection (*left*) and lateral projection (*right*). Postprocedure CT perfusion image shows resolution of perfusion deficit in the right MCA territory (*E*). On postprocedure day 2, the patient's NIHSS score had improved to 5.

around curves or at branch points, because the separator may cause arterial perforation. In addition, the largest catheter possible should be used to allow for the greatest amount of aspiration, because suction decreases with decreasing vessel diameter. Another advantage of the Penumbra system is that it can reach more distal vessels, such as proximal M3 vessels, compared with other thrombectomy devices that are difficult to manipulate in these distal vessels. The use of the Penumbra system in a patient with acute ischemic stroke is illustrated in **Fig. 2.**

A prospective, single-arm, independently monitored trial was performed to assess the efficiency and safety of the Penumbra system.[33] Twenty-three patients were enrolled, and 21 target vessels were treated in 20 patients. At baseline, the mean NIHSS score was 21. After the procedure, all 21 treated vessels (100%) were successfully revascularized to TIMI 2 or 3. At the 30-day follow-up evaluation, 9 patients (45%) had improvement of 4 points or more in NIHSS score or an mRS score of 2 or less. The all-cause mortality was 45% (9 of 20), which is lower than expected in this severe stroke cohort, in which 70% of the patients at baseline had either an NIHSS score of more than 20 or a basilar occlusion. In a prospective multicenter single-arm trial of 125 patients with acute stroke who underwent revascularization with the Penumbra device, TIMI 2 or 3 recanalization was achieved in 81.6% of patients with an SICH rate of 11.2%, although only 25% of patients achieved mRS less than or equal to 2.[72] On average, 40 minutes elapsed from the time the Penumbra device was deployed near the clot until complete flow restoration was achieved.

The investigators of the Postmarket Experience of the Penumbra System Trial (POST)[73] reviewed

157 consecutive patients with a mean presentation NIHSS score of 16. Revascularization was achieved in 87% of the treated vessels (TIMI 2, 54%; TIMI 3, 33%), compared with 82% reported in the pivotal trial. Procedure-related serious adverse events were reported 9 patients (5.7%). All-cause mortality was 20% (32 of 157 patients), and 41% had an mRS of less than or equal to 2 at 90-day follow-up, compared with only 25% in the pivotal trial. Successful Penumbra revascularization correlated with significantly better clinical outcomes.

STENT-ASSISTED REVASCULARIZATION FOR ACUTE ISCHEMIC STROKE

Several retrospective case series reported successful use of self-expanding stents for acute stroke treatment, with higher rates of recanalization than those obtained with other recanalization modalities.[74–76] A multicenter retrospective review was conducted of prospectively collected data of 20 patients with acute ischemic stroke (mean presentation NIHSS score, 17) treated with the Enterprise stent (Codman Neurovascular, Raynham, MA) placement as a bailout procedure after current embolectomy options had been used.[77] Treatment resulted in TIMI 2 or 3 recanalization in all patients (100%) and improvement in NIHSS score of greater than or equal to 4 points at discharge in 75% of patients. Adjunctive therapy included Merci retrieval (12 patients), angioplasty (7 patients), glycoprotein IIb/IIIa inhibition (12 patients), IA nitroglycerin administration (1 patient), Wingspan stent (Boston Scientific, Natick, MA) deployment (3 patients), and Xpert stent (Abbott Laboratories, Abbott Park, IL) deployment (1 patient). The Enterprise stent could be more easily navigated and deployed to the occlusion site

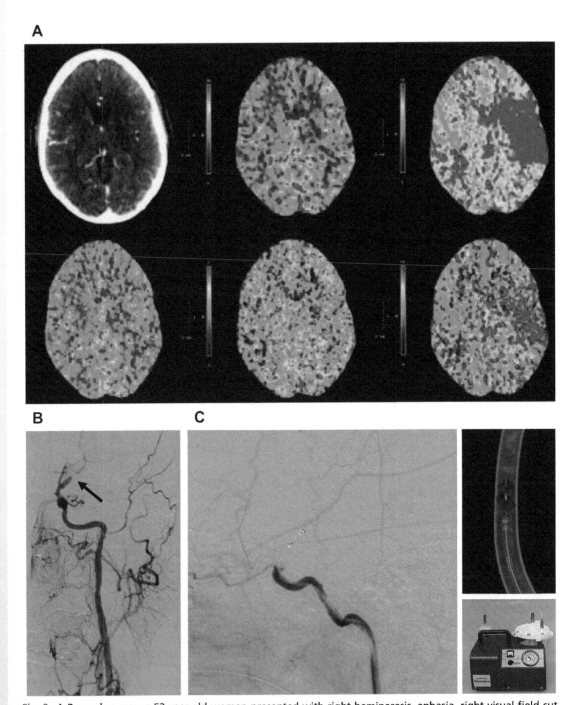

Fig. 2. A Penumbra case: a 52-year-old woman presented with right hemiparesis, aphasia, right visual field cut, and left gaze preference of 1 hour in duration (NIHSS score of 18). CT perfusion imaging shows a large perfusion deficit in the left MCA (*A*). Angiographic run, lateral view, shows left ICA terminus thrombus (*arrow*) (*B*). IV t-PA was given without improvement. A Penumbra device and separator (Penumbra Inc., Alameda, CA) were chosen to aspirate the ICA terminus thrombus (*C*). Left panel shows the lateral view of the left ICA, before the procedure, showing the same left ICA terminus thrombus. Right upper and lower panels show images of the Penumbra device.

D

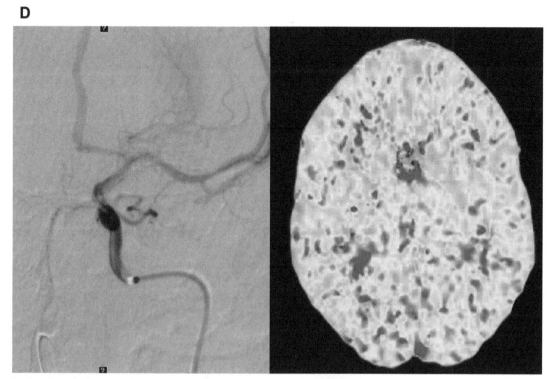

Fig. 2. After the intervention, angiographic run shows TIMI 3 flow (*D, left*, AP projection), and CT perfusion imaging shows resolution of the perfusion deficit (*D, right*). ([C] *From* Penumbra Inc., Alameda, CA; with permission.)

than the Wingspan stent, attested by its use in all 3 cases of failed Wingspan stenting. Illustrative cases of Enterprise and Wingspan stenting are provided in **Figs. 3** and **4**, respectively.

From these preliminary data, we received FDA approval for a pilot study, Stent-assisted Recanalization in Acute Ischemic Stroke (SARIS), to evaluate the Wingspan stent for revascularization in patients who did not improve after IVT or had a contraindication to IVT.[78] The mean duration from stroke onset to intervention was 5 hours and 13 minutes. Total time from procedure onset to vessel recanalization was 45 minutes. Average presenting NIHSS score was 14. Seventeen patients presented with a TIMI score of 0 and 3 patients with a TIMI score of 1. Occluded vessels included the right MCA (11 patients), left MCA (5 patients), basilar artery (3 patients), and right carotid terminus (1 patient). Intracranial stents were placed in 19 of 20 enrolled patients. One patient experienced recanalization of the occluded vessel with positioning of the Wingspan stent delivery system before stent deployment. In 2 patients, vessel tortuosity did not allow tracking of the Wingspan stent. The more navigable Enterprise stent was used in both these cases. Twelve patients had adjunctive therapies: IA eptifibatide (10 patients), IA t-PA (2 patients), angioplasty

(8 patients), and IV t-PA (2 patients). TIMI 2 or 3 recanalization was achieved in 100% of patients; 65% of patients improved by more than 4 points in NIHSS score after treatment. One patient (5%) had SICH and 2 had asymptomatic ICH. At the time of the 3-month follow-up evaluation, 12 of 20 (60%) patients had an mRS score of less than or equal to 2 and 9 (45%) had an mRS score of less than or equal to 1. Mortality at 1 month was 25% (5 patients). None of the patients enrolled in this study died of stent placement–related causes; all deaths were caused by the severity of the initial stroke and associated comorbidities. At 6 months,[79] the mRS score was less than or equal to 3 in 60% of patients (n = 12) and less than or equal to 2 in 55% (n = 11), reduced because of unrelated mortality. Mortality at the 6-month follow-up was 35% (n = 7). Follow-up angiography was performed for 85% (11 of 13) of surviving patients. All patients undergoing angiographic follow-up showed TIMI 3 flow on digital subtraction angiography or stent patency on CT angiography. None of the patients showed evidence of in-stent stenosis (ie, ≥50% vessel narrowing).

The main limitation of current stent-assisted revascularization (based on the Wingspan registries) is the theoretic risk of acute-term and midterm stent failure (within 6 months of stent

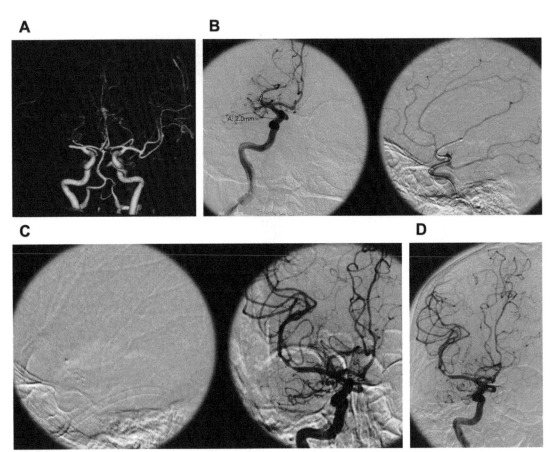

Fig. 3. Enterprise case: an 82-year-old woman presented to the emergency room 5 hours after the onset of symptoms consisting of left-sided hemiparesis, gaze deviation, and a significant left hemineglect (NIHSS score of 9). CT angiogram shows right M1 occlusion (*A*). The patient received a loading dose of aspirin and clopidogrel in anticipation of the use of an Enterprise stent (Codman Neurovascular, Raynham, MA). A guide catheter was placed high in the cervical ICA. A Prowler-Select-Plus microcatheter (Codman Neurovascular) was advanced over a gold-tip microwire (Radiofocus Guidewire M, Terumo Medical Corporation, Somerset, NJ). The microwire was used to cross the occlusion. The microcatheter was advanced across the occlusion. Right ICA angiogram, AP projection, showing guide catheter placed high in the cervical ICA (*B, left*); right ICA angiogram, lateral projection, showing the gold-tip microwire crossing the occlusion (*B, right*). Angiographic runs show stent deployed across the lesion: right ICA, lateral projection, showing the stent markers during stent deployment (*C, left*); right ICA, AP projection, showing stent deployed and flow restoration (*C, right*). After the intervention, angiographic run shows restoration of TIMI 3 flow in the right M1, with filling of the superior division of the MCA (*D*). The patient was discharged home. Her NIHSS score was 1 (mild sensory neglect).

deployment). At present, no large studies exist that have assessed stent patency and complications related to placement of a permanent implant in a patient with acute ischemic stroke beyond 1 month of stent placement. Zaidat and colleagues[76] reported 1 case (11%) of immediate in-stent restenosis after acute stroke treatment, although there were no such cases in the SARIS trial at 6 months.[79] The need for aggressive antiplatelet and/or anticoagulant therapy associated with intracranial stent placement[76,80–85] is a second major limitation if stent placement is used as a treatment technique in the setting of acute stroke because this regimen could increase the risk of hemorrhagic conversion

of the infarct. Zaidat and colleagues[76] reported an 11% hemorrhage rate associated with stent placement for acute stroke. Moreover, Levy and colleagues[75] reported an identical 11% incidence of lethal hemorrhages in patients treated with stent placement for acute stroke.

Stent Platform–based Therapies

Temporary endovascular bypass

Closed-cell stents can be used for temporary endovascular bypass with resheathing/removal of the stent after recanalization is achieved, obviating dual antiplatelet therapy. In addition, this

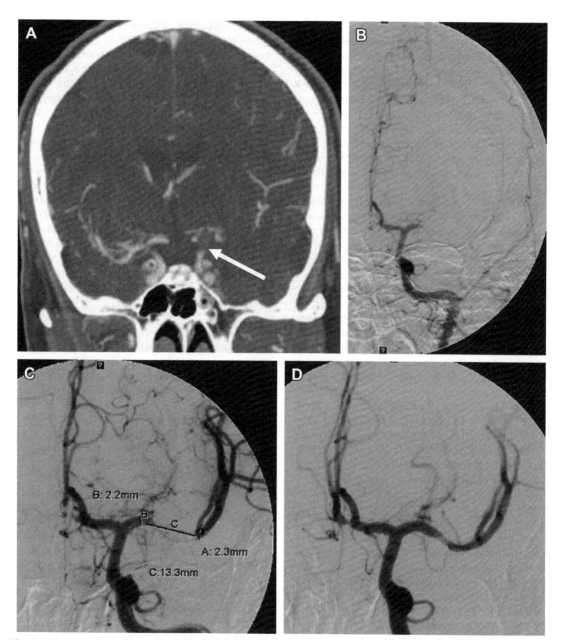

Fig. 4. Wingspan case: a 60-year-old man presented with right-sided weakness and mild aphasia (NIHSS score, 2). Medical history included atrial fibrillation (off warfarin therapy owing to a recent fall leading to development of a small subdural hematoma). CT angiogram shows left ICA terminus occlusion (*arrow*) (*A*). Treatment was initiated with aspirin, clopidogrel, and a heparin drip. Seven hours later, the patient's neurologic examination declined acutely (NIHSS of 10). CT scan (not shown) showed no change in subdural hematoma. Left ICA angiogram, AP projection, shows migration of thrombus to left M1 MCA segment (*B*). Angiographic run (left ICA, AP projection) shows length of lesion measured (*C*) for choosing the Wingspan stent and Gateway angioplasty balloon system (Boston Scientific, Natick, MA). Angiographic run (left ICA, AP projection) shows Wingspan stent (2.5 × 20 mm) deployed across the lesion (*D*). The patient was discharged home with an NIHSS score of 1.

technique should eliminate the risk of delayed in-stent stenosis. Kelly and colleagues[86] and Hauck and colleagues[87] reported the use of the closed-cell Enterprise stent as a temporary endovascular bypass in the acute stroke setting. In both cases, the Enterprise stent was partially deployed for some time and retrieved with successful recanalization of the occluded vessel.

Thrombectomy device (Stentriever)

This strategy of stent retrieval was used to great effect with use of the Solitaire stent (ev3, Irvine, CA) designed originally for assisting coil embolization of intracranial aneurysms. The Solitaire FR Revascularization Device is a recoverable self-expanding thrombectomy device.[88] This device is a fully recoverable self-expanding stent platform–based device that can be used as both a temporary endovascular bypass and a thrombectomy device. The device restores flow immediately and avoids the placement of a permanent stent and, thus, the necessary protracted antiplatelet therapy and the risk of in-stent stenosis. Moreover, it can be electrolytically detached like a coil should a permanent stent be necessary, such as in the setting of an atherothrombotic lesion. We evaluated the safety and efficacy of this device in a canine stroke model with soft and firm clots.[89] The device could be deployed and recovered easily, and TIMI 2 or 3 flow was restored immediately in all cases. Minimal residual clot in 2 of 4 instances required a second pass for complete clot retrieval. Minimal vasospasm was observed in 2 of 4 cases. Two small preliminary studies with this device have shown promising results.[90,91] The Solitaire FR With the Intention for Thrombectomy (SWIFT) trial is a multicenter randomized controlled trial that tested the ability of the Solitaire FR device versus the Merci device to achieve TIMI 2 or 3 recanalization without SICH. This trial was halted early secondary to higher mortality in the Merci arm. The results were recently reported at the 2012 International Stroke Conference.[92] The study population of 144 patients was enrolled from 18 sites across the United States. Patients were randomly assigned to treatment with the Solitaire device (n = 58) or the Merci device (n = 55). The primary efficacy outcome, successful recanalization without SICH, was achieved more often in patients treated with Solitaire than with Merci (60.7% vs 24.1%, noninferiority P<.0001, superiority P = .0001). Solitaire treatment also led to better outcomes by other measures: lower mortality at 3 months, 17.2% versus 38.2% (P = .02 for superiority); symptomatic intracranial bleeding occurred in 1.7% versus 10.9% (P<.0001 for noninferiority); good mental/motor functioning at 90 days in 58.2% versus 33.3% (P = .0001 for noninferiority). An illustrative case is provided in **Fig. 5**.

The Trevo device (Concentric Medical Inc., Mountain View, CA), another stent platform–based thrombectomy device, was tested in swine and canine models and was highly effective at achieving immediate reperfusion of occluded arteries without causing any clinically significant disruption of vascular integrity.[93] The Thrombectomy Revascularization of Large Vessel Occlusions in Acute Ischemic Stroke (TREVO 2) study was the first evaluation of Stentriever technology in a European, multicenter, prospective clinical trial (phase III) of randomization to treatment with the Trevo or Merci device. The trial began in February 2010 and completed enrollment in September 2011. The TREVO 2 trialists recruited adults aged 18–85 years with angiographically confirmed large vessel occlusion strokes and NIHSS scores of 8–29 within 8 hours of symptom onset and randomized them to receive treatment with the Trevo or Merci device.[94] The primary efficacy endpoint was Thrombolysis in Cerebral Infarction (TICI) score of 2 or greater reperfusion with the assigned device alone. A total of 76 (86%) patients in the Trevo group and 54 (60%) in the Merci group met the primary endpoint after the assigned device was used (odds ratio 4.22, 95% confidence interval 2.01–8.86; P [superiority] <0.0001).

Penumbra separator 3D and 4/5 MAX aspiration device

The main disadvantages of the aforementioned Solitaire and Trevo first-generation stentrievers are as follows: 1) although stentriever use and proximal aspiration has reduced the incidence of embolization to new territory to 9% for the Solitaire and 7% for the Trevo, when compared to a 15% incidence with only proximal aspiration, these are still relatively high numbers; 2) multiple passes increase risk of vessel injury to 8%, 3) there is a 14% incidence of vasospasm, and 4) these are devices that were not primarily developed with stroke intervention in mind (Solitaire Retrospective Study, Presented at the 2011 World Federation of Interventional and Therapeutic Neuroradiology Congress; TREVO2 Trial, Presented at the 2012 European Society of Cardiology Congress).

The new Penumbra 3D separator (Penumbra Inc.) and 4/5 MAX aspiration device (Penumbra Inc) were designed for stroke intervention. The 3D separator secures thrombus in the third or radial dimension and has four intraluminal 3D elements to aid in lesional aspiration. It is atraumatic as it has minimal wall contact. The 4 and 5 MAX catheters can be used with the 3D separator, and they improve the aspiration flow rate by 200-300% when compared to the earlier 3 MAX catheters. They come with a new pump system with larger inner diameter reinforced tubing for efficient flow and simplified set up. Thrombus is withdrawn into the 5 MAX catheter which leverages direct aspiration of the clot, thus reducing embolization to new territory and making reaccess for additional passes unnecessary.

A

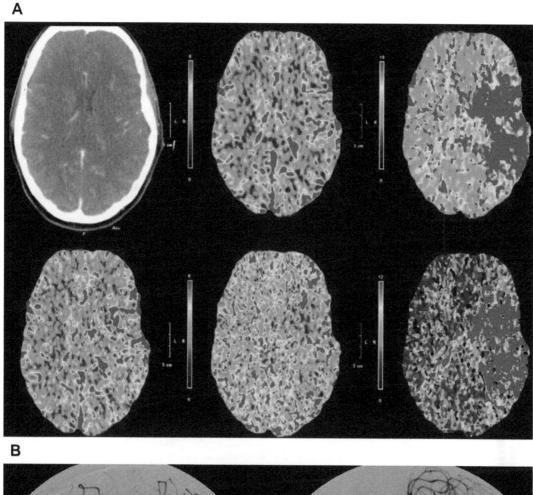

B

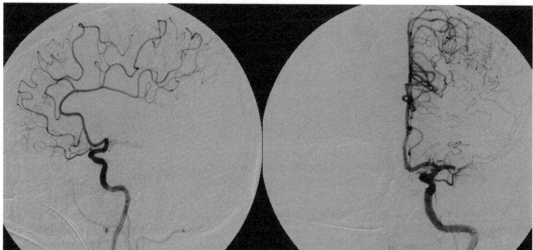

Fig. 5. Solitaire case: a 57-year-old man was found by a relative to have right hemiparesis and aphasia. He was last seen normal at 8:00 PM the previous evening (wake-up stroke). On examination, the patient had severe aphasia and right hemiparesis (NIHSS score of 14). His medical history was remarkable for hypertension, hypercholesterolemia, and diabetes. The patient was given aspirin (325 mg) at an outside hospital. CT perfusion imaging shows a large perfusion deficit in the left MCA territory (*A*). A CT angiogram showed incomplete occlusion of the left M1 (not shown). Preintervention angiographic runs show occlusion of the left M1 segment: left ICA angiogram, lateral projection (*B, left*); left ICA angiogram, AP projection (*B, right*).

C

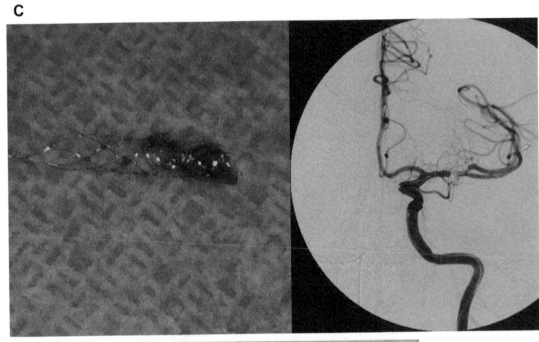

D

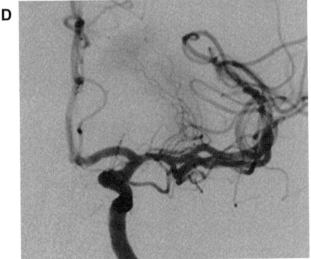

Fig. 5. The Solitaire device (ev3, Irvine, CA) was used as a temporary endovascular bypass. Clot retrieved (*C, left*). Left ICA angiogram, AP projection, shows recanalization of the left M1 segment (*C, right*). Post-Solitaire angiogram (left ICA angiogram, AP projection) shows restoration of flow (to TIMI 3) through the left MCA (*D*).

RECENT STROKE INTERVENTION TRIAL RESULTS

IMS-III

The IMS-III trialists randomized patients with acute ischemic stroke who had received IV t-PA within 3 hours after symptom onset to receive additional endovascular therapy or IV t-PA alone, in a 2:1 ratio.[95] The primary outcome measure was mRS score of 2 or less at 90 days. The study was stopped early because of futility after 656 participants had undergone randomization (434 patients to endovascular therapy and 222 to IV t-PA alone). The proportion of participants with mRS score of 2 or less at 90 days did not differ significantly according to treatment (40.8% in the endovascular therapy group and 38.7% in the IV t-PA alone group). Findings in the endovascular therapy and IV t-PA groups were similar for mortality at 90 days (19.1% and 21.6%, respectively; P = .52), and the proportion of patients with SICH within 30 hours after t-PA initiation (6.2%

and 5.9%, respectively; $P = .83$). Subgroup analysis based on NIHSS severity (NIHSS score of 8-19 and NIHSS score of >20) showed greater therapeutic benefit for endovascular therapy but did not achieve statistical significance.

The main criticism of this trial is that 20% of endovascularly treated patients did not have a large vessel occlusion. Endovascular therapy was not administered in 89 patients, as 80 had no treatable arterial occlusion, 3 lesions were not accessible, 2 had spontaneous recanalization after baseline angiogram, 2 were not target lesion responsible for the stroke, and 2 for no reasons provided. van Elteren analysis of 3-month mRS score distribution demonstrated superiority of endovascular therapy to IV-tPA alone in patients who harbored a baseline large vessel occlusion ($P = .01$). In IMS III, independent functional outcome (mRS score 0-2) was strongly associated with TICI grade 2b or 3 revascularization (current standard for endovascular intervention) ($P = .001$). A low percentage of patients in IMS III achieved this technical result due to older, inferior technologies.

MR RESCUE

The MR RESCUE trialists randomly assigned patients within 8 hours after the onset of large-vessel, anterior-circulation strokes to undergo mechanical embolectomy (Merci retriever or Penumbra system) or receive standard care (essentially IVT). All patients underwent pretreatment CT or MR imaging of the brain. Randomization was stratified according to whether the patient had a favorable penumbral pattern (substantial salvageable tissue and small infarct core) or a nonpenumbral pattern (large core or small or absent penumbra). Among all patients, mean mRS scores did not differ between embolectomy and standard care (3.9 Merci vs. 3.9 Penumbra, $P = .99$). Embolectomy was not superior to standard care in patients with either a favorable penumbral pattern (mean score, 3.9 vs. 3.4; $P = .23$) or a nonpenumbral pattern (mean score, 4.0 vs. 4.4; $P = .32$). In the primary analysis of 90-day mRS score, there was no interaction between the pretreatment imaging pattern and treatment assignment ($P = .14$). The trialists concluded that favorable penumbral pattern on neuroimaging did not identify patients who would differentially benefit from endovascular therapy for acute ischemic stroke nor was embolectomy shown to be superior to standard care.

Of importance, patients with adequate reperfusion demonstrated mean improvement in 3-month mRS score (3.2 [2.6-3.8] vs. 4.1 [3.7-4.5], $P = .04$) and reduced median absolute infarct growth (9.0 vs. 72.5 mL, $P<.001$).).[96]

IAT versus IVT in Acute Ischemic Stroke (SYNTHESIS EXPANSION)

This Italian multicenter trial randomly assigned 362 patients with acute ischemic stroke, within 4.5 hours after onset, to receive endovascular therapy (IAT with recombinant t-PA, mechanical clot disruption or retrieval, or a combination of these approaches) or IV t-PA therapy.[97] The primary outcome was mRS score of 0 or 1 at 90 days. At 3 months, 55 patients in the endovascular therapy group (30.4%) and 63 in the IV t-PA group (34.8%) achieved primary outcome measures ($P = .16$).

The main criticisms of this study are that were no preprocedural imaging studies to confirm large vessel occlusions and no lower limit NIHSS score for study inclusion. Only 165 of 180 patients randomized to IAT received an endovascular procedure, and 109 of these patients received only pharmaceutical agents or wire manipulation. Only 56 patients received advanced mechanical thrombectomy. Efficacy was not reported in terms of postprocedure TICI and time to reperfusion.

Although all these trials concluded that endovascular therapy was not superior to standard therapy, the limitations, inclusion and exclusion criteria, and subgroup analyses of their patient populations need to be taken into consideration to translate these results to those for real-world patients. The inclusion of only patient with large vessel occlusions and sufficiently high NIHSS scores with perfusion criteria (that is, those patients who are primary candidates for current endovascular stroke therapy) in future trials would increase the authenticity of these trials to evaluate the benefit of endovascular therapy, rather than randomizing patients who are chosen for IVT to endovascular therapy. Revascularization efficacy (as previously mentioned in this chapter) has been time and again proven to improve outcomes including as shown by IMS-III results and advanced technology that facilitates improved recanalization was not standardized in any of the above-mentioned trials.

Current ongoing trials that may address these issues include 1) Solitaire FR as Primary Treatment for Acute Ischemic Stroke (SWIFT PRIME) (IVT vs. IVT and the Solitaire device in patients with confirmed large vessel occlusion within 4.5 hours of stroke onset after selecting by perfusion imaging), 2) The Randomized, Concurrent Controlled Trial to Assess the Penumbra System's Safety and Effectiveness in the Treatment of Acute Stroke (The THERAPY Trial) (IVT vs. IVT and Penumbra in confirmed large vessel occlusions within 8 hours of stroke onset), and 3) Separator 3D (Penumbra aspiration vs. Penumbra separator 3D in patients with confirmed large vessel occlusion refractory to or not eligible for IVT). Although these studies use selected revascularization technologies, they include patients who are primary candidates for endovascular therapy and use advanced technology devices that have been previously shown to yield higher recanalization rates.

EXTRACRANIAL CAROTID REVASCULARIZATION

Acute strokes related to isolated proximal (extracranial) ICA occlusions typically are associated with a better prognosis than intracranial occlusions, given the compensatory collateral flow at the level of the external carotid artery–ICA anastomosis (eg, ophthalmic artery) and/or circle of Willis. However, patients with an incomplete circle of Willis or with tandem occlusions of the intracranial ICA-MCA often present with severe strokes and are potential candidates for urgent revascularization. Stent placement in the proximal cervical vessels may also be required to gain access to the intracranial thrombus with intracranial mechanical devices or catheters. Furthermore, brisk antegrade flow is essential for the maintenance of distal vascular patency, as is particularly evident in patients with severe proximal stenoses who commonly develop rethrombosis after vessel recanalization. Several case series have shown success and good outcome after endovascular treatment of acute ischemic stroke caused by proximal extracranial ICA occlusions.[98–102] In our series of 22 patients presenting with acute stroke secondary to complete cervical ICA occlusion,[103] the median age was 65 years and the mean admission NIHSS score was 14. Recanalization (TIMI 2 or 3) occurred in 17 patients (77.3%). Ten patients (45.5%) showed significant clinical improvement during hospitalization (NIHSS score improved ≥4 points). After a median follow-up of 3 months, 50% of patients had good outcomes (mRS ≤2).

FUTURE OF STROKE REVASCULARIZATION THERAPY

The establishment of endovascular stroke therapy has changed the landscape of the assessment, imaging, and selection of patients with strokes for both IV and IA revascularization. At present, there is considerable heterogeneity in the availability of imaging, expertise, and experience with respect to the novel methods for evaluating, choosing, and treating these patients. In combination with the rapid pace of advances in imaging, devices, and pharmacology of stroke therapy, this has made the assessment of these developments through randomized controlled trials and even prospective trials premature and not translatable to available technology by the time the study is completed. All these advances are complementary, and their advantages or disadvantages should be carefully analyzed before choosing the combination of methods best suited to the patient. Adjunctive methods for assessing and improving collateral supply and neuroprotective strategies before, after, and during revascularization should be evaluated in combination with revascularization outcomes. Methods to alleviate heterogeneity in the availability of resources and expertise need to be implemented. In addition, the training of personnel to meet the demand of this rapidly advancing field and the cost-effectiveness of these therapies need to be looked into carefully.

REFERENCES

1. Barber PA, Zhang J, Demchuk AM, et al. Why are stroke patients excluded from TPA therapy? An analysis of patient eligibility. Neurology 2001; 56(8):1015–20.
2. Hacke W, Kaste M, Bluhmki E, et al. Thrombolysis with alteplase 3 to 4.5 hours after acute ischemic stroke. N Engl J Med 2008;359(13):1317–29.
3. Alexandrov AV, Grotta JC. Arterial reocclusion in stroke patients treated with intravenous tissue plasminogen activator. Neurology 2002;59(6): 862–7.
4. Janjua N, Alkawi A, Suri MF, et al. Impact of arterial reocclusion and distal fragmentation during thrombolysis among patients with acute ischemic stroke. AJNR Am J Neuroradiol 2008;29(2):253–8.
5. Saqqur M, Molina CA, Salam A, et al. Clinical deterioration after intravenous recombinant tissue plasminogen activator treatment: a multicenter transcranial Doppler study. Stroke 2007;38(1):69–74.
6. Natarajan SK, Karmon Y, Snyder KV, et al. Prospective acute ischemic stroke outcomes after endovascular therapy: a real-world experience. World Neurosurg 2010;74(4–5):455–64.
7. IMS Investigators. Combined intravenous and intra-arterial recanalization for acute ischemic stroke: the Interventional Management of Stroke Study. Stroke 2004;35(4):904–11.
8. Jaillard A, Cornu C, Durieux A, et al. Hemorrhagic transformation in acute ischemic stroke. The MAST-E study. MAST-E Group. Stroke 1999;30(7): 1326–32.
9. Tanne D, Kasner SE, Demchuk AM, et al. Markers of increased risk of intracerebral hemorrhage after intravenous recombinant tissue plasminogen activator therapy for acute ischemic stroke in clinical practice: the Multicenter rt-PA Stroke Survey. Circulation 2002;105(14):1679–85.

10. Wolpert SM, Bruckmann H, Greenlee R, et al. Neuroradiologic evaluation of patients with acute stroke treated with recombinant tissue plasminogen activator. The rt-PA Acute Stroke Study Group. AJNR Am J Neuroradiol 1993;14(1): 3–13.

11. Saqqur M, Uchino K, Demchuk AM, et al. Site of arterial occlusion identified by transcranial Doppler predicts the response to intravenous thrombolysis for stroke. Stroke 2007;38(3):948–54.

12. Arnold M, Nedeltchev K, Mattle HP, et al. Intra-arterial thrombolysis in 24 consecutive patients with internal carotid artery T occlusions. J Neurol Neurosurg Psychiatry 2003;74(6):739–42.

13. Jansen O, von Kummer R, Forsting M, et al. Thrombolytic therapy in acute occlusion of the intracranial internal carotid artery bifurcation. AJNR Am J Neuroradiol 1995;16(10):1977–86.

14. Sorimachi T, Fujii Y, Tsuchiya N, et al. Recanalization by mechanical embolus disruption during intra-arterial thrombolysis in the carotid territory. AJNR Am J Neuroradiol 2004;25(8):1391–402.

15. Zaidat OO, Suarez JI, Santillan C, et al. Response to intra-arterial and combined intravenous and intra-arterial thrombolytic therapy in patients with distal internal carotid artery occlusion. Stroke 2002;33(7):1821–6.

16. Barreto AD, Albright KC, Hallevi H, et al. Thrombus burden is associated with clinical outcome after intra-arterial therapy for acute ischemic stroke. Stroke 2008;39(12):3231–5.

17. Gralla J, Burkhardt M, Schroth G, et al. Occlusion length is a crucial determinant of efficiency and complication rate in thrombectomy for acute ischemic stroke. AJNR Am J Neuroradiol 2008; 29(2):247–52.

18. Kim YS, Garami Z, Mikulik R, et al. Early recanalization rates and clinical outcomes in patients with tandem internal carotid artery/middle cerebral artery occlusion and isolated middle cerebral artery occlusion. Stroke 2005;36(4):869–71.

19. Mattle HP, Arnold M, Georgiadis D, et al. Comparison of intraarterial and intravenous thrombolysis for ischemic stroke with hyperdense middle cerebral artery sign. Stroke 2008;39(2):379–83.

20. Puetz V, Dzialowski I, Hill MD, et al. Intracranial thrombus extent predicts clinical outcome, final infarct size and hemorrhagic transformation in ischemic stroke: the clot burden score. Int J Stroke 2008;3(4):230–6.

21. Somford DM, Nederkoorn PJ, Rutgers DR, et al. Proximal and distal hyperattenuating middle cerebral artery signs at CT: different prognostic implications. Radiology 2002;223(3):667–71.

22. Fischer U, Arnold M, Nedeltchev K, et al. NIHSS score and arteriographic findings in acute ischemic stroke. Stroke 2005;36(10):2121–5.

23. Maas MB, Furie KL, Lev MH, et al. National Institutes of Health Stroke Scale score is poorly predictive of proximal occlusion in acute cerebral ischemia. Stroke 2009;40(9):2988–93.

24. Gobin YP, Starkman S, Duckwiler GR, et al. MERCI 1: a phase 1 study of mechanical embolus removal in cerebral ischemia. Stroke 2004;35(12):2848–54.

25. Smith WS, Sung G, Starkman S, et al. Safety and efficacy of mechanical embolectomy in acute ischemic stroke: results of the MERCI trial. Stroke 2005;36(7):1432–8.

26. Smith WS, Sung G, Saver J, et al. Mechanical thrombectomy for acute ischemic stroke: final results of the Multi MERCI trial. Stroke 2008;39(4):1205–12.

27. Tomsick T, Broderick J, Carrozella J, et al. Revascularization results in the Interventional Management of Stroke II trial. AJNR Am J Neuroradiol 2008;29(3):582–7.

28. Rha JH, Saver JL. The impact of recanalization on ischemic stroke outcome: a meta-analysis. Stroke 2007;38(3):967–73.

29. Lansberg MG, Bluhmki E, Thijs VN. Efficacy and safety of tissue plasminogen activator 3- to 4.5-hours after acute ischemic stroke. A metaanalysis. Stroke 2009;40:2438–41.

30. Wardlaw JM, Sandercock PA, Berge E. Thrombolytic therapy with recombinant tissue plasminogen activator for acute ischemic stroke: where do we go from here? A cumulative meta-analysis. Stroke 2003;34(6):1437–42.

31. del Zoppo GJ, Higashida RT, Furlan AJ, et al. PROACT: a phase II randomized trial of recombinant pro-urokinase by direct arterial delivery in acute middle cerebral artery stroke. PROACT Investigators. Prolyse in Acute Cerebral Thromboembolism. Stroke 1998;29(1):4–11.

32. Furlan A, Higashida R, Wechsler L, et al. Intra-arterial prourokinase for acute ischemic stroke. The PROACT II study: a randomized controlled trial. Prolyse in Acute Cerebral Thromboembolism. JAMA 1999;282(21):2003–11.

33. Bose A, Henkes H, Alfke K, et al. The Penumbra System: a mechanical device for the treatment of acute stroke due to thromboembolism. AJNR Am J Neuroradiol 2008;29(7):1409–13.

34. Hacke W, Albers G, Al-Rawi Y, et al. The Desmoteplase in Acute Ischemic Stroke Trial (DIAS): a phase II MRI-based 9-hour window acute stroke thrombolysis trial with intravenous desmoteplase. Stroke 2005;36(1):66–73.

35. Furlan AJ, Eyding D, Albers GW, et al. Dose Escalation of Desmoteplase for Acute Ischemic Stroke (DEDAS): evidence of safety and efficacy 3 to 9 hours after stroke onset. Stroke 2006;37(5): 1227–31.

36. Thomalla G, Schwark C, Sobesky J, et al. Outcome and symptomatic bleeding complications of

intravenous thrombolysis within 6 hours in MRI-selected stroke patients: comparison of a German multicenter study with the pooled data of ATLANTIS, ECASS, and NINDS tPA trials. Stroke 2006;37(3):852–8.

37. Kohrmann M, Juttler E, Fiebach JB, et al. MRI versus CT-based thrombolysis treatment within and beyond the 3 h time window after stroke onset: a cohort study. Lancet Neurol 2006;5(8):661–7.

38. Davis SM, Donnan GA, Parsons MW, et al. Effects of alteplase beyond 3 h after stroke in the Echoplanar Imaging Thrombolytic Evaluation Trial (EPITHET): a placebo-controlled randomised trial. Lancet Neurol 2008;7(4):299–309.

39. Hacke W, Furlan AJ, Al-Rawi Y, et al. Intravenous desmoteplase in patients with acute ischaemic stroke selected by MRI perfusion-diffusion weighted imaging or perfusion CT (DIAS-2): a prospective, randomised, double-blind, placebo-controlled study. Lancet Neurol 2009;8(2):141–50.

40. Jovin TG, Liebeskind DS, Gupta R, et al. Imaging-based endovascular therapy for acute ischemic stroke due to proximal intracranial anterior circulation occlusion treated beyond 8 hours from time last seen well: retrospective multicenter analysis of 237 consecutive patients. Stroke 2011;42(8):2206–11.

41. Bozzao L, Fantozzi LM, Bastianello S, et al. Early collateral blood supply and late parenchymal brain damage in patients with middle cerebral artery occlusion. Stroke 1989;20(6):735–40.

42. Hendrikse J, Hartkamp MJ, Hillen B, et al. Collateral ability of the circle of Willis in patients with unilateral internal carotid artery occlusion: border zone infarcts and clinical symptoms. Stroke 2001; 32(12):2768–73.

43. Liebeskind DS. Collateral circulation. Stroke 2003; 34(9):2279–84.

44. Shuaib A, Butcher K, Mohammad AA, et al. Collateral blood vessels in acute ischaemic stroke: a potential therapeutic target. Lancet Neurol 2011; 10(10):909–21.

45. Liebeskind DS, Kim D, Starkman S, et al. Collateral failure? Late mechanical thrombectomy after failed intravenous thrombolysis. J Neuroimaging 2010; 20(1):78–82.

46. The National Institute of Neurological Disorders and Stroke rt-PA Stroke Study Group. Tissue plasminogen activator for acute ischemic stroke. N Engl J Med 1995;333(24):1581–7.

47. Barber PA, Demchuk AM, Zhang J, et al. Validity and reliability of a quantitative computed tomography score in predicting outcome of hyperacute stroke before thrombolytic therapy. ASPECTS Study Group. Alberta Stroke Programme Early CT Score. Lancet 2000;355(9216):1670–4.

48. Parsons MW, Pepper EM, Chan V, et al. Perfusion computed tomography: prediction of final infarct extent and stroke outcome. Ann Neurol 2005; 58(5):672–9.

49. Albers GW, Thijs VN, Wechsler L, et al. Magnetic resonance imaging profiles predict clinical response to early reperfusion: the Diffusion and Perfusion Imaging Evaluation for Understanding Stroke Evolution (DEFUSE) study. Ann Neurol 2006;60(5):508–17.

50. Loh Y, Towfighi A, Liebeskind DS, et al. Basal ganglionic infarction before mechanical thrombectomy predicts poor outcome. Stroke 2009;40(10): 3315–20.

51. Lui YW, Tang ER, Allmendinger AM, et al. Evaluation of CT perfusion in the setting of cerebral ischemia: patterns and pitfalls. AJNR Am J Neuroradiol 2010;31(9):1552–63.

52. Abou-Chebl A. Endovascular treatment of acute ischemic stroke may be safely performed with no time window limit in appropriately selected patients. Stroke 2010;41(9):1996–2000.

53. Natarajan SK, Snyder KV, Siddiqui AH, et al. Safety and effectiveness of endovascular therapy after 8 hours of acute ischemic stroke onset and wake-up strokes. Stroke 2009;40(10):3269–74.

54. Hellier KD, Hampton JL, Guadagno JV, et al. Perfusion CT helps decision making for thrombolysis when there is no clear time of onset. J Neurol Neurosurg Psychiatry 2006;77(3):417–9.

55. Wintermark M, Fischbein NJ, Smith WS, et al. Accuracy of dynamic perfusion CT with deconvolution in detecting acute hemispheric stroke. AJNR Am J Neuroradiol 2005;26(1):104–12.

56. Eastwood JD, Lev MH, Azhari T, et al. CT perfusion scanning with deconvolution analysis: pilot study in patients with acute middle cerebral artery stroke. Radiology 2002;222(1):227–36.

57. Miles KA, Griffiths MR. Perfusion CT: a worthwhile enhancement? Br J Radiol 2003;76(904):220–31.

58. Wintermark M, Albers GW, Alexandrov AV, et al. Acute stroke imaging research roadmap. Stroke 2008;39(5):1621–8.

59. Wintermark M, Flanders AE, Velthuis B, et al. Perfusion-CT assessment of infarct core and penumbra: receiver operating characteristic curve analysis in 130 patients suspected of acute hemispheric stroke. Stroke 2006;37(4):979–85.

60. Murphy BD, Fox AJ, Lee DH, et al. Identification of penumbra and infarct in acute ischemic stroke using computed tomography perfusion-derived blood flow and blood volume measurements. Stroke 2006;37(7):1771–7.

61. Sanelli PC, Lev MH, Eastwood JD, et al. The effect of varying user-selected input parameters on quantitative values in CT perfusion maps. Acad Radiol 2004;11(10):1085–92.

62. Meyers PM, Schumacher HC, Higashida RT, et al. Indications for the performance of intracranial endovascular neurointerventional procedures: a

scientific statement from the American Heart Association Council on Cardiovascular Radiology and Intervention, Stroke Council, Council on Cardiovascular Surgery and Anesthesia, Interdisciplinary Council on Peripheral Vascular Disease, and Interdisciplinary Council on Quality of Care and Outcomes Research. Circulation 2009;119(16): 2235–49.

63. Inoue T, Kimura K, Minematsu K, et al. A case-control analysis of intra-arterial urokinase thrombolysis in acute cardioembolic stroke. Cerebrovasc Dis 2005;19(4):225–8.

64. Ogawa A, Mori E, Minematsu K, et al. Randomized trial of intraarterial infusion of urokinase within 6 hours of middle cerebral artery stroke: the Middle Cerebral Artery Embolism Local Fibrinolytic Intervention Trial (MELT) Japan. Stroke 2007;38(10): 2633–9.

65. Urbach H, Hartmann A, Pohl C, et al. Local intra-arterial thrombolysis in the carotid territory: does recanalization depend on the thromboembolus type? Neuroradiology 2002;44(8):695–9.

66. IMS Investigators. The Interventional Management of Stroke (IMS) II Study. Stroke 2007;38(7):2127–35.

67. Khatri P, Hill MD, Palesch YY, et al. Methodology of the Interventional Management of Stroke III Trial. Int J Stroke 2008;3(2):130–7.

68. Barnwell SL, Clark WM, Nguyen TT, et al. Safety and efficacy of delayed intraarterial urokinase therapy with mechanical clot disruption for thromboembolic stroke. AJNR Am J Neuroradiol 1994;15(10): 1817–22.

69. Gralla J, Schroth G, Remonda L, et al. A dedicated animal model for mechanical thrombectomy in acute stroke. AJNR Am J Neuroradiol 2006;27(6): 1357–61.

70. Gralla J, Schroth G, Remonda L, et al. Mechanical thrombectomy for acute ischemic stroke: thrombus-device interaction, efficiency, and complications in vivo. Stroke 2006;37(12):3019–24.

71. Flint AC, Duckwiler GR, Budzik RF, et al. Mechanical thrombectomy of intracranial internal carotid occlusion: pooled results of the MERCI and Multi MERCI Part I trials. Stroke 2007; 38(4):1274–80.

72. Penumbra Pivotal Stroke Trial Investigators. The penumbra pivotal stroke trial: safety and effectiveness of a new generation of mechanical devices for clot removal in intracranial large vessel occlusive disease. Stroke 2009;40(8):2761–8.

73. Tarr R, Hsu D, Kulcsar Z, et al. The POST trial: initial post-market experience of the Penumbra system: revascularization of large vessel occlusion in acute ischemic stroke in the United States and Europe. J Neurointerv Surg 2010;2(4):341–4.

74. Brekenfeld C, Schroth G, Mattle HP, et al. Stent placement in acute cerebral artery occlusion: use of a self-expandable intracranial stent for acute stroke treatment. Stroke 2009;40(3):847–52.

75. Levy EI, Mehta R, Gupta R, et al. Self-expanding stents for recanalization of acute cerebrovascular occlusions. AJNR Am J Neuroradiol 2007;28(5): 816–22.

76. Zaidat OO, Wolfe T, Hussain SI, et al. Interventional acute ischemic stroke therapy with intracranial self-expanding stent. Stroke 2008;39(8):2392–5.

77. Mocco J, Hanel RA, Sharma J, et al. Use of a vascular reconstruction device to salvage acute ischemic occlusions refractory to traditional endovascular recanalization methods. J Neurosurg 2010;112(3):557–62.

78. Levy EI, Siddiqui AH, Crumlish A, et al. First Food and Drug Administration-approved prospective trial of primary intracranial stenting for acute stroke: SARIS (Stent-Assisted Recanalization in Acute Ischemic Stroke). Stroke 2009;40(11):3552–6.

79. Levy EI, Rahman M, Khalessi AA, et al. Midterm clinical and angiographic follow-up for the first Food and Drug Administration-approved prospective, single-arm trial of primary stenting for stroke: SARIS (Stent-Assisted Recanalization for Acute Ischemic Stroke). Neurosurgery 2011; 69(4):915–20.

80. Bose A, Hartmann M, Henkes H, et al. A novel, self-expanding, nitinol stent in medically refractory intracranial atherosclerotic stenoses: the Wingspan study. Stroke 2007;38(5):1531–7.

81. Chiam PT, Samuelson RM, Mocco J, et al. Navigability trumps all: stenting of acute middle cerebral artery occlusions with a new self-expandable stent. AJNR Am J Neuroradiol 2008;29(10):1956–8.

82. Fiorella D, Levy EI, Turk AS, et al. US multicenter experience with the Wingspan stent system for the treatment of intracranial atheromatous disease: periprocedural results. Stroke 2007;38(3):881–7.

83. Hahnel S, Ringleb P, Hartmann M. Treatment of intracranial stenoses using the Neuroform stent system: initial experience in five cases. Neuroradiology 2006;48(7):479–85.

84. Kurre W, Berkefeld J, Sitzer M, et al. Treatment of symptomatic high-grade intracranial stenoses with the balloon-expandable Pharos stent: initial experience. Neuroradiology 2008;50(8):701–8.

85. Sauvageau E, Levy EI. Self-expanding stent-assisted middle cerebral artery recanalization: technical note. Neuroradiology 2006;48(6):405–8.

86. Kelly ME, Furlan AJ, Fiorella D. Recanalization of an acute middle cerebral artery occlusion using a self-expanding, reconstrainable, intracranial microstent as a temporary endovascular bypass. Stroke 2008; 39(6):1770–3.

87. Hauck EF, Mocco J, Snyder KV, et al. Temporary endovascular bypass: a novel treatment for acute stroke. AJNR Am J Neuroradiol 2009;30:1532–3.

88. Yavuz K, Geyik S, Pamuk AG, et al. Immediate and midterm follow-up results of using an electrode-tachable, fully retrievable SOLO stent system in the endovascular coil occlusion of wide-necked cerebral aneurysms. J Neurosurg 2007;107(1):49–55.

89. Natarajan SK, Siddiqui AH, Hopkins LN, et al. Retrievable, detachable stent-platform-based clot-retrieval device (Solitaire™ FR) for acute stroke revascularization: first demonstration of feasibility in a canine stroke model. Vascular Disease Management 2010;7:E120–5.

90. Cohen JE, Gomori JM, Leker RR, et al. Preliminary experience with the use of self-expanding stent as a thrombectomy device in ischemic stroke. Neurol Res 2011;33(4):439–43.

91. Miteff F, Faulder KC, Goh AC, et al. Mechanical thrombectomy with a self-expanding retrievable intracranial stent (Solitaire AB): experience in 26 patients with acute cerebral artery occlusion. AJNR Am J Neuroradiol 2011;32:1078–81.

92. Saver JL, Jahan R, Levy EI, et al. Solitaire flow restoration device versus the Merci Retriever in patients with acute ischaemic stroke (SWIFT): a randomised, parallel-group, non-inferiority trial. Lancet 2012;380:1241–9.

93. Nogueira RG, Levy EI, Gounis M, et al. The Trevo device: preclinical data of a novel stroke thrombectomy device in two different animal models of arterial thrombo-occlusive disease. J Neurointerv Surg 2012;4(4):295–300.

94. Nogueira RG, Lutsep HL, Gupta R, et al. Trevo versus Merci retrievers for thrombectomy revascularisation of large vessel occlusions in acute ischaemic stroke (TREVO 2): a randomised trial. Lancet 2012;380:1231–40.

95. Broderick JP, Palesch YY, Demchuk AM, et al. Endovascular therapy after intravenous t-PA versus t-PA alone for stroke. N Engl J Med 2013;368:893–903.

96. Kidwell CS, Jahan R, Gornbein J, et al. A trial of imaging selection and endovascular treatment for ischemic stroke. N Engl J Med 2013;368:914–23.

97. Ciccone A, Valvassori L, Nichelatti M, et al. Endovascular treatment for acute ischemic stroke. N Engl J Med 2013;368:904–13.

98. Dabitz R, Triebe S, Leppmeier U, et al. Percutaneous recanalization of acute internal carotid artery occlusions in patients with severe stroke. Cardiovasc Intervent Radiol 2007;30(1):34–41.

99. Jovin TG, Gupta R, Uchino K, et al. Emergent stenting of extracranial internal carotid artery occlusion in acute stroke has a high revascularization rate. Stroke 2005;36(11):2426–30.

100. Lavallee PC, Mazighi M, Saint-Maurice JP, et al. Stent-assisted endovascular thrombolysis versus intravenous thrombolysis in internal carotid artery dissection with tandem internal carotid and middle cerebral artery occlusion. Stroke 2007;38(8):2270–4.

101. Miyamoto N, Naito I, Takatama S, et al. Urgent stenting for patients with acute stroke due to atherosclerotic occlusive lesions of the cervical internal carotid artery. Neurol Med Chir (Tokyo) 2008;48(2):49–56.

102. Nikas D, Reimers B, Elisabetta M, et al. Percutaneous interventions in patients with acute ischemic stroke related to obstructive atherosclerotic disease or dissection of the extracranial carotid artery. J Endovasc Ther 2007;14(3):279–88.

103. Hauck EF, Natarajan SK, Ohta H, et al. Emergent endovascular recanalization for cervical internal carotid artery occlusion in patients presenting with acute stroke. Neurosurgery 2011;69(4):899–907.

Intracranial Endovascular Balloon Test Occlusion
Indications, Methods, and Predictive Value

Augusto E. Elias, DDS, MD[a],
Neeraj Chaudhary, MD, MRCS, FRCR[b], Aditya S. Pandey, MD[b],
Joseph J. Gemmete, MD, FSIR[c],*

KEYWORDS

- Balloon test occlusion • Carotid artery occlusion • Cerebral ischemia • Hemodynamics • Outcome
- Permanent vessel occlusion

KEY POINTS

- Parent vessel occlusion (PVO) may be required in wide-neck giant aneurysms, pseudoaneurysms, traumatic vascular injuries, carotid blowout, and carotid fistulas.
- Clinical tolerance of PVO can be assessed by a balloon test occlusion (BTO) with several variables, including the clinical examination, angiographic assessment, stump pressure, induced hypotension, perfusion scanning, transcranial Doppler ultrasonography, and neurophysiologic monitoring.
- A good rule of thumb is to place the balloon at or near the level of the proposed occlusion.
- Two of the most useful variables during a BTO to determine whether a patient will tolerate a PVO are the clinical examination and venous phase assessment on the angiogram.
- Primary collaterals are those related to the circle of Willis (anterior communicating artery and posterior communicating artery), whereas secondary collaterals consist of retrograde flow within the ophthalmic artery, external carotid artery branches, and leptomeningeal collaterals.

INTRODUCTION

The evolution of endovascular technology has allowed for the treatment of complex vascular pathologies. Advances in stent and coil technology are at the heart of this treatment; however, parent vessel occlusion (PVO) remains a viable option in treating certain vascular diseases. Endovascular PVO with detachable balloons dates back to the early 1970s and was first reported by Serbinenko.[1,2]

Wide-neck giant aneurysms, pseudoaneurysms, traumatic vascular injuries, carotid blowout, and carotid fistulas are examples of conditions that may require PVO. A patient harboring a head

and neck cancer may also require PVO as preoperative preparation before tumor resection. Carotid artery occlusion is a simple procedure, but avoiding immediate or delayed hemodynamic cerebral ischemia remains a challenge.

The main complications associated with PVO are thromboembolic or related to immediate or delayed hemodynamic ischemia. Linskey and colleagues[3] reported 254 patients who underwent PVO without a balloon test occlusion (BTO). The ischemic complication rates were high, with 26% of patients suffering a cerebral infarct and 12% of the patients experiencing mortality related to the infarct. Thromboembolic complications are

[a] Division of Interventional Neuroradiology, Department of Radiology, University of Michigan Health System, 1500 East Medical Center Drive, Ann Arbor, MI 48109-5030, USA; [b] Division of Interventional Neuroradiology, Departments of Neurosurgery and Radiology, University of Michigan Health System, 1500 East Medical Center Drive, Ann Arbor, MI 48109-5030, USA; [c] Division of Interventional Neuroradiology and Cranial Base Surgery, Departments of Neurosurgery, Radiology and Otolaryngology, University of Michigan Health System, 1500 East Medical Center Drive, Ann Arbor, MI 48109, USA
* Corresponding author.
E-mail address: gemmete@med.umich.edu

Neuroimag Clin N Am 23 (2013) 695–702
http://dx.doi.org/10.1016/j.nic.2013.03.015
1052-5149/13/$ – see front matter © 2013 Elsevier Inc. All rights reserved.

treated with anticoagulation; however, immediate or delayed hemodynamic ischemia is best treated by determination of which patients will develop this state before PVO. BTO is one method by which an interventionalist can evaluate whether a patient is able to tolerate a PVO. Those patients who fail the BTO require a revascularization procedure before PVO. This review discusses the indications, methods, predictive value, and complications of BTO.

TECHNIQUE FOR BTO

Several techniques have been described for performing a BTO. The underlying principle is to evaluate the efficacy of the intracranial collateral circulation in maintaining perfusion of the affected vascular territory during temporary occlusion of the main arterial supply. Clinical tolerance of PVO can be assessed by a BTO with several variables including: the clinical examination, angiographic assessment, stump pressure, induced hypotension, perfusion scanning, transcranial Doppler (TCD) ultrasonography, and neurophysiologic monitoring. Most centers use several of these variables in assessing the clinical safety of PVO.

STANDARD TECHNIQUE

Informed consent is obtained from the patient. In cases in which clinical examination is to be assessed, the patient is awake and the procedure is performed under local anesthetic. Benzodiazepines should not be used because they can interfere with memory functions and related tasks. The patient is told that they will be asked questions evaluating their memory, speech, motor, sensory, and analytical skills (calculations) while the procedure is being performed.

A 6-French femoral sheath is introduced into the femoral artery using a single wall puncture technique. Although either femoral artery can be used for access, we prefer to puncture the femoral artery opposite to the side of disease. This precaution ensures that any complication associated with the BTO, PVO, or femoral sheath placement affects only 1 extremity. A baseline activated clotting time (ACT) is drawn, and the patient is given 70 to 100 units per kilogram (U/kg) of heparin. An ACT is drawn 10 minutes after administration of heparin and then every 15 minutes as needed. The goal ACT is approximately 2.5 times the patients' baseline to prevent procedure-related thromboembolic complications.

A 4-French diagnostic catheter is used to perform a 4-vessel cervical and cerebral angiogram in the anteroposterior and lateral projections.

Next, a 6-French guide catheter is introduced into the common carotid artery (CCA). A nondetachable balloon catheter is then introduced and positioned in the distal cervical segment of the internal carotid artery (ICA). A good rule of thumb is to place the balloon at or near the level of the proposed occlusion. Low position of the balloon can cause a carotid sinus reflex, leading to significant bradycardia. This is the main reason BTO is not performed from the CCA, because this leads to a decreased pressure within the carotid sinus, which reflexively causes an increase in arterial blood pressure (ABP). Such a reflex can give a confounding clinical result because the ABP could be lower in a normal state. Although we have not experienced significant alteration in ABP or heart rate during a BTO, we are always prepared with temporary pacer wires as well as atropine in case the situation were to arise.

The balloon is inflated with angiographic confirmation of complete occlusion of the vessel in question. The balloon is inflated for a total duration of 30 minutes and a neurologic examination is performed by the operator every 5 minutes (**Fig. 1**). If there are any changes in the patient's neurologic examination, then the balloon is immediately deflated and cerebral angiography is performed. If the patient is under general anesthesia for the procedure, 12-lead electroencephalogram (EEG) monitoring maybe helpful. Some investigators puncture the contralateral femoral artery and perform a cerebral angiogram of the contralateral ICA and 1 vertebral artery to evaluate the collateral circulation with the balloon inflated.

The technique for vertebral artery occlusion is similar to that described for the ICA. For tumor disease and posttraumatic lesions of the vertebral artery, BTO is performed proximal to the level of the lesion. For vertebral arteriovenous fistulae, BTO is performed over the site of the fistula or just proximal to it (**Fig. 2**). In the case of an aneurysm, the level of occlusion depends on the location of the aneurysm and whether the therapeutic goal is to reduce flow in the aneurysm or occlude the parent vessel.

At the end of the procedure, the balloon is deflated and an angiogram is performed to ensure normal patency of the vessel and its distal territory. The catheter and sheath are removed. Hemostasis at the puncture is obtained by manual compression. If there is no change in the patient's neurologic examination during the 30 minutes of BTO, then the vessel in question can be occluded. Before discharge, the patient is observed for 4 hours, with a neurologic examination performed every 15 minutes in the recovery unit.

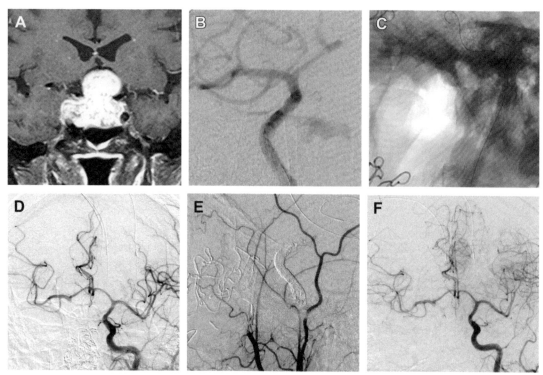

Fig. 1. 77-year-old man with a large pituitary macroadenoma who suffered an injury of the right internal carotid artery during endoscopic resection of the tumor. (*A*) Coronal fat-saturated contrast-enhanced T1-weighted MRI show a large enhancing mass centered in the pituitary fossa. (*B*) Frontal right internal carotid angiogram shows contrast extravasation from the cavernous segment of the right internal carotid artery. (*C*) Lateral spot fluoroscopic image shows balloon position for BTO. (*D*) Frontal left internal carotid angiogram with balloon inflated in the right internal carotid artery shows flow through the ACOM filling the right anterior circulation. (*E*) Lateral right common carotid angiogram after PVO of the right internal carotid artery shows no intracranial filling of the right internal carotid artery. (*F*) Repeat left internal carotid angiogram after PVO of the right internal carotid artery again shows excellent filling of the right anterior circulation through the ACOM.

MODIFICATIONS TO BASIC TECHNIQUE
Venous Phase Assessment: Predictive Value of PVO Tolerance

Venous phase comparison of the 2 hemispheres can be useful in evaluation of the patient's collateral circulation before PVO. This comparison is based on the assumption that patients who have symmetry within the venous phase during a BTO harbor enough intracranial collateral circulation to tolerate a PVO procedure. This comparison can be accomplished by performing angiography through the vertebral and contralateral ICA while the balloon is inflated. Van Rooij and colleagues performed angiographic assessment as well as clinical evaluation during BTO procedures. The angiographic assessment compared the venous phase between hemispheres of the supratentorial and infratentorial structures, depending on whether the collateral flow was from the anterior communicating artery or the posterior communicating artery. A delay of more than 0.5 seconds

was considered a high ischemic risk for PVO. Of the 49 surviving patients in this series who passed the angiographic evaluation and had undergone PVO, 1 patient developed a delayed ischemic event, thus giving this evaluation a positive predictive value of 98%.

Abud and colleagues[4] tested this hypothesis on 60 patients who underwent a PVO procedure. All of these patients were tested with angiographic venous state evaluation during the BTO procedure. Clinical evaluation was not performed, because the procedure was performed under general anesthesia. Carotid sacrifice was found to be possible when the delay was not greater than 2 seconds. Fifty-seven of the 60 patients had a delay of less than 2 seconds and none of these patients suffered an ischemic complication after PVO. Of the 3 patients who had a delay of 3 seconds, 1 suffered an ischemic complication.[4] The predictive value of this technique is powerful; however, the procedure requires puncture of both femoral arteries

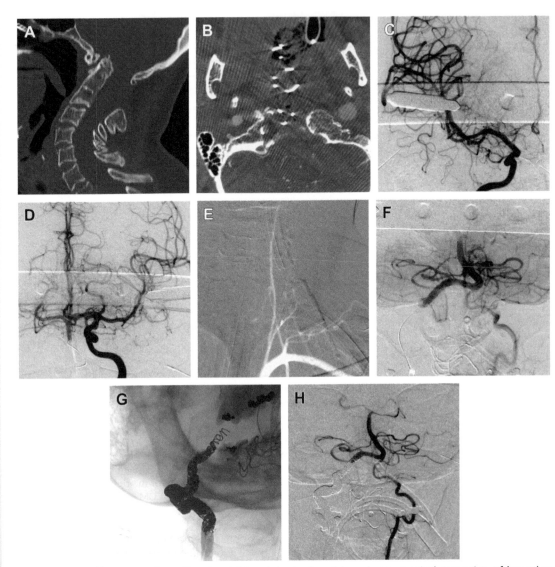

Fig. 2. 37-year-old woman who suffered a right vertebral artery injury during surgical correction of her atlantoaxial instability. (A) Sagittal CT cervical spine shows atlantoaxial instability. (B) Axial DynaCT shows injury to the V3 segment of the right vertebral artery. (C) Frontal right internal carotid angiogram shows no posterior communicating artery. (D) Frontal left internal carotid angiogram shows a large left posterior communicating artery filling the top of the basilar artery. (E) Frontal left subclavian angiogram shows a patent left vertebral artery within the neck. (F) Frontal left vertebral angiogram centered over the head with a balloon in the V3 segment of the right vertebral shows filling of the left vertebral artery, both V4 segments right and left PICA, along with the basilar artery. There is washout at the top of the basilar from the left posterior communicating artery. (G) Frontal spot fluoroscopic images shows coils and Onyx (eV3, Irvine, CA) within the right vertebral artery to the right V3/V4 junction. (H) Left vertebral angiogram after occlusion of the right vertebral artery shows adequate filling of the posterior circulation.

and additional catheterization of the cervical vasculature. Both of these series did not report a periprocedural complication; however, this method is more invasive, requiring further intravascular manipulation and theoretically increasing the probability of vessel dissection or thromboembolism.

Measurement of Stump Pressures

Arterial pressure can be measured with a double-lumen balloon catheter. The second lumen is connection to a pressure transducer to measure the pressure within the artery above the level of the balloon. Morishima and colleagues[5] reported that maintenance of a stump pressure ratio (initial mean stump pressure/preocclusion mean arterial pressure) of 60% or more during BTO is a useful marker of an adequate intracranial collateral circulation. The usefulness of this technique is controversial, because although several studies have found a significant correlation between stump pressures and measures of cerebral perfusion, such as single-photon emission computed tomography (SPECT),[6] others have not found such a correlation.[7]

Induced Hypotension

Inducing hypotension during a BTO can provide further information about whether the patient's intracranial collateral circulation will provide adequate blood flow after PVO. Twenty minutes after the start of the BTO, the mean arterial pressure is decreased 30% lower than baseline. This decrease is maintained for an additional 15 to 20 minutes with a repeat neurologic examination. Dare and colleagues[8] studied 13 patients who underwent BTO with a hypotensive challenge. Using this technique, Standard and colleagues[9] identified an additional 19% of patients with limited intracranial collateral circulation. The false-negative rate was 5%. However, Dare and colleagues[8] reported a false-negative rate of 15%. They suggested that the direct vasodilator effect of nitroprusside on the cerebral circulation could increase the false-negative rate of the test. Overall, the literature does not show that a hypotensive challenge is superior to a traditional BTO.

BTO and Perfusion Assessment

SPECT

Technetium 99m hexamethylpropylene-amine oxime (HMPAO) is a radiotracer injected after 2 minutes of asymptomatic BTO. A SPECT study is performed 1 to 6 hours later. The sensitivity of this type of imaging is high and the specificity is poor. In 1 study, all patients with focal defects on SPECT immediately after BTO returned to normal on a repeat SPECT examination at 24 hours.[10] There are also reports of use of ^{15}O, H_2O positron emission tomography (PET) for quantitative measurements of cerebral blood flow (CBF) during BTO.[11] This test is performed during BTO and then after deflation of the balloon.

Computed tomography perfusion with acetazolamide challenge

Computed tomography (CT) perfusion before and after the injection of acetazolamide has been reported in the literature as a useful adjunct to a BTO in determining which patients tolerate a PVO. A CT perfusion examination is performed as a baseline before the BTO. The patient is administered acetazolamide, and a BTO is performed, followed by a repeat CT perfusion scan.[12] Acetazolamide penetrates the blood-brain barrier slowly by means of diffusion and inhibits carbonic anhydrase, thus causing acidosis. This increase in acidity leads to compensatory dilation of small arterioles. It is believed that the increase in CBF induced by acetazolamide is reduced if compensatory vasodilation associated with a decrease in CBF from BTO has already occurred.[13] However, at institutions in which there is no CT scanner within the angiography suite, this procedure involves the transfer of the patient to the CT scanner with a balloon within the ICA, which may increase the risk of carotid artery injury.

Xenon CT perfusion

Xenon CT perfusion is another modality to quantify CBF in patients who have clinically tolerated a BTO.[3,14,15] The patient inhales a gas mixture of 33% xenon and 67% oxygen. A baseline image is obtained. The balloon is inflated for 30 minutes, if tolerated by the patient. Repeat imaging is performed. Xenon uptake in the middle cerebral artery territory is used to estimate regional CBF with the threshold to predict delayed ischemic stroke set at less than 30 mL/100 g/min.

MR perfusion

MR perfusion imaging with dynamic gadolinium enhancement can be performed during BTO when magnetic resonance (MR) is available in the angiography suite. A bolus injection of gadolinium is administered at a dose of 0.1 mmol/kg and various parameters such as cerebral blood volume, mean transit time, and regional CBF (rCBF) can be calculated. Reports in the literature have shown perfusion delays, asymmetry in contrast enhancement, and parenchymal signal intensity in the areas of hypoperfusion in patients who have clinically failed a BTO.[16,17]

TCD ultrasonography

The use of TCD ultrasonography to evaluate flow in the middle cerebral artery is well documented in the literature. This technique can be used as an adjunct in the evaluation of collateral flow in a BTO. TCD has the advantage of being noninvasive; however, the correlation between CBF and mean velocity in the middle cerebral artery is not linear because mean velocity can be affected by vessel caliber, hematocrit, and viscosity.[14] Eckert and colleagues[18] reported that a reduction in mean blood flow velocity and pulsatility index of less than 30% is a good predictor of clinical tolerance to occlusion, whereas a reduction of more than 50% indicates failure of the BTO.

Neurophysiologic monitoring

The use of neurophysiologic monitoring (NPM) electroencephalography (EEG), somatosensory-evoked potentials (SSEPs), and brain stem-evoked potentials is well documented as an important adjunct in performing endovascular procedures. NPM is certainly of value when clinical assessment cannot be performed, as in a patient under general anesthesia. An rCBF of less than 15 mL/100 g/min appears to be the critical value in which cortical SSEP amplitude is reduced, central conduction time is prolonged, and cerebral infarction is likely to occur. Liu and colleagues[19] claim that although this technique has limitations, in their series of 35 patients, 5 patients had their treatment decisions altered because of NPM. Hence, they believe that NPM is a useful adjunct to clinical neurologic testing during BTO.

DISCUSSION

Despite technological advances in neurointerventional surgery, PVO remains an important option in the treatment of certain vascular diseases. Sudden ligation of the ICA is not ideal because it leads to a significant risk of ischemic stroke. Linskey and colleagues[3] reported a 26% risk of ischemia with abrupt ICA occlusion compared with a 13% risk when BTO was used before permanent occlusion. Many techniques, including venous phase evaluation, stump pressure, hypotensive challenge, perfusion measurements, TCD, and NPM, have been evaluated as adjuncts to a clinical BTO evaluation. These techniques were developed to enhance the predictive value of a successful BTO and subsequent PVO.[8,11,16,20–22]

Complications in patients undergoing PVO are either thromboembolic or a result of an immediate or delayed hemodynamic infarction. Although anticoagulation can decrease the incidence of thromboembolic complications, immediate or delayed hemodynamic infarction is best treated with a cerebral bypass procedure. The goal of BTO procedures is to identify those individuals who would benefit from cerebral bypass before PVO and thereby reduce the risk of complications related to an immediate or delayed hemodynamic infarction.

A BTO evaluates the efficacy of the intracranial collateral circulation. Primary intracranial collaterals are those related to the circle of Willis (anterior communicating artery [ACOM] and posterior communicating artery [PCOM]) whereas secondary intracranial collaterals consist of retrograde flow within the ophthalmic artery (OA), external carotid artery branches, and leptomeningeal collaterals. The presence of a primary collateral from the ACOM complex leads to a decrease in the incidence and volume of internal zone infarcts (corona radiata, centrum semiovale), as reported by Bisschops and colleagues.[23] Primary intracranial collaterals are tested with a BTO; however, secondary intracranial collaterals are difficult to evaluate because they can take months to develop. Rutgers and colleagues[24] showed that secondary intracranial collaterals are more important than primary intracranial collaterals. These investigators followed 62 patients who were initially symptomatic from an ICA occlusion. Over a 2-year follow-up period, all patients remained asymptomatic. Angiographic follow-up showed no change in flow directionality across the ACOM/PCOM, and the flow within the OA became antegrade. The investigators thus concluded that leptomeningeal collaterals must have prevented delayed hemodynamic infarction.

The various adjunctive techniques described earlier in combination with a clinical BTO have improved the immediate and delayed hemodynamic ischemic risk associated with a PVO. Comparison of the venous filling phase between the occluded and the normal contralateral side seems to be most useful.[4] This evaluation can be performed with or without a clinical examination. If performed without a clinical examination, the procedure is shortened (20–30 minutes), because only angiographic data are evaluated. This technique can be performed under general anesthesia and thus is more comfortable for the patient as well as potentially shortening the procedure. In addition, the PVO can be performed immediately after the BTO because the patient is already under general anesthesia and under full anticoagulation. This technique needs to be studied as a part of a larger prospective trial to verify its positive predictive value and long-term outcome.

Angiographic description and quantification of cross flow were found to have no predictive value for tolerance of an ICA occlusion, nor could the presence of cerebral ischemia be associated with specific patterns of flow within the circle of Willis.[25,26] The same is true for hypotensive challenge, which failed to improve long-term outcome of patients undergoing PVO. The HMPAO SPECT technique requires 24 to 48 hours before results can be obtained; a repeat examination within this period is required because of the half-life of this isotope. The CT perfusion method described is cumbersome and involves knowledge of image postprocessing. At institutions in which there is no CT within the angiography suite, it involves the transfer of the patient to the CT suite with a balloon catheter in the carotid artery. The addition of stable xenon-enhanced CT reduced postoperative infarction and mortality; however, it was not significant when compared with a clinical BTO alone.[3] In addition, xenon inhalation has severe limitations such as patient motion, spontaneous respiratory depression, and induction of rapid changes in CBF.[3,27–29] The TCD method is a user-friendly and convenient adjunct to a clinical BTO, but needs trained personnel and provides no further improvement in outcome.[29] The patients at risk for a delayed hemodynamic infarct identified by BTO with additional NPM corresponded to those identified by clinical BTO alone.[3]

SUMMARY

BTO performed with clinical assessment is a powerful tool in assessing a patient's ability to tolerate a PVO. The balloon should be placed at or near the level of the proposed occlusion. Clinical tolerance of PVO can be assessed by a BTO with several variables, including the clinical examination, angiographic assessment, stump pressure, induced hypotension, perfusion scanning, TCD ultrasonography, and neurophysiologic monitoring. The 2 most useful variables are the clinical examination and venous phase assessment on the angiogram.

REFERENCES

1. Serbinenko FA. Catheterization and occlusion of major cerebral vessels and prospects for the development of vascular neurosurgery. Vopr Neirokhir 1971;35:17–27 [in Russian].
2. Serbinenko FA. Balloon catheterization and occlusion of major cerebral vessels. J Neurosurg 1974; 41:125–45.
3. Linskey ME, Jungreis CA, Yonas H, et al. Stroke risk after abrupt internal carotid artery sacrifice: accuracy of preoperative assessment with balloon test occlusion and stable xenon-enhanced CT. AJNR Am J Neuroradiol 1994;15:829–43.
4. Abud DG, Spelle L, Piotin M, et al. Venous phase timing during balloon test occlusion as a criterion for permanent internal carotid artery sacrifice. AJNR Am J Neuroradiol 2005;26:2602–9.
5. Morishima H, Kurata A, Miyasaka Y, et al. Efficacy of the stump pressure ratio as a guide to the safety of permanent occlusion of the internal carotid artery. Neurol Res 1998;20:732–6.
6. Tomura N, Omachi K, Takahashi S, et al. Comparison of technetium Tc 99m hexamethylpropylene-amine oxime single-photon emission tomograph with stump pressure during the balloon occlusion

test of the internal carotid artery. AJNR Am J Neuroradiol 2005;26:1937–42.
7. Barker DW, Jungreis CA, Horton JA, et al. Balloon test occlusion of the internal carotid artery: change in stump pressure over 15 minutes and its correlation with xenon CT cerebral blood flow. AJNR Am J Neuroradiol 1993;14:587–90.
8. Dare AO, Chaloupka JC, Putman CM, et al. Failure of the hypotensive provocative test during temporary balloon test occlusion of the internal carotid artery to predict delayed hemodynamic ischemia after therapeutic carotid occlusion. Surg Neurol 1998;50: 147–55 [discussion: 55–6].
9. Standard SC, Ahuja A, Guterman LR, et al. Balloon test occlusion of the internal carotid artery with hypotensive challenge. AJNR Am J Neuroradiol 1995;16:1453–8.
10. Simonson TM, Ryals TJ, Yuh WT, et al. MR imaging and HMPAO scintigraphy in conjunction with balloon test occlusion: value in predicting sequelae after permanent carotid occlusion. AJR Am J Roentgenol 1992;159:1063–8.
11. Brunberg JA, Frey KA, Horton JA, et al. [15O]H2O positron emission tomography determination of cerebral blood flow during balloon test occlusion of the internal carotid artery. AJNR Am J Neuroradiol 1994;15:725–32.
12. Jain R, Hoeffner EG, Deveikis JP, et al. Carotid perfusion CT with balloon occlusion and acetazolamide challenge test: feasibility. Radiology 2004; 231:906–13.
13. Okudaira Y, Arai H, Sato K. Cerebral blood flow alteration by acetazolamide during carotid balloon occlusion: parameters reflecting cerebral perfusion pressure in the acetazolamide test. Stroke 1996; 27:617–21.
14. Kofke WA, Brauer P, Policare R, et al. Middle cerebral artery blood flow velocity and stable xenon-enhanced computed tomographic blood flow during balloon test occlusion of the internal carotid artery. Stroke 1995;26:1603–6.
15. Johnson DW, Stringer WA, Marks MP, et al. Stable xenon CT cerebral blood flow imaging: rationale for and role in clinical decision making. AJNR Am J Neuroradiol 1991;12:201–13.
16. Michel E, Liu H, Remley KB, et al. Perfusion MR neuroimaging in patients undergoing balloon test occlusion of the internal carotid artery. AJNR Am J Neuroradiol 2001;22:1590–6.
17. Ma J, Mehrkens JH, Holtmannspoetter M, et al. Perfusion MRI before and after acetazolamide administration for assessment of cerebrovascular reserve capacity in patients with symptomatic internal carotid artery (ICA) occlusion: comparison with 99mTc-ECD SPECT. Neuroradiology 2007;49:317–26.
18. Eckert B, Thie A, Carvajal M, et al. Predicting hemodynamic ischemia by transcranial Doppler

monitoring during therapeutic balloon occlusion of the internal carotid artery. AJNR Am J Neuroradiol 1998;19:577–82.

19. Liu AY, Lopez JR, Do HM, et al. Neurophysiological monitoring in the endovascular therapy of aneurysms. AJNR Am J Neuroradiol 2003;24:1520–7.

20. Eskridge JM. Xenon-enhanced CT: past and present. AJNR Am J Neuroradiol 1994;15:845–6.

21. van der Schaaf IC, Brilstra EH, Buskens E, et al. Endovascular treatment of aneurysms in the cavernous sinus: a systematic review on balloon occlusion of the parent vessel and embolization with coils. Stroke 2002;33:313–8.

22. Vazquez Anon V, Aymard A, Gobin YP, et al. Balloon occlusion of the internal carotid artery in 40 cases of giant intracavernous aneurysm: technical aspects, cerebral monitoring, and results. Neuroradiology 1992;34:245–51.

23. Bisschops RH, Klijn CJ, Kappelle LJ, et al. Collateral flow and ischemic brain lesions in patients with unilateral carotid artery occlusion. Neurology 2003;60: 1435–41.

24. Rutgers DR, Klijn CJ, Kappelle LJ, et al. A longitudinal study of collateral flow patterns in the circle of Willis and the ophthalmic artery in patients with a symptomatic internal carotid artery occlusion. Stroke 2000;31:1913–20.

25. Beatty RA, Richardson AE. Predicting intolerance to common carotid artery ligation by carotid angiography. J Neurosurg 1968;28:9–13.

26. Jawad K, Miller D, Wyper DJ, et al. Measurement of CBF and carotid artery pressure compared with cerebral angiography in assessing collateral blood supply after carotid ligation. J Neurosurg 1977;46: 185–96.

27. Latchaw RE, Yonas H, Pentheny SL, et al. Adverse reactions to xenon-enhanced CT cerebral blood flow determination. Radiology 1987;163:251–4.

28. Giller CA, Mathews D, Walker B, et al. Prediction of tolerance to carotid artery occlusion using transcranial Doppler ultrasound. J Neurosurg 1994;81:15–9.

29. Giller CA, Purdy P, Lindstrom WW. Effects of inhaled stable xenon on cerebral blood flow velocity. AJNR Am J Neuroradiol 1990;11:177–82.

Endovascular Methods for the Treatment of Vascular Anomalies

Joseph J. Gemmete, MD, FSIR[a],*, Aditya S. Pandey, MD[b],
Steven J. Kasten, MD[c], Neeraj Chaudhary, MD, MRCS, FRCR[b]

KEYWORDS

- Vascular malformations • Vascular anomalies • Venous malformation • Lymphatic malformation
- Capillary malformation • Hemangioma • Arteriovenous malformation

KEY POINTS

- Venous malformations can be treated percutaneously by injecting a sclerosing agent. The most commonly used sclerosing agents include alcohol, sodium tetradecol, Ethibloc, polidocanol, and bleomycin.
- Multiple sclerosing agents have been used effectively for the treatment of lymphatic malformations, including absolute alcohol, sodium tetradecyl sulfate, doxycycline, Ethibloc, OK 432, and bleomycin.
- Approximately 8% of capillary malformations (CMs) are associated with Sturge-Weber syndrome and unilateral glaucoma. CMs are also associated with Klippel-Trenaunay, Parkes-Weber, macrocephaly CM, and CM-arteriovenous malformation (AVM) syndromes.
- Treatment of AVMs is difficult. Endovascular embolization is often the first treatment option with or without surgical resection. The main goal of any form of treatment is to eradicate the nidus.
- Endovascular treatment of an AVM can be performed from a transarterial approach, direct percutaneous puncture of the nidus, or a retrograde transvenous approach with alcohol, N-butyl-2-cyanoacrylate (n-BCA), or Onyx.
- Congenital hemangioma is a vascular lesion that completes the proliferative phase before birth. Two forms exist: the rapidly involuting congenital hemangioma (RICH) and the noninvoluting congenital hemangioma (NICH). RICHs involute more rapidly than hemangiomas of infancy, usually within the first 14 months of life. NICHs do not involute but grow in proportion to the child.

INTRODUCTION

In 1982, John Mulliken and Julie Glowacki proposed a classification of vascular anomalies based on clinical behavior, histology, and histochemistry.[1] The International Society for the Study of Vascular Anomalies (ISSVA) accepted this classification in 1992.[2–4] The classification divides vascular anomalies into 2 groups: tumors (eg, hemangiomas), the cause of which is endothelial cell proliferation, and vascular malformations, in which developmental error has resulted in abnormally formed vascular channels. In the tumor group, this article

[a] Division of Interventional Neuroradiology and Cranial Base Surgery, Departments of Radiology, Neurosurgery, and Otolaryngology, University of Michigan Health System, UH B1D 328, 1500 East Medical Center Drive, Ann Arbor, MI 48109–5030, USA; [b] Division of Interventional Neuroradiology, Departments of Neurosurgery and Radiology, University of Michigan Health System, 1500 East Medical Center Drive, Ann Arbor, MI 48109–5030, USA; [c] Department of Plastic Surgery, University of Michigan Health System, 1500 East Medical Center Drive, Ann Arbor, MI 48109-5030, USA
* Corresponding author.
E-mail address: gemmete@med.umich.edu

Neuroimag Clin N Am 23 (2013) 703–728
http://dx.doi.org/10.1016/j.nic.2013.03.016
1052-5149/13/$ – see front matter © 2013 Elsevier Inc. All rights reserved.

focuses on hemangiomas; the other tumor subtypes are beyond the scope of this review. Vascular malformations can be further subdivided into lesions consisting of arterial, capillary, lymphatic, venous, and fistulous networks. Furthermore, they can be further subdivided functionally based on the flow characteristics (ie, high-flow vs low-flow lesions).[5] This article discusses the clinical features, natural history and epidemiology, and presents the diagnostic imaging features of vascular anomalies of the head and neck. The percutaneous/endovascular treatment of each of the vascular anomalies are presented. Additional treatment options, such as surgery are discussed briefly. Finally, the clinical outcomes of the main forms of treatment and level of evidence are presented.

VENOUS MALFORMATIONS
Clinical Features

Venous malformations (VMs) can occur anywhere in the body, but are most frequently located in the head and neck. They can be solitary, small, well circumscribed, large, superficial, or infiltrative involving multiple tissue planes. The lesion is nonpulsatile, may have a light blue to deep purple color, and can be associated with telangiectasias, varicosities, or ecchymosis. The mass may increase in size in a dependent position, with a tourniquet, or during a Valsalva maneuver. Superficial lesions are soft and compressible and can usually be emptied of blood. Patients usually present with pain associated with compression on the surrounding nerves or thrombosis of a portion of the mass. An increased level of D-dimer has been determined to be highly specific for a VM and can help to distinguish VMs from lymphatic malformations and slow-flow Klippel-Trenaunay syndrome from high-flow Parks-Weber syndrome.[6]

VMs are usually isolated findings; however, they may be associated with the following syndromes (Table 1):

Klippel-Trenaunay syndrome
Blue rubber bleb nevus (BRBN) syndrome
Mucocutaneous familial VMs
Glomuvenous malformation
Maffucci syndrome
Proteus syndrome
Bannayan-Riley-Ruvalcaba syndrome
CLOVES/S syndrome

Natural History/Epidemiology

VMs are present at birth. They are not always clinically apparent and tend to grow in proportion to the growth of the child. The growth is most pronounced during puberty and pregnancy. These are congenital lesions that affect boys and girls with equal frequency with a reported incidence of 1 to 2 per 100,000 births and a prevalence of 1%.[7]

Most VMs (95%) are sporadic, but can be seen in several heritable conditions. The molecular basis for sporadic occurrence has yet to be discovered, however there are familial cases where the genetic defect has been localized on a specific chromosome. In 1994/1995, 2 families were identified to have autosomal dominant inherited cutaneous and mucosal VMs. Genetic analysis mapped a locus for both of these families to chromosome 9p21.[8,9] These families shared a mutation resulting in an arginine to tryptophan substitution R849W in the gene that encodes for the kinase domain of the endothelial cell receptor Tie2.[10] In 1999, 4 more families with autosomal dominant inherited VMs were identified.[11] Only 1 of those families shared the same mutation as the previous 2 reports. The second family had a novel hyperphosphorylating Y897S mutation in the TIE2 gene. The other families showed no evidence of linkage to 9p21, which suggests genetic heterogeneity. Multifocal VMs are most commonly seen in the familial forms of VM, including the following: BRBN syndrome, mucocutaneous familial VMs, glomuvenous malformation, and Maffucci syndrome.[12]

Diagnostic Imaging

Ultrasonography

On grayscale imaging, VMs are usually hypoechoic to anechoic with the shape of tubular structures.[13] Some lesions can have a heterogeneous echotexture if phleboliths or different forms of thrombus are present within the lesion. Doppler flow is usually a monophasic low-velocity flow. Sometimes flow can only be seen with compression and release of the lesion.[14]

Computed tomography

On noncontrast computed tomography (CT), VMs are usually hypoattentuating, however they can be heterogeneous depending on the amount of fatty tissue within the lesion. Phleboliths or dystrophic calcifications can be seen within the lesion. After the administration of contrast, the lesion usually enhances on the periphery and then fills in centrally on the delay images.[14] CT is excellent at looking for boney involvement from the lesion. Magnetic resonance (MR) imaging is better at characterizing the relationship of the lesion with surrounding soft tissue structures.

MR imaging

VMs usually appear as hypointense to isointense on T1-weighted imaging. They can, however,

Table 1
Syndromes associated with vascular anomalies

Syndromes	Vascular Tumors — Infantile Hemangioma	Venous	Capillary	Lymphatic	Arterial or Arteriovenous
PHACES	●				
LUMBAR	●				●
Kasabach-Merritt				●	
Maffucci		●		●	
Klippel-Trenaunay	●	●	●	●	●
Gorham-Stout		●	●	●	
Proteus		●	●	●	
Parkers-Weber		●	●		●
Sturge-Weber	●	●	●		
CM-AVM		●			●
Familial cerebral VM		●			
Familial cutaneomucosal VM		●			
Blue rubber bleb nevus		●			
Bockenheimer		●			
Cobb			●		●
Osler-Weber-Rendu	●		●		●
Beckwith-Wiedemann	●		●		
Louis-Barr			●		
Down				●	
Turner				●	
Wyburn-Mason					●
Dandy-Walker	●				
Von Hippel-Lindau	●				

This table is intended to generalize common associations. For example, there are at least 6 case reports of AVM in PHACES syndrome, but the association is uncommon, and thus is not included in the table. Syndromes with multiple malformation subtypes (eg, Proteus) often involve mixed-type malformations.
Abbreviations: AVM, arteriovenous malformation; CM, capillary malformation; VM, venous malformation.

have areas of bright signal on T1-weighted images if the lesion has fat, subacute blood products, or certain types of calcifications contained within the lesion.[15] On T2-weighted images, VMs have high signal intensity. Gradient echo sequences usually show areas of low signal corresponding to calcification, hemosiderin, or thrombus. The best sequence to determine the full extent of the lesion and its relationship with surrounding soft tissue structures is the T2-weighted sequence.[16] On T1-weighted postcontrast imaging, the lesions usually demonstrate early peripheral enhancement that later fills in centrally on delayed imaging.[17]

Diagnostic venography
Contrast venography is helpful in the anatomic characterization of a VM. It is performed to determine the full extent of the malformation and its draining veins. It is also helpful in confirming patency of the deep venous system in the extremity. Venography is also performed to determine the volume of contrast needed to fill the malformation before it empties into normal draining veins.

Based on the pattern of venous drainage, VMs can be divided into 4 types.[18–20] This drainage pattern is a reflection of the response to treatment and rates of complications. Types I and II respond best to sclerotherapy with a better control rate and fewer sessions to achieve control. Types III and IV have a higher rate of complications.[20]

Type I: isolated malformation without discernible venous drainage
Type II: lesion draining into normal veins
Type III: lesion draining into dysplastic veins
Type IV: lesion consists primarily of venous ectasia

Treatment

VMs can be treated percutaneously by injecting a sclerosing agent. The most commonly described sclerosing agents (**Box 1**) include alcohol, sodium tetradecol, Ethibloc, polidocanol, and bleomycin.[19,21–24] The procedure is performed under general anesthesia because injection of the sclerosing agent can be extremely painful. A Foley catheter is placed in the bladder to monitor urine output and color because some patients may develop hemoglobinuria. This is most likely to happen in younger patients and in patients with large lesions. In addition, if an extremity is being treated, we start an intravenous (IV) line distal to the lesion to infuse saline and heparin overnight to flush out the sclerosing agent and prevent acute deep venous thrombosis.[12] Sclerotherapy is performed by cannulating the lesion percutaneously under ultrasonography or fluoroscopy (**Fig. 1**). Contrast material is injected to define the extent of the lesion, determine the flow rate within the lesion, the communication with normal veins, and the presence of a possible arterial component, and to give an estimate of the volume of sclerosing agent needed to fill the lesion. If a large draining vein is visualized, this can be treated with embolization using coils, liquid embolic agents, or with temporary balloon occlusion to increase the contact time of the sclerosing agent with the VM and to prevent egress of the agent into the systemic circulation.[12] This may also be performed with a tourniquet, blood pressure cuff, or manual compression. The sclerosant is then injected under fluoroscopic guidance to decrease the risk of extravasation and overfilling of the lesion, and to limit undesired egress of the sclerosing agent into the normal deep veins. Overfilling of the lesion may also be prevented by the 2-needle access technique, which allows decompression of the lesion through the second needle access. Cone beam CT can be performed to evaluate the anatomic distribution of the sclerosant

administered and compare the distribution with the preprocedure imaging.[25] After the needles are removed, a 20 to 30 mm Hg compression stocking is placed over the area of concern so that the veins do not refill with blood. Compression allows maximum contact of the damaged endothelium of the vein wall, promoting fibrosis and scarring. The procedure is then repeated at intervals of 8 to 10 weeks until there is no recanalization, swelling, or pain from the lesion. Diffuse VMs are much more difficult to treat. The area of maximum symptomatology is usually targeted because these lesions cannot be completely obliterated.

After sclerotherapy the lesion should feel firm to palpation. Swelling is generally maximum 24 hours after the procedure. We recommend placing a custom-fitted class II compression garment over the lesion as soon as possible. If the lesion involves the airway, the patient may need to be kept intubated overnight in the intensive care unit. The patient is given IV steroids in the hospital and then sent home on a tapered dose pack. The affected area is kept elevated above the heart with ice packs applied to minimize swelling. Patients receive IV fluids at twice the maintenance dose before, during, and after the sclerotherapy for 24 hours. Urine output is closely monitored for hemoglobinuria. Appropriate IV and oral analgesics and antiinflammatory agents are prescribed in the hospital and for 7 days after discharge.

Patients with extensive limb lesions should be instructed from childhood in the proper use of compression garments. Compression helps to decrease the discomfort associated with the lesion, protects the overlying skin, limits swelling, and improves localized intravascular coagulation.

In patients with extensive VMs in whom a low fibrinogen level is present, the use of low-molecular-weight heparin is recommended for 2 weeks pretreatment and possible cryoprecipitate transfusion if still low on the day of the procedure. This therapy reduces the consumptive coagulopathy of the extensive VM and potentially lowers the recanalization rate.[12]

Sclerosant drugs

Absolute ethanol (95%–98%) is probably the most common agent used for sclerotherapy. It is the most effective sclerosant agent available, however it is also the most toxic.[12] Ethanol works by causing instant precipitation of endothelial cell proteins and rapid thrombosis. It may also cause transmural vessel necrosis resulting in diffusion into the surrounding tissues. Serious side effects from ethanol injection include massive swelling, tissue necrosis, hypoglycemia, peripheral nerve injury,

---

Box 1
Common sclerosing agents

- Alcohol
- Sodium tetradecol
- Alcoholic solution of zein (Ethibloc)
- Polidocanol
- Bleomycin
- OK-432 (picibanil)
- Doxycycline

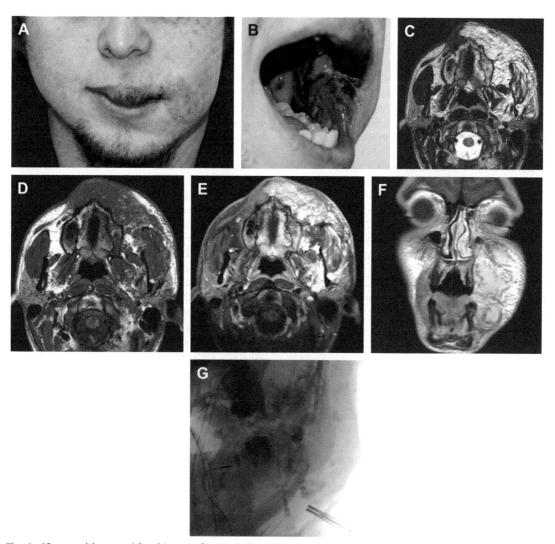

Fig. 1. 19-year-old man with a history of pain and swelling on the left side of his face since birth. The mass increases in size when he is in a dependent position. (*A*) Dilated superficial veins involving the left upper lip and face. (*B*) The buccal surface of the left mouth shows multiple dilated veins. (*C*) Axial MR T2-weighted image at the level of the maxilla shows multiple tubular structures with abnormal high signal within the left face. (*D*) Corresponding axial MR T1-weighted image at the same level as (*C*) shows that these tubular structures have the same signal as muscle. (*E*) Corresponding axial MR postgadolinium T1-weighted fat-saturated image at the same level as (*C, D*) shows uniform enhancement of the tubular structures. (*F*) Coronal MR postgadolinium T1-weighted image shows the cranial caudal extent of the lesion involving the left face. (*G*) Frontal spot fluoroscopy image shows contrast mixed with alcohol filling the VM. Multiple phleboliths are identified with the soft tissues.

central nervous system depression, hemolysis, pulmonary vasospasm, cardiac arrhythmias, and electromechanical disassociation.[26–33] Given the serious side effects, patients must be closely monitored during procedures involving ethanol. Some practitioners even suggest monitoring of pulmonary artery pressure during and for a short period after the procedure. Ethanol blood levels correlate directly with the amount of ethanol injected.[34] Mason and colleagues[35] demonstrated that a level of more than 1 mL/kg may put patients at increased risk of respiratory depression, cardiac arrhythmias, seizures, and rhabdomyolysis. A total dose of 1 mL/kg (or 60 mL) per session should never be exceeded. In pediatric patients, a maximum dose of 0.5 mg/kg per session is recommended. Ethanol can be injected in an undiluted form; however we believe this is dangerous because the agent cannot be identified under fluoroscopy. We usually dilute alcohol with water-soluble liquid or oily contrast medium during injection. Alcohol should not be mixed with Visipaque because this causes precipitation of the contrast medium. In a series of 60 patients with VM involving the head and neck treated with ethanol, Su and colleagues[36] reported 68% complete response (>90% volume reduction), 25% marked response (>50% volume reduction), and 7% moderate response (<50% volume decrease) with a 10% complication rate (level IV evidence). In a series of 158 patients with VM, 16% of patients had a good response defined by clinical examination and a decrease in size of 30% or greater on MR imaging; unfortunately 27% of these patients experienced a complication (level IV evidence).[37] In another series of 87 patients with craniofacial VMs treated with ethanol sclerotherapy, 32% had an excellent response (>75% volume reduction), 52% a good response (>25% volume reduction), and 16% a poor response (25% volume decrease) with a 5% complication rate (level IV evidence).[38]

Detergents

Detergents used for sclerotherapy of VMs include sodium tetradecyl sulfate, polidocanol, sodium morrhuate, and ethanolamine.[39–43] Sodium tetradecyl sulfate, is approved in the United States for treatment of varicose veins.[44] Polidocanol has US Food and Drug Administration approval for sclerosis of spider and reticular veins.[45] Similar to ethanol, all of the drugs damage the endothelial cells, resulting in thrombosis and fibrosis. Detergents may be mixed with water-soluble or oily contrast medium before injection. These agents are believed to have a low rate of complications compared with ethanol, but a greater tendency toward recanalization. Reported complications include cardiovascular collapse, skin pigmentation, skin necrosis, anaphylaxis, and hemoglobinuria.[46] Foaming the sclerosant by mixing the drug with air has also become popular.[42,47] The theory is that the foam probably results in better contact between the drug and vein wall along with prolonged displacement of the blood with the lesion. Foam is made easily by mixing 10 mL of sclerosant with 3 mL of Ethiodol and 5 to 10 mL of air through a 3-way stopcock. Patients receiving large volumes of detergent sclerosants may need aggressive hydration and alkalization of the urine to treat hemoglobinuria.[39] In a prospective randomized controlled trial comparing foamed versus liquid polidocanol or ethanolamine in 89 patients with VMs, 90% of patients had partial or complete response in the foamed group versus 63% in the liquid group (P = .002) (level I evidence).[48] In another series of 50 patients with VMs treated with polidocanol foam, complete resolution

occurred in 38% of patients, a reduction in size of 50% or more in 30% of patients, a reduction in size of between 0% and 50% in 26% of patients, and no change in 8% of patients (level IV evidence).[49] Reported complications were noted in 8% of the patients. Furthermore, in a series involving 26 patients with VM, use of ethanolamine oleate showed 49% excellent, 39% good, 12% fair, and 0% poor results based on clinical examination (level IV evidence).[50]

Bleomycin

Bleomycin, an antibiotic and antitumor agent originally derived from Streptomyces verticillus in 1966, causes an inflammatory response in endothelial cells.[21] Bleomycin can be mixed with water-soluble liquid or oily contrast medium. There is some concern about the use of this agent because of the association with pulmonary fibrosis in the setting of chemotherapy. The threshold dose for pulmonary fibrosis and interstitial fibrosis is 450 mg; doses for sclerotherapy are typically 0.5 to 1 mg/kg for pediatric patients and 1 to 15 mg in adults.[21] Reported complications include skin ulceration, skin pigmentation, laryngeal edema, flu-like symptoms, cellulitis, nausea and vomiting, and focal alopecia.[21,51] In a series of 31 patients with VM treated with percutaneous injection of bleomycin, complete resolution occurred in 0%, marked decrease (≥50%) in size in 34%, minimal decrease (≤50%) in size in 31%, stable size in 34%, and increase in size in 0% on postprocedure MR imaging (level IV evidence).[51] Complications were seen in 12.5% of patients and consisted predominantly of transient skin pigmentation and cellulitis. In another series of 32 patients treated with percutaneous bleomycin sclerotherapy, complete resolution of the lesion was found in 32% of patients and significant improvement in 52% of patients by clinical examination (level IV evidence).[21]

Liquid embolic agents

BCA has a limited role in the treatment of vascular malformations because of its high cost, limited reabsorption, and the formation of a hard mass after injection that may last for many months. Burrows and colleagues[12] suggest this form of treatment for preoperative embolization before surgical resection. BCA is most commonly used in the treatment of intra-articular VMs because injection of a sclerosing agent could cause damage to the articular cartilage. This form of treatment has also been described for an orbital VM (level IV evidence).[52] Ethylene vinyl alcohol copolymer (Onyx), a newer liquid polymer, may also be useful for preoperative embolization of VMs before resection.

Other forms of treatment

Endovascular diode laser therapy has been reported in a small series of VMs with a good response rate at 14-month follow-up (level IV evidence).[53] In patients with Klippel-Trenaunay syndrome, endovenous laser ablation of the marginal vein may be a useful alternative therapy. Percutaneous, interstitial (nonendovascular) laser photocoagulation of VM using the diode or neodymium:yttrium-aluminum-garnet (Nd:YAG) lasers via a fiber-optic delivery system has also been reported with reasonable success (level IV evidence).[54–58] Because of the controlled delivery of energy, and with external cooling, this modality may be useful for extensive superficial cutaneous/subcutaneous lesions or isolated anatomic locations such as the digit or tongue where sclerosis or embolization may carry a higher risk of surrounding tissue necrosis.

Surgical resection of VMs is indicated only when complete resection without a resulting functional or anatomic deficit is possible. Surgery plays a limited role in the management of extremity lesions, but if performed, localized coagulopathy must be controlled before surgery.[19,59,60] Surgery may also help to avoid joint distention from repeat hemarthrosis if joint involvement with a VM of the synovium is present.

LYMPHATIC MALFORMATION
Clinical Features

Lymphatic malformations (LMs) are present at birth and are composed of abnormal dilated lakes of lymphatic tissue that result from defective embryologic development of the primordial lymphatic channels. LMs can be classified radiographically as macrocystic (cysts ≥ 2 cm), microcystic (cysts <2 cm) or mixed, which has important implications for treatment. Macrocystic lesions are most commonly located in the neck, axilla, and chest wall, and, when large, may interfere with the birth process. Microcystic lesions usually present as diffuse soft tissue thickening, often associated with vesicles of the skin and mucosa with an overlying capillary malformation. The lesions grow in proportion to the patient. They may undergo periodic swelling often associated with signs of inflammation, which may be spontaneous or related to a regional infection. Acute swelling of the lesion may also be related to hemorrhage or lymphatic obstruction. Symptoms caused by LMs are typically related to the localized mass effect on adjacent structures. On physical examination, LMs are mobile and have a boggy or cystic consistency. The lesions cannot be decompressed and do not distend with the Valsalva maneuver like VMs. The presence of lymphatic endothelium can be confirmed by staining with D2-40 antibody.[61]

Infection is usually common in suprahyoid LMs with mucosal involvement. Patients with airway involvement can present with stridor and sleep apnea. In one series, tracheostomy placement occurred in 5% of patients with airway compromise at birth. Orbit LMs can present with pain, swelling, proptosis, blepharoptosis, and emblyopia. An underlying cerebral developmental anomaly is seen in 45% of patients with orbital involvement.

Natural History/Epidemiology

Developmental defects during embryonic lymphangiogenesis result in LMs.[7,62] They tend to grow in proportion with the growth of the child. The growth is most pronounced during puberty and pregnancy. The incidence is reported at between 0.02% and 0.05%, and represents approximately 3 of 100,000 hospital admissions.[63,64] More than 50% of LMs are identified at birth, with 80% to 90% usually identified by 2 years of age.[65] Approximately 75% of the lesions occur in the head and neck region.[64] Spontaneous regression is rare and has been report in less than 4% of cases.[63,66] Multiple genes have been described in the process of lymph angiogenesis including VEGFR3, VEGFC, Ang2, Lyve1, Nrp2, and podoplanin.[7] No evidence exists for heritable LM. Cervical LMs do occur in association with Klippel-Trenaunay, Turner, and Noonan syndromes, as well as trisomy 13 and 18.[67]

Diagnostic Imaging

Ultrasonography
Macrocystic lesions appear on grayscale imaging as multiple anechoic or hypoechoic cystic spaces with internal septations and debri. Microcystic lesions appear as an ill-defined hyperechoic mass on grayscale imaging.[68]

CT
LMs appear as fluid-filled low-attenuation lesions, with occasional fluid/fluid levels that represent hemorrhage into the cystic structure. Peripheral enhancement of the walls may occur, however there is no central filling of the lesion on delayed images like a VM.[69] The internal septations are commonly not seen.

MR imaging
Macrocystic LMs appear as fluid-filled lesions with a single locule or multiple loculations, displaying high signal on T2-weighted images and low signal on T1-weighted images.[70] Occasionally, a fluid/fluid level can be seen in the setting of internal hemorrhage. Postgadolinium T1-weighted images show minimal or absent septal enhancement.

Microcystic lesions demonstrate intermediate signal intensity on magnetic resonance imaging (MRI) T1 and T2 spin echo sequences.[18]

Treatment

Multiple sclerosing agents have been used effectively for the treatment of LMs, including absolute alcohol, sodium tetradecyl sulfate, doxycycline, Ethibloc, OK 432, and bleomycin.[71–76]

The technique for sclerotherapy of LMs consists of cannulation of each cyst with a standard angiocatheter under ultrasonographic guidance. As much fluid as possible is aspirated from the cyst. Contrast is injected under fluoroscopic guidance to identify the size of the lesion. The sclerosing agent is mixed with a contrast medium and the cyst injected under fluoroscopic guidance (**Fig. 2**). Smaller macrocystic lesions can be treated with aspiration and sclerotherapy without catheter drainage.[76] For large lesions, a pigtail catheter may be placed into the cyst and the lesion drained and injected over several days. Microcystic lesions are a challenge to treat and generally require multiple injections. Treatment is continued until imaging identifies no treatable cysts or the patient is satisfied with the clinical outcome.

Doxycycline
Doxycycline is generally instilled into the cyst as a solution of 10 mg/mL. The dose of doxycycline can range from 150 mg to 1000 mg depending on the size of the lesion. In neonates, the maximum recommend dose at 1 time is 150 mg, because higher doses may cause hemolytic anemia, hypoglycemia, and metabolic acidosis.[77] Blood glucose is monitored 2 hours after the procedure in neonates. If the patient develops hypoglycemia, IV dextrose can be administered. A few small series have described a 93% to 100% complete radiographic response for treatment of macrocystic LMs (type IV evidence).[73,78] Lower response rates are noted for microcystic LMs.

Detergents
There is limited literature on the used of detergents as sclerosant agents for LMs. One study described the use of 98% ethanol and 3% sodium tetradecyl sulfate, with a 100% complete radiographic response rate (level IV evidence).[73] A second series described the use of foamed sodium tetradecyl sulfate, for the treatment of 6 intraorbital LMs with a reduction in lesion size in all patients (level IV evidence).[79]

OK-432 (picibanil)
OK-432 (picibanil) is a lyophilized mixture of group A *Streptococcus pyogenes* initially developed as an immunotherapeutic agent in the treatment of gastric and lung carcinoma with the first use as a sclerosant in the treatment of an LM described in a case report in 1987 (level IV evidence).[80] OK-432 is not approved in the United States. Direct injection of the solution into an LM has been shown to increase intralesional cytokine levels, namely tumor necrosis factor, interleukin 6 (IL-6), IL-8, interferon-α, and vascular endothelial growth factor in patients with a response to treatment with OK-432.[81,82] A review of the literature by Poldervaart and colleagues[83] showed an 88% excellent response rate for macrocystic lesions. Microcystic lesions demonstrated an excellent response rate in 27%, good in 33%, and poor in 40% of cases.[83] Adverse side effects were mild and consisted of fever, lethargy, and local inflammation. A phase II trial was conducted in the United States on 182 patients with LMs. In this trial, 94% of the patients with macrocystic disease had a response to treatment, 63% of the patients with mixed macrocystic/microcystic disease had a response to treatment, and 0% of the patients with microcystic disease responded to treatment (level I evidence).[66] In 2 other series, complete response rates of 76% and 83.5% were noted (level IV evidence).[82,84]

Alcohol solution of zein
Alcoholic solution of zein (Ethibloc; Ethicon, Norderstedt, Germany) is a biodegradable thrombogenic solution consisting of a combination of zein (corn protein), sodium diaatrizoate, and oleum in ethanol. It has been used in Canada and Europe but is currently not approved in the United States. Dubois and colleagues[75] reported a more than 95% volumetric regression by CT in 64% of lesions and more than 50% in the remainder of macrocystic and microcystic lesions (level IV evidence). Reported complications in this series included a minor local inflammatory reaction and an initial increase in size of the lesion in all patients. In another study of 65 patients with LMs treated with Ethibloc equal to 10% of the lesion volume, 49% achieved excellent results, 35% showed satisfactory results, and 16% had poor results (level IV evidence).[85] Complications included a localized inflammatory reaction and self-limiting external leakage of the Ethiobloc at a mean of 2 months after therapy.

Bleomycin
Bleomycin is also used for sclerotherapy of LMs. The previous discussion on the use of bleomycin for VMs also holds true for LMs. In a series of 70 patients with LM treated with intralesional injection of bleomycin, 47% of patients achieved excellent

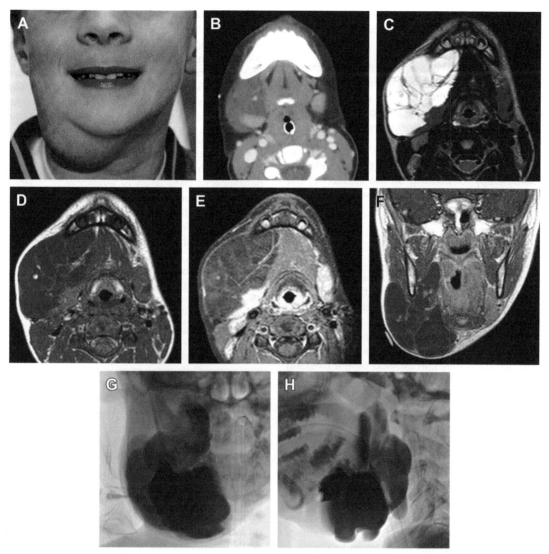

Fig. 2. 4-year-old boy with a large mass involving his right neck. The mass has been present since birth and periodically becomes swollen with signs of inflammation. (*A*) The mass involving the right neck. (*B*) Axial CT contrast-enhanced image of the neck shows a fluid-filled mass with no enhancement within the submandibular space. (*C*) Axial MR fat-saturated T2-weighted image of the neck shows a large mass with high signal and multiple internal septations within the submandibular space. (*D*) Axial MR fat-saturated T1-weighted image of the neck at the same level as (*C*) shows a large mass with low signal and multiple internal septations within the submandibular space. (*E*) Axial MR postgadolinium fat-saturated T1-weighted image of the neck at the same level as (*C*, *D*) shows some septal and peripheral enhancement of the mass. (*F*) Coronal MR postgadolinium fat-saturated T1 weighted image of the neck shows the cranial caudal extent of the mass. (*G*, *H*) Spot fluoroscopy images in the anterior posterior and lateral projections show contrast mixed with doxycycline filling the entire mass.

results, 36% achieved good results, and 17% had poor results. Seven percent of the group had recurrence (level IV evidence).[86] Mild side effects consisted of fever, pain, swelling, and leukopenia. In another series of 200 patients with LM treated with intralesional injection of bleomycin-A5, 87% of patients demonstrated complete lesion resolution with a recurrence rate of 13% (level IV evidence).[87] Complications were mild; anorexia and fever were the most common complications reported.

Laser therapy
Laser therapy is generally reserved for lesions with superficial cutaneous/mucosal vesicles. Microcystic lesions of the oral cavity and tongue have also

been treated with the carbon dioxide laser and the Nd:YAG with success (level IV evidence).[54,88]

Radiofrequency ablation

In a series of 11 patients, Grimmer and colleagues[89] reported a response rate of 62% with radiofrequency ablation in patients with microcystic lesions of the lips, tongue, buccal mucosa, and floor of the mouth (level IV evidence).

Surgery

Surgery is usually performed after an attempt at sclerotherapy. Depending on the location of the lesion, removal can be disfiguring with a high incidence of recurrence.

CAPILLARY MALFORMATIONS
Clinical Presentation

Capillary malformations (CMs) are present at birth and grow commensurately with the child. CMs may be single or multiple, involve only the dermis, are well demarcated, and appear pink in infancy and may become dark purple with age.[90] Symptoms related to sporadic CM are primarily cosmetic although they can develop severe bleeding after minor trauma.[44] CMs can be associated with overgrowth of the affected limb or face with certain syndromes.[91]

Natural History/Epidemiology

CM, also termed port-wine stain, capillary hemangioma, nevus flammeus, angel's kiss, and stork's bite, are common vascular malformations with an incidence of 0.3%.[44,90] CM is usually sporadic, but families with a dominant inheritance pattern with incomplete penetrance have been reported. CM-AVM syndrome has been linked to chromosome 5q14-21, with a defect in the RASA1 gene that encodes a p120 RasGTPase-activating protein, which is involved in cell adhesion and angiogenesis.[92,93] Most CMs in the head and neck occur in the V1 and V2 distribution of the trigeminal nerve. Approximately 8% of CMs are associated with Sturge-Weber syndrome and unilateral glaucoma.[94] CMs are also associated with Klippel-Trenaunay, Parkes-Weber, macrocephaly CM, and CM-AVM syndromes.[7]

Diagnostic Imaging

There is little role for imaging except to exclude more serious disorders associated with CMs such as in Sturge-Weber syndrome. Ultrasonography may reveal areas of hyperechogenicity on grayscale images with minimal flow on Doppler imaging. Given the superficial location of these lesions, a high-frequency ultrasound probe (>10 MHz) is necessary to fully characterize the lesion. CT imaging findings are usually minimal even with extensive disease. On MR imaging, the skin may appear thickened with abnormal signal in the superficial soft tissue. The lesion may enhance after IV contrast administration. The value of CT and MR imaging for diagnosing CM is in ruling out more serious syndromes.

Treatment

Photocoagulation with pulsed dye laser (PDL) has been shown to be effective in improving the appearance of CMs (level IV evidence).[95–97] However, controversy exists on whether PDL provides long-term benefit (level IV evidence).[96,97]

There is no indication for embolization of these lesions, except in reconstruction of a hyperemic facial skeleton. Preoperative particulate embolization of the lesion may decrease blood loss during surgical reconstruction (Fig. 3).

AVMS
Clinical Presentation

An AVM consists of an abnormal nidus of vascular channels with feeding arteries and draining veins with no normal intervening capillary network. Except for rare high-flow lesions, which may present with cardiac overload in neonates and infants, most AVMs are asymptomatic in the first 2 decades of life. On physical examination, an AVM may show local erythema and hyperthermia with prominent pulsations, a palpable thrill, and an audible bruit. Growth of these lesions is often precipitated by hormonal factors (puberty, pregnancy, and hormone therapy), trauma, infection, or iatrogenic causes (surgery, embolization). If venous hypertension develops, this may result in tissue ischemia leading to pain and skin ulceration, often associated with bleeding. In 1990, the Schobinger clinical staging system documenting the natural history of AVMs was introduced at the International Workshop for the Study of Vascular Anomalies in Amsterdam.[98]

Natural History/Epidemiology

AVMs can be detected at birth in 40% of cases and most commonly occur in the pelvis or extremities.[7] Rapid growth is not characteristic of the lesion's natural history. AVMs are usually sporadic with no genetic predisposition. There is a relationship between CMs and high-flow lesions, such as arterial venous fistulas and AVMs, and Parkes-Weber syndrome associated with RASA-1 mutations.[92]

There are also numerous reports in the literature of phosphatase and tension homolog (PTEN) mutations associated with cerebral and peripheral

AVMs. PTEN is a tumor suppressive gene located on chromosome 10q. Mutations of this gene are associated with various syndromes including Bannayan-Riley-Ruvalcaba syndrome and Cowden syndrome.[99–101] Screening of patients with this mutation is recommended.

Mutations in endoglin and activin receptor-like kinase 1 (ALK1) are associated with hereditary hemorrhagic telangiectasia (HHT). AVMs in HHT can be seen in the brain, liver, lung, and gastrointestinal tract.[102]

Diagnostic Imaging

AVMs are high-flow lesions without a normal capillary bed between the arteries and veins. These features contribute to their imaging characteristics.

Ultrasonography

Grayscale ultrasonography shows a poorly defined heterogeneous structure. Fat is often seen around the AVM. Doppler ultrasonography shows a network of multiple arteries with increased diastolic flow and arterialized draining veins with a biphasic waveform.[68]

CT

AVMs appear as multiple, enlarged, enhancing, feeding arteries filling a cluster of grapelike structures (ie, the nidus) with enlarged surrounding draining veins. CT may show hypertrophy of the adjacent bone. CT is important for delineating bone involvement of the axial skeleton, mandible, maxilla, skull base, and orbits.

MR imaging

MR imaging is the modality of choice to image an AVM given its excellent soft tissue resolution and ability to characterize the flow characteristics and hemodynamics. T2-weighted spin echo sequence shows multiple flow voids from enlarged feeding arteries, the AVM nidus, and draining outflow veins. On contrast-enhanced gradient echo images, the corresponding flow voids show enhancement.[68] 4D-TRAKS (four-dimensional time-resolved angiography using keyhole) can give an idea of the flow characteristics and hemodynamics of the lesion.[103]

Angiography

Angiography is only necessary when intervention is considered or MR imaging/MR angiography examination is equivocal. The classic angiographic appearance of an AVM is that of multiple enlarged feeding arteries rapidly shunting into a nidus and then into dilated draining veins. Direct arteriovenous fistulous components and intralesional aneurysms may be identified.

Treatment

Treatment of AVMs is difficult. Endovascular embolization is often the first treatment option with or without surgical resection. The main goal of any form of treatment is to eradicate the nidus. From an endovascular approach, this can be performed using a transarterial approach, direct percutaneous puncture of the nidus, or a retrograde transvenous approach.

Flow reduction techniques can be used to increase the concentration of the embolic agent within the AVM nidus. This can be performed using balloon catheters to temporarily occlude the arterial inflow or venous outflow. If the lesion involves an extremity, a tourniquet or pneumatic cuff can be placed upstream or downstream from the lesion. In addition, coils or liquid adhesive agents may be placed in the draining vein to assist in flow reduction.

Cho and colleagues[104] proposed an angiographic classification of AVMs based on nidal morphology with implication for a therapeutic approach and outcome.

Type I: arteriovenous fistulae
Type II: arteriolovenous fistulae
Type IIIa: arteriolovenulous fistulae with nondilated fistula
Type IIIb: arteriolovenulous fistulae with dilated fistula

Eradication of the nidus is necessary for proper treatment of an AVM. This requires placement of a permanent agent within the nidus. Surgical ligation or occlusion of the feeding artery with coils should not be performed because the lesion will develop collateral arterial feeders that will make treatment of the lesion more difficult. The authors also believe that polyvinyl alcohol (PVA) particles have a limited role in the embolization of an AVM, because of there nonpermanent nature.

Alcohol

Alcohol is the agent most often used for embolization of peripheral AVMs, given that it is permanent and probably the most effective. The maximum recommend volume is 1.0 mL/kg, however Mason and colleagues[35] suggested the dose should be reduced to 0.5 mL/kg given the increased serum alcohol levels and potential negative side effects. Success rates of up to 68% have been published with multiple treatment sessions and complications noted in 52% of patients (level IV evidence).[105] Response rates of up to 82% have been reported with extremity bone AVMs (level IV evidence).[106] In a series of 66 AVMs, Cho and colleagues[104] found alcohol most effective for type II (100%), and more

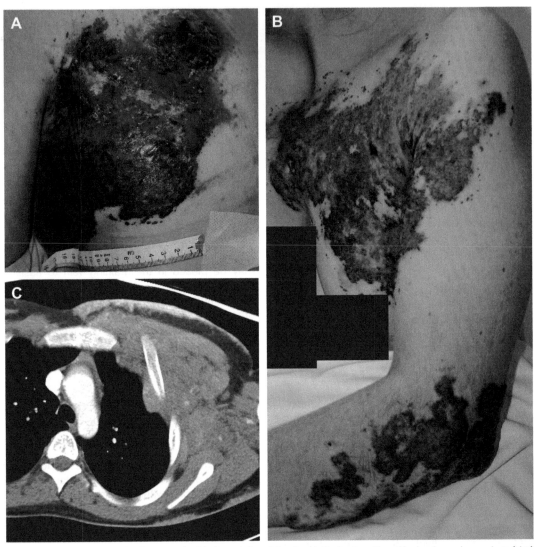

Fig. 3. 16-year-old girl with a history of a birthmark involving her left chest wall, axilla, back, and arm since birth. (*A, B*) A large flat patch partially raised with purple and red color skin, and well-demarcated borders involving the left chest wall, axilla, back, and arm. (*A*) The back shows an area of ulceration with drainage of serosanguinous fluid. (*C*) Axial CT contrast-enhanced image of the chest shows multiple lobulated enhancing masses within the left axilla. There is also thickening of the superficial skin of the anterior chest wall and back with enhancement.

effective for type IIIb (83%) than for type IIIa or mixed types (≤50%) (level IV evidence). Despite the use of the transarterial approach, direct puncture and transvenous approaches were more relevant for treating type II AVMs. Only the transarterial approach was used for treating type IIIa; both direct puncture and transarterial approaches were used for treating the other types. In a retrospective review of absolute alcohol use in soft tissue AVMs involving a series of 32 patients (142 total sessions), Shin and colleagues[105] concluded that dose limitations of less than 0.5 to 1 mg/kg and a maximum dose per injection of 10 mL do not cause an overall increase in pulmonary artery pressure.

The most common complications reported with alcohol include skin and peripheral nerve injury. Less common complications include cardiopulmonary collapse, end-organ damage, and renal failure.[104–107]

n-BCA

BCA belongs to a group of cyanoacrylates or adhesive glues. Because BCA is a clear substance, it mixed with Ethiodol and tantalum to provide radiopacity during fluoroscopic injection. The amount of Ethiodol mixed with the glue controls the rate of polymerization. When the glue is exposed to the anions in blood, it polymerizes and

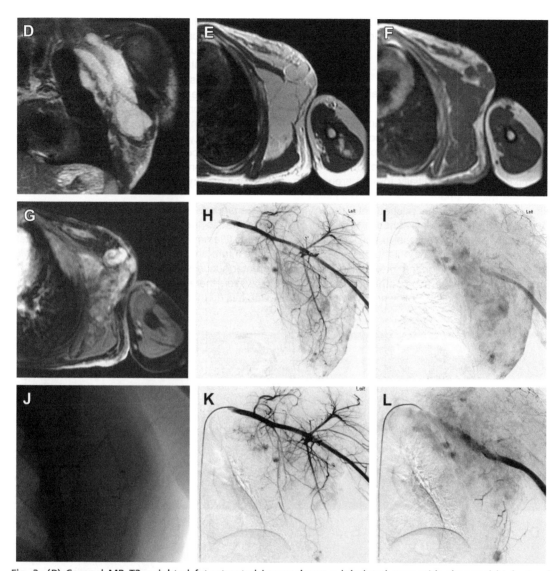

Fig. 3. (D) Coronal MR T2-weighted fat-saturated image shows a lobulated mass with abnormal high signal within the left axilla. (E) Axial MR T2-weighted image of the chest shows a large lobulated mass with high signal involving the left lateral chest wall. (F) Axial MR T1-weighted image of the chest at the same level as (E) shows a large lobulated mass with the same signal as muscle involving the left lateral chest wall. Note the thickening of the superficial skin involving the left back. (G) Axial MR postgadolinium fat-saturated T1-weighted image of the chest at the same level as (E, F) shows enhancement of the mass and skin. (H, I) Left subclavian arteriogram in the arterial phase (H) and the late venous phase (I) shows a large area of hypervascularity involving the left lateral chest wall with pooling of contrast in the late venous phase. (J) Spot fluoroscopy image shows injection of particulate material mixed with contrast material through a microcatheter placed within the left lateral thoracic artery. (K, L) Left subclavian arteriogram after embolization of the left lateral thoracic artery in the arterial phase (K) and the late venous phase (L) shows no filling of the inferior portion of the mass involving the left lateral chest wall.

forms a cast, which adheres to the vessel wall. To prevent polymerization within the catheter, 5% dextrose in water (D5W) is infused before the injection. Once the glue refluxes retrograde around the tip of the microcatheter, it is removed to prevent gluing of the catheter within the vessel. The glue causes an acute fibrotic inflammatory reaction that progresses over several weeks as a foreign-body giant-cell granulomatous reaction. There are limited reports in the literature describing its use in peripheral AVMs. Reports on the use of BCA have mostly involved embolization of cerebral AVMs (level I evidence).[108] Complications of its use include pulmonary embolism, catheter retention, formation of a glue mass that can be a source of infection, tissue erosion, or muscle dysfunction.[107,109,110]

Ethylene vinyl alcohol (Onyx)

Ethylene vinyl alcohol copolymer (Onyx) is a nonadhesive liquid embolic agent. It is dissolved in dimethyl sulfoxide (DMSO). Tantalum powder is added to the mixture for fluoroscopic visualization. The risk of catheter retention is less than with BCA given the nonadhesive properties of the mixture. A plug is initially formed around the tip of the microcatheter acting as a backstop to allow the mixture to be pushed into the AVM. The concentration of Onyx chosen is based on the rapidity of flow within the tumor vasculature. Embolization is continued until the desired degree of tumor penetrance or the maximal degree of Onyx reflux along the microcatheter is reached. Suction is then applied, followed by withdrawal of the microcatheter. Embolization of other feeding pedicles then proceeds in a similar manner (Fig. 4). Reports of its use have mostly involved embolization of cerebral AVMs. There are a few small case series on its use in peripheral AVMs (level IV evidence).[111] The published literature reports cure rates for cerebral AVM lesions up to 24%, and an average lesion volume reduction of 70% with 3.8% morbidity and 2.5% mortality (level IV and level I evidence).[112,113] Complications of its use include pulmonary embolism, catheter retention, and nerve injury.

Gamma knife

Stereotactic radiosurgery with a cobalt x-ray source (Gamma knife) may be successful in obliterating intracranial AVM in up to 80% of cases, with greater success in lesions less than 4 cm.[114–116] However, there is lack of certainty of obliteration with this method.

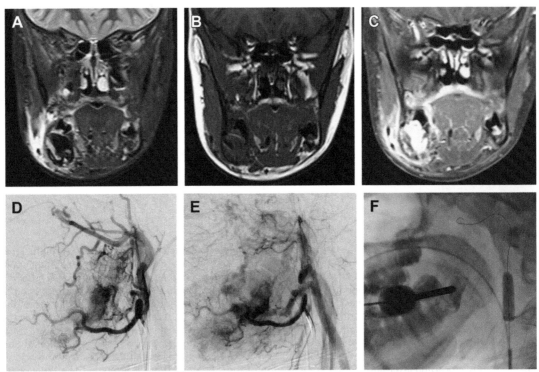

Fig. 4. 9-year-old girl with a history of bleeding from her right lower teeth. (A) Coronal MR fat-saturation T2-weighted image of the face shows multiple flow voids within and surrounding the right mandible with abnormal high signal in the adjacent soft tissues. (B) Coronal MR T1-weighted image of the face at the same level as (A) shows enlargement of the right mandible with multiple flow voids. (C) Coronal MR postgadolinium fat-saturated T1-weighted image of the face at the same level as (A, B) shows enhancement within the corresponding flow voids with additional enhancement of the surrounding soft tissues. (D, E) Lateral right external carotid angiogram in the arterial phase (D) and the late venous phase (E) shows an AVM within right ramus and angle of the mandible. The arterial supply is from the inferior alveolar artery and proximal branches from the facial artery. A large venous pouch is seen within the ramus and angle of the mandible. (F) Lateral spot fluoroscopy image shows an occlusion balloon with the main trunk of the right external carotid artery for flow control with alcohol mixed with contrast injected through a needle placed within the venous pouch.

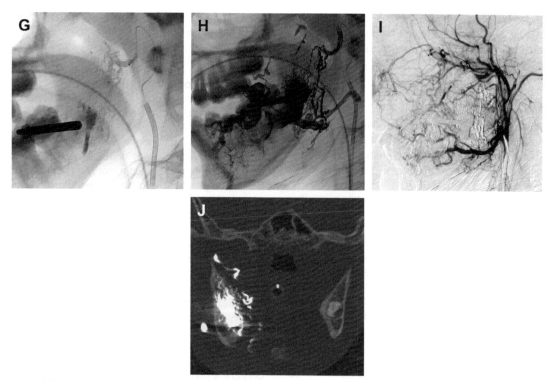

Fig. 4. (*G*) Lateral inferior alveolar arteriogram shows multiple small arterial branches off the main trunk filling the venous pouch. (*H*) Lateral spot fluoroscopy image shows the Onyx (eV3, Irvine, CA) cast after embolization. (*I*) Lateral right external carotid angiogram after embolization shows the Onyx cast with no arterial venous shunt. (*J*) Coronal DynaCT image after embolization shows the Onyx cast within the mandible and the surrounding arterial feeders to the AVM.

Surgery

Surgery alone in not generally effective for treatment of AVM, with significant risk of recurrence. When surgery is indicated, it should be preceded by embolization of the lesion and/or feeding vessels 48 to 72 hours prior to surgery; whenever possible to reduce intraoperative blood loss.

HEMANGIOMAS
Clinical Presentation

The clinical appearance of the lesion depends mainly on the depth of the lesion with 2 classic presentations described for an infantile hemangioma. Superficial hemangioma (previously called strawberry hemangioma) describes an infantile hemangioma that is superficial in location and generally bright red in color. In contrast, deep hemangiomas (previously called mixed or cavernous hemangioma) describes a deeper lesion that may be colorless or have a bluish hue.[98] Most infantile hemangiomas are not visible at birth, but present within the first several weeks of infancy. The proliferative phase, which begins in infancy, involves rapid growth and may last up to 18 months at which point growth reaches a plateau. The hemangiomas then undergo an involution phase with complete regression seen in about 70% of cases by 7 years of age.[117]

Superficial hemangiomas are easy to diagnose on physical examination because of their characteristic red, raised, strawberrylike appearance. The lesions are soft on palpation and warm to the touch, and may be pulsatile, with an audible bruit during the proliferative phase. Skin color may appear blue due to dilated draining veins beneath the skin. Other characteristic physical features include a pale halo around the lesion and superficial telangiectasias. Usually, the first sign of the involution phase is marked by a change from the bright reddish, purplish, or crimson color of the cutaneous component to a grayish, patchy, less intense vascular soft tissue, with decrease or absent pulsations. Involuting lesions have a soft fatty consistency.

Congenital hemangiomas

Congenital hemangiomas have a similar physical appearance to infantile hemangiomas, however these lesions are present at birth and do not undergo a proliferative phase. Two forms exist: the rapidly involuting congenital hemangioma (RICH) and the noninvoluting congenital hemangioma (NICH).[118]

Natural History/Epidemiology

Infantile hemangioma

Infantile hemangiomas are the most prevalent benign tumor of infancy, appearing in as many as 10% to 12% of children less than 1 year of age, with double this incidence in preterm infants weighing less than 1000 g.[119,120] In the children of mothers who have undergone chorionic villus sampling, the incidence of hemangiomas has been report to be 10 times higher.[121] The female-to-male predominance is about 4:1.

Hemangiomas are usually first noticed after birth and present as a small, irregular, red or blue cutaneous mark. They quickly undergo a proliferative phase that is variable in length and intensity, but usually lasts for 3 to 9 months[59] In most cases, endothelial cell hyperplasia plateaus, which leads to spontaneous regression. This involuting period usually occurs when the child is between 7 to 8 months and 7 to 9 years of age.[120,122,123] To date, no evidence-based algorithm exists to stratify which tumors will likely involute versus those likely to remain unchanged. Even though a lesion may involute, more than 50% will leave stigmata as evident by telangiectasias, scarring from ulceration, hypoelastic patches, facial discoloration, pitting, or fibrofatty replacement of tissue.[124–126]

Several syndromes have been associated with hemangiomas including PHACES (posterior fossa malformations, hemangiomas, arterial anomalies, coarctation of the aorta and other cardiac defects, and eye abnormalities), Dandy-Walker, Klippel-Trenaunay, Sturge-Weber, Beckwith-Wiedeman, von Hippel-Lindau, and Osler-Weber-Rendu syndromes.[98] Despite contradictions in the literature, the Kasabach-Merritt phenomenon (consumptive coagulopathy and thrombocytopenia) does not have an association with true hemangiomas. Current evidence suggests that the discolored raised cutaneous lesions believed to be hemangiomas in Kasabach-Merritt syndrome are kaposiform hemangioendotheliomas or tufted angiomas.[127]

Congenital hemangiomas

Congenital hemangioma is a vascular lesion that completes the proliferative phase before birth. A specific glucose transport protein GLUT-1 has been identified as specific to hemangiomas of infancy but is not expressed by congenital hemangiomas or vascular malformations.[5,118,128] Two forms exist: RICH and NICH.[118] RICHs involute more rapidly than hemangiomas of infancy, usually within the first 14 months of life.[98] NICHs do not involute but grow in proportion to the child.

Diagnostic Imaging

The hallmark of hemangiomas on imaging is the combination of a homogeneous, solid, parenchymal mass with evidence of increased vascularity.

Grayscale ultrasonography depicts a well-demarcated mass with variable echogenicity. Color-flow Doppler shows a highly vascular mass. During the proliferative phase, hemangiomas demonstrate high flow velocities, which become normal during the involutional phase.

On nonenhanced CT images, the mass is homogeneous and isodense to muscle in the proliferative phase and becomes heterogeneous with areas of low attenuation consistent with fat in the involutional phase. Contrast-enhanced CT demonstrates uniform enhancement of the mass. Phleboliths are uncommon in true hemangiomas.

MR imaging shows a well-demarcated soft tissue mass. T1-weighted imaging shows a homogeneous mass with intermediate signal intensity during the proliferative phase. During the involution phase, the mass has a more heterogeneous signal appearance with focal areas of fat replacement. On T2-weighted images, the mass is homogeneous and moderately hyperintense during the proliferative phase and more heterogeneous during involution. High-flow vessels are frequently seen at the periphery of the mass. On the postcontrast images during the proliferative phase, the mass enhances homogeneously. Phleboliths produce areas of low signal within the mass on the gradient echo sequence and are commonly not seen in hemangiomas.

Conventional angiography demonstrates a hypervascular mass with parenchymal enhancement and enlarged arterial feeding vessels along with prominent draining veins.

Treatment

Knowledge of the natural history of hemangiomas is important in determining the proper treatment options. Because most hemangiomas involute with time, observation is usually the recommended treatment unless the patient has symptoms related to the lesion. A recent Cochrane Database Systemic Review on interventions for infantile hemangiomas of the skin found limited evidence from individual randomized controlled trials to support existing interventions (corticosteroids and PDL) for infantile hemangiomas.[129] For patients with symptoms related to the lesion, surgical resection is the standard of care because this lets the child reach a normal appearance during the critical years of development.[130] Early intervention is gaining wider acceptance.[130]

Medical

Corticosteroids

Steroid therapy is a long-established first-line treatment. This may be administered intralesionally (triamcinolone 25 mg/mL, 3–5 mg/kg) or orally (prednisolone 2 mg/kg/d tapered down every 2 weeks), and has been shown to induce a dramatic response in about one-third of cases, an equivocal response in one-third, and continued growth in the remaining one-third (level IV evidence).[131,132] Steroids are effective in the early, active, proliferating phase of a hemangioma, which occurs in the first 6 to 8 months.[133–135]

Potential complications of corticosteroid use include immunosuppression leading to an increased risk of infection.[136] Cushingoid changes, increased appetite, irritability, and failure to thrive are reversible.[137] In an effort to overcome the systemic side effects and the risk with intralesion injections, topical steroids have been used.[138,139] Systemic or local steroids are not always effective in capillary hemangiomas, with the exception of Kasabach-Merritt syndrome.[140] It may take 1 to 2 weeks to observe a response to the steroids; sometimes involution can occur too rapidly with necrosis and bleeding leading to difficulty in the reconstruction. For those hemangiomas that are resistant to steroid therapy, other treatment modalities can be used.

Interferon-α2a, vincristine, and others

Interferon-α2a has been used in the treatment of life-threatening hemangiomas with excellent response rates, but is no longer recommended because of the high incidence of severe spastic diplegia, which is usually irreversible and sometimes presents months after treatment (level IV evidence).[141,142]

Vincristine

Vincristine has been described as an alternative treatment in cases that are resistant to steroids, and is believed to act as an antiangiogenic through its effect on vascular endothelial growth factor.[143] Vincristine has been shown to have a low incidence of side effects in children, but it is a vesicant and therefore extravasation must be avoided otherwise skin necrosis may ensue (level IV evidence).[144]

Propanolol

Propanolol therapy has recently been reported to be a highly effective treatment of infantile hemangioma and is emerging as a first-line therapy.[145,146] Approximately 95% to 100% of patients show a response to this type of treatment with minimal side effects.[147–150] In a retrospective study, propranolol was superior to oral prednisone in inducing a more rapid and greater clinical improvement in patients with infantile hemangioma (level IV evidence).[148] β-Blockers have well-known side effects that include transient bradycardia, hypotension, and bronchospasm. Reduction in lipolysis, glycogenolysis, and gluconeogenesis by β-blockers predispose patients to hypoglycemia, with potential adverse neurologic sequelae.[151,152]

Bleomycin

Bleomycin is a glycooligopeptide antibiotic that has antineoplastic activity, an apoptotic effect on immature cells with a high turnover, and a sclerosing effect on vascular endothelium.[21,153–155] The indications for bleomycin injection include painful lesions, bleeding, ulceration, and lesions with a lower incidence of spontaneous resolution.[156] Injection is described through adjacent nonaffected tissue into subcutaneous and deep tissue planes or by advancing the needle into the hemangioma and injecting radially.[157] Concentrations of 0.5 to 2 mg/mL are recommended with lower doses recommended for infants and superficial lesions.[21,155] A maximum dose of 15 mg per session is advised. Injections should be performed at intervals of 2 to 8 weeks and 4 to 8 injections are usually required depending on the size of the lesion and the response.[155,157] Complications include hypopigmentation, hyperpigmentation, scarring, local ulceration, flulike symptoms, and partial hair loss.[21,157] Complete resolution was found to occur in 56% of patients, with an overall response rate of 93%, and 82% of lesions demonstrated complete response or significant improvement (level IV evidence).[158]

Radiation

Hemangiomas are responsive to radiation therapy, however this therapy is no longer favored because of long-term side effects, which include malignancy, regional growth impairment, and scarring (level IV evidence).[159–161]

Laser

Lasers are commonly used to treat hemangiomas for 3 distinct indications: treatment of the proliferative phase, treatment of ulcerations, and the treatment of residual telangiectasias after involution is complete.[162] Various devices can be used to treat hemangiomas, including PDL, Nd:YAG, alexandrite, and potassium titanyl phosphate (KTP) platforms.

The most commonly used device is the PDL, which is regarded as the treatment of choice for superficial lesions. It does not penetrate as deeply as long-wavelength lasers. It is particularly useful in photocoagulating ulcerated lesions leading to improved reepithelization and decreasing pain.[163]

Thicker deep lesions may have an increased deoxyhemoglobin/oxyhemoglobin ratio, thereby shifting the absorption curve of these lesions to the near-infrared range (700–1200 nm). The deeper penetrating lasers are less commonly used in the treatment of deep hemangiomas because of the increased risk of deep thermal injury and subsequent scarring. Oxyhemoglobin strongly absorbs at 532 nm, but when a laser applies this wavelength transcutaneously, its poor penetration limits its effect on deeper hemangiomas. The 532-nm platform has been shown to be inferior to PDL in treating hemangiomas.[164] Intralesional bare-fiber KTP treatment of hemangiomas has been reported as an option for treating the deeper components of cutaneous hemangiomas (level IV evidence).[165,166]

Embolization

Arterial embolization can produce ischemia and necrosis of a hemangioma, which can expedite involution.[167–169] This approach is usually performed before surgical excision, however this can also be applied in patients for whom drug treatment has failed, when rapid mass reduction is required, or in cases of cardiac failure.[170–172] Embolization of at least 70% of the arterial supply is necessary to produce a clinical response.[173] The mass decreases in size in about 1 week and then stabilizes before following a regressive course (Fig. 5).

Careful examination of the angiogram is necessary before embolization of a hemangioma in the head and neck region given that the external carotid to internal carotid arterial anastomosis is open in infants and children. Volume overload, radiation, and contrast dose are issues when performing an embolization in small children. Therefore, glue (BCA) is the preferred embolic agent of choice given that this can be used with less contrast and radiation dose to the child.

Direct percutaneous embolization of the lesion can also be performed with alcohol, Onyx, or glue alone or in combination with transarterial embolization.[174] Better penetration of the lesion can be obtained with direct percutaneous embolization of the lesion, however confirmation of an intravascular location is absolutely necessary to

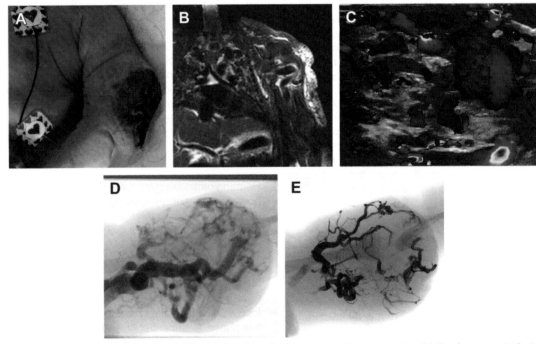

Fig. 5. 12-day-old boy with a large RICH involving the left upper extremity present since birth who presented with high cardiac output failure. (*A*) The large mass involving the left upper extremity with a central area of necrosis. (*B*) Coronal MR fat-saturation T2-weighted image of the chest and left upper extremity shows a hyperintense mass within the left upper extremity with enlarged arterial flow voids within the adjacent soft tissues supplying the mass. (*C*) Color Doppler ultrasonography image shows the hypervascularity of the mass. (*D*) Left brachial arteriogram shows an enlarged brachial artery with multiple arterial feeders filling the hypervascular mass with early venous drainage. (*E*) Spot fluoroscopy image shows the Onyx cast within the lesion after embolization.

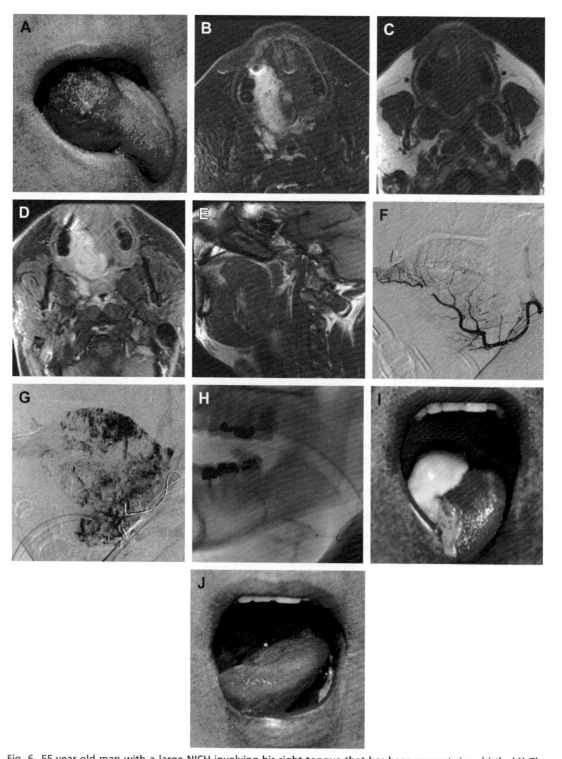

Fig. 6. 55-year-old man with a large NICH involving his right tongue that has been present since birth. (*A*) The large mass involving the right tongue. Note the normal tongue is deviated to the left. (*B*) Axial MR fat-saturation T2-weighted image of the face shows an area of abnormal high signal within the right tongue with small central round areas of low signal. (*C*) Axial MR T1-weighted image of the face at the same level as (*B*) shows a mass with the same signal as muscle involving the right tongue. (*D*) Axial MR postgadolinium fat-saturated T1-weighted image of the face at the same level as (*B, C*) shows uniform enhancement of the mass. (*E*) Sagittal MR T1-weighted image of the face shows the cranial caudal extent of the mass involving the right tongue. (*F, G*) Lateral right lingual arteriogram in the arterial phase (*F*) and the late venous phase (*G*) shows a hypervascular mass with pooling of contrast on the late venous phase. (*H*) Spot fluoroscopy images shows injection of alcohol mixed with contrast material through a microcatheter placed within the right lingual artery. (*I*) Two weeks after embolization shows complete necrosis of the mass embolized with alcohol. (*J*) A relatively normal tongue after removal of the necrotic mass. Note the uvula and tonsils are now visible.

prevent complications (**Fig. 6**). Furthermore, intralesional bleomycin has been shown to be effective in treating infantile hemangiomas (level IV evidence).[155,158]

Surgery

Surgical resection of hemangiomas is indicated when complete resection without a resulting functional or anatomic deficit is possible. For patients with symptoms related to the lesion, surgical resection is the standard of care because this lets the child reach a normal appearance during the critical years of development.[130]

SUMMARY

Vascular malformations are congenital lesions secondary to errors in the development of arteries, capillaries, veins, or lymphatics. Most of these lesions are sporadic, however a certain percentage present with syndromes, which the treating physician should be aware of. These lesions are best treated by a multidisciplinary team comprising pediatricians, plastic surgeons, dermatologists, radiologists, otolaryngologists, and oral maxillary facial surgeons. Minimal invasive percutaneous therapies play a vital role in the treatment of vascular malformations as a sole therapy of choice or as an adjunct to surgery. Currently, a wide variety of embolic agents are used in the treatment of vascular malformations, however to date there are no published randomized control trials comparing the efficacy of the different agents. Further animal and clinical studies are needed to help optimize the treatment for each type of vascular malformation.

REFERENCES

1. Mulliken JB, Glowacki J. Classification of pediatric vascular lesions. Plast Reconstr Surg 1982;70: 120–1.
2. Legiehn GM, Heran MK. Venous malformations: classification, development, diagnosis, and interventional radiologic management. Radiol Clin North Am 2008;46:545–97, vi.
3. Tucci FM, De Vincentiis GC, Sitzia E, et al. Head and neck vascular anomalies in children. Int J Pediatr Otorhinolaryngol 2009;73(Suppl 1):S71–6.
4. Burrows PE, Mulliken JB, Fellows KE, et al. Childhood hemangiomas and vascular malformations: angiographic differentiation. AJR Am J Roentgenol 1983;141:483–8.
5. Mulliken JB, Glowacki J. Hemangiomas and vascular malformations in infants and children: a classification based on endothelial characteristics. Plast Reconstr Surg 1982;69:412–22.
6. Dompmartin A, Ballieux F, Thibon P, et al. Elevated D-dimer level in the differential diagnosis of venous malformations. Arch Dermatol 2009;145: 1239–44.
7. Brouillard P, Vikkula M. Genetic causes of vascular malformations. Hum Mol Genet 2007;16(Spec No. 2):R140–9.
8. Boon LM, Mulliken JB, Vikkula M, et al. Assignment of a locus for dominantly inherited venous malformations to chromosome 9p. Hum Mol Genet 1994;3:1583–7.
9. Gallione CJ, Pasyk KA, Boon LM, et al. A gene for familial venous malformations maps to chromosome 9p in a second large kindred. J Med Genet 1995;32:197–9.
10. Vikkula M, Boon LM, Carraway KL 3rd, et al. Vascular dysmorphogenesis caused by an activating mutation in the receptor tyrosine kinase TIE2. Cell 1996;87:1181–90.
11. Calvert JT, Riney TJ, Kontos CD, et al. Allelic and locus heterogeneity in inherited venous malformations. Hum Mol Genet 1999;8:1279–89.
12. Burrows PE, Mason KP. Percutaneous treatment of low flow vascular malformations. J Vasc Interv Radiol 2004;15:431–45.
13. Trop I, Dubois J, Guibaud L, et al. Soft-tissue venous malformations in pediatric and young adult patients: diagnosis with Doppler US. Radiology 1999;212:841–5.
14. Dubois J, Soulez G, Oliva VL, et al. Soft-tissue venous malformations in adult patients: imaging and therapeutic issues. Radiographics 2001;21: 1519–31.
15. Moukaddam H, Pollak J, Haims AH. MRI characteristics and classification of peripheral vascular malformations and tumors. Skeletal Radiol 2009;38: 535–47.
16. Fayad LM, Hazirolan T, Carrino JA, et al. Venous malformations: MR imaging features that predict skin burns after percutaneous alcohol embolization procedures. Skeletal Radiol 2008;37:895–901.
17. van Rijswijk CS, van der Linden E, van der Woude HJ, et al. Value of dynamic contrast-enhanced MR imaging in diagnosing and classifying peripheral vascular malformations. AJR Am J Roentgenol 2002;178:1181–7.
18. Puig S, Casati B, Staudenherz A, et al. Vascular low-flow malformations in children: current concepts for classification, diagnosis and therapy. Eur J Radiol 2005;53:35–45.
19. Dubois JM, Sebag GH, De Prost Y, et al. Soft-tissue venous malformations in children: percutaneous sclerotherapy with Ethibloc. Radiology 1991;180: 195–8.
20. Puig S, Aref H, Chigot V, et al. Classification of venous malformations in children and implications for sclerotherapy. Pediatr Radiol 2003;33:99–103.

21. Muir T, Kirsten M, Fourie P, et al. Intralesional bleomycin injection (IBI) treatment for haemangiomas and congenital vascular malformations. Pediatr Surg Int 2004;19:766–73.

22. Lee BB. New approaches to the treatment of congenital vascular malformations (CVMs)–a single centre experience. Eur J Vasc Endovasc Surg 2005;30:184–97.

23. O'Donovan JC, Donaldson JS, Morello FP, et al. Symptomatic hemangiomas and venous malformations in infants, children, and young adults: treatment with percutaneous injection of sodium tetradecyl sulfate. AJR Am J Roentgenol 1997;169:723–9.

24. Chen Y, Li Y, Zhu Q, et al. Fluoroscopic intralesional injection with pingyangmycin lipiodol emulsion for the treatment of orbital venous malformations. AJR Am J Roentgenol 2008;190:966–71.

25. Wallace MJ, Kuo MD, Glaiberman C, et al. Three-dimensional C-arm cone-beam CT: applications in the interventional suite. J Vasc Interv Radiol 2008;19:799–813.

26. Berenguer B, Burrows PE, Zurakowski D, et al. Sclerotherapy of craniofacial venous malformations: complications and results. Plast Reconstr Surg 1999;104:1–11 [discussion: 2–5].

27. Lee BB, Do YS, Byun HS, et al. Advanced management of venous malformation with ethanol sclerotherapy: mid-term results. J Vasc Surg 2003;37:533–8.

28. Mason KP, Neufeld EJ, Karian VE, et al. Coagulation abnormalities in pediatric and adult patients after sclerotherapy or embolization of vascular anomalies. AJR Am J Roentgenol 2001;177:1359–63.

29. Wong GA, Armstrong DC, Robertson JM. Cardiovascular collapse during ethanol sclerotherapy in a pediatric patient. Paediatr Anaesth 2006;16:343–6.

30. Donnelly LF, Bisset GS 3rd, Adams DM. Marked acute tissue swelling following percutaneous sclerosis of low-flow vascular malformations: a predictor of both prolonged recovery and therapeutic effect. Pediatr Radiol 2000;30:415–9.

31. Anadon MJ, Almendral J, Gonzalez P, et al. Alcohol concentration determines the type of atrial arrhythmia induced in a porcine model of acute alcoholic intoxication. Pacing Clin Electrophysiol 1996;19:1962–7.

32. Chi LM, Wu WG. Mechanism of hemolysis of red blood cell mediated by ethanol. Biochim Biophys Acta 1991;1062:46–50.

33. Behnia R. Systemic effects of absolute alcohol embolization in a patient with a congenital arteriovenous malformation of the lower extremity. Anesth Analg 1995;80:415–7.

34. Hammer FD, Boon LM, Mathurin P, et al. Ethanol sclerotherapy of venous malformations: evaluation of systemic ethanol contamination. J Vasc Interv Radiol 2001;12:595–600.

35. Mason KP, Michna E, Zurakowski D, et al. Serum ethanol levels in children and adults after ethanol embolization or sclerotherapy for vascular anomalies. Radiology 2000;217:127–32.

36. Su L, Fan X, Zheng L, et al. Absolute ethanol sclerotherapy for venous malformations in the face and neck. J Oral Maxillofac Surg 2010;68:1622–7.

37. Yun WS, Kim YW, Lee KB, et al. Predictors of response to percutaneous ethanol sclerotherapy (PES) in patients with venous malformations: analysis of patient self-assessment and imaging. J Vasc Surg 2009;50:581–9, 589.e1.

38. Lee IH, Kim KH, Jeon P, et al. Ethanol sclerotherapy for the management of craniofacial venous malformations: the interim results. Korean J Radiol 2009;10:269–76.

39. de Lorimier AA. Sclerotherapy for venous malformations. J Pediatr Surg 1995;30:188–93 [discussion: 94].

40. Gelbert F, Enjolras O, Deffrenne D, et al. Percutaneous sclerotherapy for venous malformation of the lips: a retrospective study of 23 patients. Neuroradiology 2000;42:692–6.

41. Siniluoto TM, Svendsen PA, Wikholm GM, et al. Percutaneous sclerotherapy of venous malformations of the head and neck using sodium tetradecyl sulphate (sotradecol). Scand J Plast Reconstr Surg Hand Surg 1997;31:145–50.

42. Cabrera J, Cabrera J Jr, Garcia-Olmedo MA. Sclerosants in microfoam. A new approach in angiology. Int Angiol 2001;20:322–9.

43. Yamaki T, Nozaki M, Fujiwara O, et al. Duplex-guided foam sclerotherapy for the treatment of the symptomatic venous malformations of the face. Dermatol Surg 2002;28:619–22.

44. Choi DJ, Alomari AI, Chaudry G, et al. Neurointerventional management of low-flow vascular malformations of the head and neck. Neuroimaging Clin N Am 2009;19:199–218.

45. Hussar DA, Stevenson T. New drugs: denosumab, dienogest/estradiol valerate, and polidocanol. J Am Pharm Assoc 2010;50:658–62.

46. Marrocco-Trischitta MM, Guerrini P, Abeni D, et al. Reversible cardiac arrest after polidocanol sclerotherapy of peripheral venous malformation. Dermatol Surg 2002;28:153–5.

47. Tessari L, Cavezzi A, Frullini A. Preliminary experience with a new sclerosing foam in the treatment of varicose veins. Dermatol Surg 2001;27:58–60.

48. Yamaki T, Nozaki M, Sakurai H, et al. Prospective randomized efficacy of ultrasound-guided foam sclerotherapy compared with ultrasound-guided liquid sclerotherapy in the treatment of symptomatic venous malformations. J Vasc Surg 2008;47:578–84.

49. Cabrera J, Cabrera J Jr, Garcia-Olmedo MA, et al. Treatment of venous malformations with

sclerosant in microfoam form. Arch Dermatol 2003;139:1409–16.

50. Kaji N, Kurita M, Ozaki M, et al. Experience of sclerotherapy and embolosclerotherapy using ethanolamine oleate for vascular malformations of the head and neck. Scand J Plast Reconstr Surg Hand Surg 2009;43:126–36.

51. Spence J, Krings T, terBrugge KG, et al. Percutaneous sclerotherapy for facial venous malformations: subjective clinical and objective MR imaging follow-up results. AJNR Am J Neuroradiol 2010;31:955–60.

52. Lacey B, Rootman J, Marotta TR. Distensible venous malformations of the orbit: clinical and hemodynamic features and a new technique of management. Ophthalmology 1999;106:1197–209.

53. Sidhu MK, Perkins JA, Shaw DW, et al. Ultrasound-guided endovenous diode laser in the treatment of congenital venous malformations: preliminary experience. J Vasc Interv Radiol 2005;16:879–84.

54. Werner JA, Lippert BM, Gottschlich S, et al. Ultrasound-guided interstitial Nd:YAG laser treatment of voluminous hemangiomas and vascular malformations in 92 patients. Laryngoscope 1998;108:463–70.

55. Chang CJ, Fisher DM, Chen YR. Intralesional photocoagulation of vascular anomalies of the tongue. Br J Plast Surg 1999;52:178–81.

56. Vesnaver A, Dovsak DA. Treatment of vascular lesions in the head and neck using Nd:YAG laser. J Craniomaxillofac Surg 2006;34:17–24.

57. Scherer K, Waner M. Nd:YAG lasers (1,064 nm) in the treatment of venous malformations of the face and neck: challenges and benefits. Lasers Med Sci 2007;22:119–26.

58. Sarig O, Kimel S, Orenstein A. Laser treatment of venous malformations. Ann Plast Surg 2006;57:20–4.

59. Enjolras O, Mulliken JB. The current management of vascular birthmarks. Pediatr Dermatol 1993;10:311–3.

60. Burrows PE, Fellows KE. Techniques for management of pediatric vascular anomalies. In: Cope C, editor. Current techniques in interventional radiology. Philadelphia: Current Medicine; 1994. p. 11–7.

61. Al-Adnani M, Williams S, Rampling D, et al. Histopathological reporting of paediatric cutaneous vascular anomalies in relation to proposed multidisciplinary classification system. J Clin Pathol 2006;59:1278–82.

62. North PE, Waner M, Buckmiller L, et al. Vascular tumors of infancy and childhood: beyond capillary hemangioma. Cardiovasc Pathol 2006;15:303–17.

63. Smith RJ. Lymphatic malformations. Lymphat Res Biol 2004;2:25–31.

64. Perkins JA, Manning SC, Tempero RM, et al. Lymphatic malformations: review of current

treatment. Otolaryngol Head Neck Surg 2010;142:795–803, 803.e1.

65. de Serres LM, Sie KC, Richardson MA. Lymphatic malformations of the head and neck. A proposal for staging. Arch Otolaryngol Head Neck Surg 1995;121:577–82.

66. Smith MC, Zimmerman MB, Burke DK, et al. Efficacy and safety of OK-432 immunotherapy of lymphatic malformations. Laryngoscope 2009;119:107–15.

67. Abernethy LJ. Classification and imaging of vascular malformations in children. Eur Radiol 2003;13:2483–97.

68. Dubois J, Alison M. Vascular anomalies: what a radiologist needs to know. Pediatr Radiol 2010;40:895–905.

69. Dubois J, Garel L. Imaging and therapeutic approach of hemangiomas and vascular malformations in the pediatric age group. Pediatr Radiol 1999;29:879–93.

70. Burrows PE, Laor T, Paltiel H, et al. Diagnostic imaging in the evaluation of vascular birthmarks. Dermatol Clin 1998;16:455–88.

71. Mathur NN, Rana I, Bothra R, et al. Bleomycin sclerotherapy in congenital lymphatic and vascular malformations of head and neck. Int J Pediatr Otorhinolaryngol 2005;69:75–80.

72. Shiels WE 2nd, Kenney BD, Caniano DA, et al. Definitive percutaneous treatment of lymphatic malformations of the trunk and extremities. J Pediatr Surg 2008;43:136–9 [discussion: 40].

73. Shiels WE 2nd, Kang DR, Murakami JW, et al. Percutaneous treatment of lymphatic malformations. Otolaryngol Head Neck Surg 2009;141:219–24.

74. Okazaki T, Iwatani S, Yanai T, et al. Treatment of lymphangioma in children: our experience of 128 cases. J Pediatr Surg 2007;42:386–9.

75. Dubois J, Garel L, Abela A, et al. Lymphangiomas in children: percutaneous sclerotherapy with an alcoholic solution of zein. Radiology 1997;204:651–4.

76. Alomari AI, Karian VE, Lord DJ, et al. Percutaneous sclerotherapy for lymphatic malformations: a retrospective analysis of patient-evaluated improvement. J Vasc Interv Radiol 2006;17:1639–48.

77. Cahill AM, Nijs EL. Pediatric vascular malformations: pathophysiology, diagnosis, and the role of interventional radiology. Cardiovasc Intervent Radiol 2011;34:691–704.

78. Nehra D, Jacobson L, Barnes P, et al. Doxycycline sclerotherapy as primary treatment of head and neck lymphatic malformations in children. J Pediatr Surg 2008;43:451–60.

79. Svendsen PA, Wikholm G, Rodriguez M, et al. Direct puncture and sclerotherapy with sotradecol ((r)). Orbital lymphatic malformations. Interv Neuroradiol 2001;7:193–9.

80. Ogita S, Tsuto T, Tokiwa K, et al. Intracystic injection of OK-432: a new sclerosing therapy for cystic hygroma in children. Br J Surg 1987;74:690–1.

81. Ogita S, Tsuto T, Nakamura K, et al. OK-432 therapy for lymphangioma in children: why and how does it work? J Pediatr Surg 1996;31:477–80.

82. Ohta N, Fukase S, Watanabe T, et al. Effects and mechanism of OK-432 therapy in various neck cystic lesions. Acta Otolaryngol 2010;130:1287–92.

83. Poldervaart MT, Breugem CC, Speleman L, et al. Treatment of lymphatic malformations with OK-432 (Picibanil): review of the literature. J Craniofac Surg 2009;20:1159–62.

84. Yoo JC, Ahn Y, Lim YS, et al. OK-432 sclerotherapy in head and neck lymphangiomas: long-term follow-up result. Otolaryngol Head Neck Surg 2009;140:120–3.

85. Emran MA, Dubois J, Laberge L, et al. Alcoholic solution of zein (Ethibloc) sclerotherapy for treatment of lymphangiomas in children. J Pediatr Surg 2006;41:975–9.

86. Niramis R, Watanatittan S, Rattanasuwan T. Treatment of cystic hygroma by intralesional bleomycin injection: experience in 70 patients. Eur J Pediatr Surg 2010;20:178–82.

87. Zhong PQ, Zhi FX, Li R, et al. Long-term results of intratumorous bleomycin-A5 injection for head and neck lymphangioma. Oral Surg Oral Med Oral Pathol Oral Radiol Endod 1998;86:139–44.

88. Wiegand S, Eivazi B, Zimmermann AP, et al. Microcystic lymphatic malformations of the tongue: diagnosis, classification, and treatment. Arch Otolaryngol Head Neck Surg 2009;135:976–83.

89. Grimmer JF, Mulliken JB, Burrows PE, et al. Radiofrequency ablation of microcystic lymphatic malformation in the oral cavity. Arch Otolaryngol Head Neck Surg 2006;132:1251–6.

90. Elluru RG, Azizkhan RG. Cervicofacial vascular anomalies. II. Vascular malformations. Semin Pediatr Surg 2006;15:133–9.

91. Geronemus RG, Ashinoff R. The medical necessity of evaluation and treatment of port-wine stains. J Dermatol Surg Oncol 1991;17:76–9.

92. Eerola I, Boon LM, Mulliken JB, et al. Capillary malformation-arteriovenous malformation, a new clinical and genetic disorder caused by RASA1 mutations. Am J Hum Genet 2003;73:1240–9.

93. Frech M, John J, Pizon V, et al. Inhibition of GTPase activating protein stimulation of Ras-p21 GTPase by the Krev-1 gene product. Science 1990;249:169–71.

94. Tallman B, Tan OT, Morelli JG, et al. Location of port-wine stains and the likelihood of ophthalmic and/or central nervous system complications. Pediatrics 1991;87:323–7.

95. Geronemus RG, Quintana AT, Lou WW, et al. High-fluence modified pulsed dye laser photocoagulation with dynamic cooling of port-wine stains in infancy. Arch Dermatol 2000;136:942–3.

96. van der Horst CM, Koster PH, de Borgie CA, et al. Effect of the timing of treatment of port-wine stains with the flash-lamp-pumped pulsed-dye laser. N Engl J Med 1998;338:1028–33.

97. Cordoro KM, Speetzen LS, Koerper MA, et al. Physiologic changes in vascular birthmarks during early infancy: mechanisms and clinical implications. J Am Acad Dermatol 2009;60:669–75.

98. Enjolras O, Mulliken JB. Vascular tumors and vascular malformations (new issues). Adv Dermatol 1997;13:375–423.

99. Srinivasa RN, Burrows PE. Dural arteriovenous malformation in a child with Bannayan-Riley-Ruvalcaba Syndrome. AJNR Am J Neuroradiol 2006;27:1927–9.

100. Naidich JJ, Rofsky NM, Rosen R, et al. Arteriovenous malformation in a patient with Bannayan–Zonana syndrome. Clin Imaging 2001;25:130–2.

101. Tan WH, Baris HN, Burrows PE, et al. The spectrum of vascular anomalies in patients with PTEN mutations: implications for diagnosis and management. J Med Genet 2007;44:594–602.

102. Seki T, Yun J, Oh SP. Arterial endothelium-specific activin receptor-like kinase 1 expression suggests its role in arterialization and vascular remodeling. Circ Res 2003;93:682–9.

103. Taschner CA, Gieseke J, Le Thuc V, et al. Intracranial arteriovenous malformation: time-resolved contrast-enhanced MR angiography with combination of parallel imaging, keyhole acquisition, and k-space sampling techniques at 1.5 T. Radiology 2008;246:871–9.

104. Cho SK, Do YS, Shin SW, et al. Arteriovenous malformations of the body and extremities: analysis of therapeutic outcomes and approaches according to a modified angiographic classification. J Endovasc Ther 2006;13:527–38.

105. Shin BS, Do YS, Lee BB, et al. Multistage ethanol sclerotherapy of soft-tissue arteriovenous malformations: effect on pulmonary arterial pressure. Radiology 2005;235:1072–7.

106. Do YS, Park KB, Park HS, et al. Extremity arteriovenous malformations involving the bone: therapeutic outcomes of ethanol embolotherapy. J Vasc Interv Radiol 2010;21:807–16.

107. Yakes WF, Rossi P, Odink H. How I do it. Arteriovenous malformation management. Cardiovasc Intervent Radiol 1996;19:65–71.

108. n-BCA Trail Investigators. N-Butyl cyanoacrylate embolization of cerebral arteriovenous malformations: results of a prospective, randomized, multicenter trial. AJNR Am J Neuroradiol 2002;23:748–55.

109. Pollak JS, White RI Jr. The use of cyanoacrylate adhesives in peripheral embolization. J Vasc Interv Radiol 2001;12:907–13.

110. De Luca D, Piastra M, Pietrini D, et al. "Glue lung": pulmonary micro-embolism caused by the glue used during interventional radiology. Arch Dis Child 2008;93:263.

111. Arat A, Cil BE, Vargel I, et al. Embolization of high-flow craniofacial vascular malformations with onyx. AJNR Am J Neuroradiol 2007;28:1409–14.

112. Panagiotopoulos V, Gizewski E, Asgari S, et al. Embolization of intracranial arteriovenous malformations with ethylene-vinyl alcohol copolymer (Onyx). AJNR Am J Neuroradiol 2009;30:99–106.

113. Loh Y, Duckwiler GR. A prospective, multicenter, randomized trial of the Onyx liquid embolic system and N-butyl cyanoacrylate embolization of cerebral arteriovenous malformations. Clinical article. J Neurosurg 2010;113:733–41.

114. Pollock BE, Flickinger JC, Lunsford LD, et al. Factors associated with successful arteriovenous malformation radiosurgery. Neurosurgery 1998;42:1239–44 [discussion: 44–7].

115. Pollock BE, Gorman DA, Coffey RJ. Patient outcomes after arteriovenous malformation radiosurgical management: results based on a 5- to 14-year follow-up study. Neurosurgery 2003;52:1291–6 [discussion: 6–7].

116. Friedman WA. Radiosurgery versus surgery for arteriovenous malformations: the case for radiosurgery. Clin Neurosurg 1999;45:18–20.

117. Bingham HG. Predicting the course of a congenital hemangioma. Plast Reconstr Surg 1979;63:161–6.

118. Berenguer B, Mulliken JB, Enjolras O, et al. Rapidly involuting congenital hemangioma: clinical and histopathologic features. Pediatr Dev Pathol 2003;6:495–510.

119. Amir J, Metzker A, Krikler R, et al. Strawberry hemangioma in preterm infants. Pediatr Dermatol 1986;3:331–2.

120. Mueller BU, Mulliken JB. The infant with a vascular tumor. Semin Perinatol 1999;23:332–40.

121. Burton BK, Schulz CJ, Angle B, et al. An increased incidence of haemangiomas in infants born following chorionic villus sampling (CVS). Prenat Diagn 1995;15:209–14.

122. Fishman SJ, Mulliken JB. Hemangiomas and vascular malformations of infancy and childhood. Pediatr Clin North Am 1993;40:1177–200.

123. Razon MJ, Kraling BM, Mulliken JB, et al. Increased apoptosis coincides with onset of involution in infantile hemangioma. Microcirculation 1998;5:189–95.

124. Esterly NB. Cutaneous hemangiomas, vascular stains and associated syndromes. Curr Probl Pediatr 1987;17:1–69.

125. Esterly NB. Cutaneous hemangiomas, vascular stains and malformations, and associated syndromes. Curr Probl Pediatr 1996;26:3–39.

126. Maleville J, Taieb A, Roubaud E, et al. Immature cutaneous hemangiomas. Epidemiologic study of 351 cases. Ann Dermatol Venereol 1985;112:603–8 [in French].

127. Enjolras O, Wassef M, Mazoyer E, et al. Infants with Kasabach-Merritt syndrome do not have "true" hemangiomas. J Pediatr 1997;130:631–40.

128. Navarro OM, Laffan EE, Ngan BY. Pediatric soft-tissue tumors and pseudo-tumors: MR imaging features with pathologic correlation: part 1. Imaging approach, pseudotumors, vascular lesions, and adipocytic tumors. Radiographics 2009;29:887–906.

129. Leonardi-Bee J, Batta K, O'Brien C, et al. Interventions for infantile haemangiomas (strawberry birthmarks) of the skin. Cochrane Database Syst Rev 2011;(5):CD006545.

130. Waner M, Suen JY. Treatment Options for the management of hemangiomas. In: Waner M, Suen JY, editors. Hemangiomas and vascular malformations of the head and neck. New York: Wiley-Liss; 1999. p. 233–61.

131. Zarem HA, Edgerton MT. Induced resolution of cavernous hemangiomas following prednisolone therapy. Plast Reconstr Surg 1967;39:76–83.

132. Chim H, Gosain AK. Discussion: oral prednisolone for infantile hemangioma: efficacy and safety using a standardized treatment protocol. Plast Reconstr Surg 2011;128:753–4.

133. Greene AK, Couto RA. Oral prednisolone for infantile hemangioma: efficacy and safety using a standardized treatment protocol. Plast Reconstr Surg 2011;128:743–52.

134. Zhou Q, Yang XJ, Zheng JW, et al. Short-term high-dose oral prednisone on alternate days is safe and effective for treatment of infantile hemangiomas. Oral Surg Oral Med Oral Pathol Oral Radiol Endod 2010;109:166–7.

135. Pandey A, Gangopadhyay AN, Gopal SC, et al. Twenty years' experience of steroids in infantile hemangioma–a developing country's perspective. J Pediatr Surg 2009;44:688–94.

136. Gunn T, Reece ER, Metrakos K, et al. Depressed T cells following neonatal steroid treatment. Pediatrics 1981;67:61–7.

137. Sadan N, Wolach B. Treatment of hemangiomas of infants with high doses of prednisone. J Pediatr 1996;128:141–6.

138. Pandey A, Gangopadhyay AN, Sharma SP, et al. Evaluation of topical steroids in the treatment of superficial hemangioma. Skinmed 2010;8:9–11.

139. Serra AM, Soares FM, Cunha Junior AG, et al. Therapeutic management of skin hemangiomas in children. An Bras Dermatol 2010;85:307–17.

140. Haik BG, Jakobiec FA, Ellsworth RM, et al. Capillary hemangioma of the lids and orbit: an analysis of the clinical features and therapeutic results in 101 cases. Ophthalmology 1979;86:760–92.

141. Egbert JE, Nelson SC. Neurologic toxicity associated with interferon alfa treatment of capillary hemangioma. J AAPOS 1997;1:190.

142. Barlow CF, Priebe CJ, Mulliken JB, et al. Spastic diplegia as a complication of interferon Alfa-2a treatment of hemangiomas of infancy. J Pediatr 1998;132:527–30.

143. Enjolras O, Breviere GM, Roger G, et al. Vincristine treatment for function- and life-threatening infantile hemangioma. Arch Pediatr 2004;11:99–107 [in French].

144. Fawcett SL, Grant I, Hall PN, et al. Vincristine as a treatment for a large haemangioma threatening vital functions. Br J Plast Surg 2004;57:168–71.

145. Sans V, de la Roque ED, Berge J, et al. Propranolol for severe infantile hemangiomas: follow-up report. Pediatrics 2009;124:e423–31.

146. Leaute-Labreze C, Dumas de la Roque E, Hubiche T, et al. Propranolol for severe hemangiomas of infancy. N Engl J Med 2008;358:2649–51.

147. Schupp CJ, Kleber JB, Gunther P, et al. Propranolol therapy in 55 infants with infantile hemangioma: dosage, duration, adverse effects, and outcome. Pediatr Dermatol 2011;28(6):640–4.

148. Bertrand J, McCuaig C, Dubois J, et al. Propranolol versus prednisone in the treatment of infantile hemangiomas: a retrospective comparative study. Pediatr Dermatol 2011;28(6):649–54.

149. Zaher H, Rasheed H, Hegazy RA, et al. Oral propranolol: an effective, safe treatment for infantile hemangiomas. Eur J Dermatol 2011;21: 558–63.

150. Schiestl C, Neuhaus K, Zoller S, et al. Efficacy and safety of propranolol as first-line treatment for infantile hemangiomas. Eur J Pediatr 2011;170: 493–501.

151. Tan ST, Itinteang T, Leadbitter P. Low-dose propranolol for infantile haemangioma. J Plast Reconstr Aesthet Surg 2011;64:292–9.

152. Siegfried EC, Keenan WJ, Al-Jureidini S. More on propranolol for hemangiomas of infancy. N Engl J Med 2008;359:2846 [author reply: 7].

153. Shastri S, Slayton RE, Wolter J, et al. Clinical study with bleomycin. Cancer 1971;28:1142–6.

154. Kullendorff CM. Efficacy of bleomycin treatment for symptomatic hemangiomas in children. Pediatr Surg Int 1997;12:526–8.

155. Luo QF, Zhao FY. The effects of Bleomycin A5 on infantile maxillofacial haemangioma. Head Face Med 2011;7:11.

156. Omidvari S, Nezakatgoo N, Ahmadloo N, et al. Role of intralesional bleomycin in the treatment of complicated hemangiomas: prospective clinical study. Dermatol Surg 2005;31:499–501.

157. Pienaar C, Graham R, Geldenhuys S, et al. Intralesional bleomycin for the treatment of hemangiomas. Plast Reconstr Surg 2006;117:221–6.

158. Sainsbury DC, Kessell G, Fall AJ, et al. Intralesional bleomycin injection treatment for vascular birthmarks: a 5-year experience at a single United kingdom unit. Plast Reconstr Surg 2011;127: 2031–44.

159. Breit A. Problem of the irradiation treatment of hemangioma. Experiences with 3,000 patients. Strahlentherapie 1970;139:1–8 [in German].

160. Gross E, Luger A. Results of hemangioma treatment with contact irradiation. Dermatol Wochenschr 1967;153:142–59 [in German].

161. Huang KC, Cheng KL, Liu CH, et al. Capillary hemangioma treated by radioactive P32. Chin Med J 1960;80:170–5.

162. Bruckner AL, Frieden IJ. Hemangiomas of infancy. J Am Acad Dermatol 2003;48:477–93 [quiz: 94–6].

163. David LR, Malek MM, Argenta LC. Efficacy of pulse dye laser therapy for the treatment of ulcerated haemangiomas: a review of 78 patients. Br J Plast Surg 2003;56:317–27.

164. Raulin C, Greve B. Retrospective clinical comparison of hemangioma treatment by flashlamp-pumped (585 nm) and frequency-doubled Nd:YAG (532 nm) lasers. Lasers Surg Med 2001;28:40–3.

165. Burstein FD, Williams JK, Schwentker AR, et al. Intralesional laser therapy treatment for hemangiomas: technical evolution. J Craniofac Surg 2006; 17:756–60.

166. Stier MF, Glick SA, Hirsch RJ. Laser treatment of pediatric vascular lesions: port wine stains and hemangiomas. J Am Acad Dermatol 2008;58:261–85.

167. Canter HI, Vargel I, Mavlll ME, et al. Tissue response to N-butyl-2-cyanoacrylate after percutaneous injection into cutaneous vascular lesions. Ann Plast Surg 2002;49:520–6.

168. Wolfe SQ, Farhat H, Elhammady MS, et al. Transarterial embolization of a scalp hemangioma presenting with Kasabach-Merritt syndrome. J Neurosurg Pediatr 2009;4:453–7.

169. Enomoto Y, Yoshimura S, Egashira Y, et al. Transarterial embolization for cervical hemangioma associated with Kasabach-Merritt syndrome. Neurol Med Chir 2011;51:375–8.

170. Li W, Feng B, Wang J, et al. Observe the curative effect of n-Butyl cyanoacrylate injection in treating laryngopharynx hemangioma. Lin Chung Er Bi Yan Hou Tou Jing Wai Ke Za Zhi 2008;22:1120–2 [in Chinese].

171. Syal R, Tyagi I, Goyal A, et al. Multiple intraosseous hemangiomas-investigation and role of N-butylcyanoacrylate in management. Head Neck 2007;29: 512–7.

172. Kaneko R, Tohnai I, Ueda M, et al. Curative treatment of central hemangioma in the mandible by direct puncture and embolisation with n-butyl-cyanoacrylate (NBCA). Oral Oncol 2001; 37:605–8.

173. Lasjuanias P, ter Brugge KG, Berenstein A. 2nd edition. Surgical neuroangiography, clinical and interventional aspects in children, vol. 3. Berlin: Springer-Verlag; 2006.

174. Liu XJ, Qin ZP, Tai MZ. Angiographic classification and sclerotic therapy of maxillofacial cavernous haemangiomas: a report of 204 cases. J Int Med Res 2009;37:1285–92.

Endovascular Treatment of Adult Spinal Arteriovenous Lesions

Neeraj Chaudhary, MD, MRCS, FRCR[a],*,
Aditya S. Pandey, MD[a], Joseph J. Gemmete, MD, FSIR[b]

KEYWORDS

- Spinal arteriovenous lesions • Spinal angiography • Spinal cord arteriovenous malformation
- Spinal arteriovenous fistula • Spinal dural arteriovenous fistula • Epidural arteriovenous fistula

KEY POINTS

- Spinal arteriovenous lesions (SAVLs) are rare.
- Spinal dural arteriovenous fistulas (SDAVFs) are the most common SAVLs.
- Diagnosis is difficult, and a high clinical index of suspicion is recommended.
- Magnetic resonance imaging should be the noninvasive imaging modality of choice to confirm the diagnosis.
- Selective spinal angiography remains the gold standard for the evaluation of SAVLs.
- The optimal treatment modality, either endovascular or surgical, remains to be established.

INTRODUCTION

Spinal arteriovenous lesions (SAVLs) are rare.[1] SAVLs represent only 3% to 4% of all spinal cord lesions, and can be associated with considerable morbidity and mortality if left untreated.[2] Elsberg[3] was the first person to surgically treat an SAVL in 1914. He successfully treated a spinal dural arteriovenous fistula (SDAVF) with medullary venous drainage. In the early 1960s in the United States, Di Chiro and colleagues[4] pioneered selective spinal arteriography, which led to real-time recognition of the spinal cord vascular anatomy and pathology. At the same time in France, Djindjian[5] was the first to describe the technique of selective spinal angiography. Since this time, there has been an evolution in imaging, endovascular, and surgical techniques.

These technological advancements and a better understanding of spinal cord pathophysiology now allow us to manage SAVLs more effectively within the context of a multidisciplinary approach involving neurointerventional radiology and cerebrovascular neurosurgery. However, there is still a lack of a comprehensive understanding of spinal cord pathophysiology, consensus in the clinical classification of the various types of SAVLs, and ambiguity in anatomic spinal cord terminology. Moreover, there are conflicting reports in the literature advocating either an endovascular technique or surgery as the first line of treatment. This article discusses the anatomy, epidemiology, presentation, natural history, pathophysiology, and endovascular treatment of the various types of SAVLs in adults.

[a] Division of Interventional Neuroradiology, Departments of Neurosurgery and Radiology, University of Michigan Health System, 1500 East Medical Center Drive, Ann Arbor, MI 48109-5030, USA; [b] Division of Interventional Neuroradiology and Cranial Base Surgery, Departments of Radiology, Neurosurgery, and Otolaryngology, University of Michigan Health System, UH B1D 328, 1500 East Medical Center Drive, Ann Arbor, MI 48109-5030, USA
* Corresponding author.
E-mail address: neerajc@med.umich.edu

Neuroimag Clin N Am 23 (2013) 729–747
http://dx.doi.org/10.1016/j.nic.2013.03.017
1052-5149/13/$ – see front matter © 2013 Elsevier Inc. All rights reserved.

ANGIOARCHITECTURE OF NORMAL BLOOD SUPPLY OF THE SPINAL CORD
Arterial Supply

The neural plate starts development during the third gestational week and is derived from the embryologic ectoderm. The process is induced by the underlying notochord, and derives arterial blood supply from individual metameric/mesodermal segmental vessels that originate from the corresponding dorsal and ventral aortic arches at around the third week of gestation.[6,7] Neural-tube formation commences early in the fourth week (days 22–23), with closure of the cranial and caudal neuropores by days 25 to 27, which coincides with establishment of the intrinsic circulation to the spinal cord.[8] Cellular differentiation and proliferation of the arterial supply to the spinal cord in an embryo closely resembles that of an adult-type pattern by the 10th week of gestation.[7]

In the adult, segmental arteries from the vertebral, deep, and ascending cervical arteries, intercostal and lumbar arteries, median and lateral sacral arteries, and iliolumbar arteries supply the spinal cord, meninges, vertebral bodies, paraspinal muscles, and soft tissues at each level of the spinal column.[9] As the primitive notochord elongates the segmental vessels coalesce in the midline, with the developing anterior spinal artery typically originating from the V4 segment of both vertebral arteries. The individual segmental artery branches supplying the spinal cord regress in their proximal portion in response to the dominant developing longitudinal ventral arterial axis (anterior spinal artery) (ASA) that annexes the distal portion. However, there is usually more than 1 persistent segmental arterial branch that remains patent throughout its length and forms the radiculomedullary artery, which typically follows the course of the radicular nerve root sleeve.[10] The radiculomedullary artery supplements the anterior and posterior spinal arterial supply to the spinal cord (Fig. 1A). The dominant radiculomedullary artery in the lower thoracic or lumbar region is called the artery of Adamkiewicz, or arteria radicularis magna. The number and location of the radiculomedullary arteries are unpredictable in a given patient. The course of the radiculomedullary artery has a very typical appearance of a smaller ascending and larger descending branch, with a characteristic "hairpin" loop at the point of entrance to the anterior fissure of the spinal cord.[11] The branchlet from the radicular artery at each segmental level supplying the dura is called the radicular/radiculomeningeal artery, and usually accompanies the corresponding nerve root in its dural sleeve to reach its destination. There are often separate sub-branches supplying the pial surface called the radiculopial arteries.

The most common pattern of arterial supply to the posterior spinal cord is via 2 parasagittal arterial axes called the posterior spinal arteries, which are smaller in comparison with their anterior counterparts and form a more discontinuous arcade of vessels. There is free communication between these posterior networks and the sulcocommissural branches from the anterior spinal arterial axis around the lateral aspects of the spinal cord. From these rings (vasa corona) there are penetrating vessels (rami perforantes) supplying the spinal cord parenchyma, with communication from the adjacent level branches.[12]

Venous Drainage

Unlike the brain, the venous drainage of the spinal cord is important in understanding the etiology of the clinical manifestations of SAVLs. Arterial

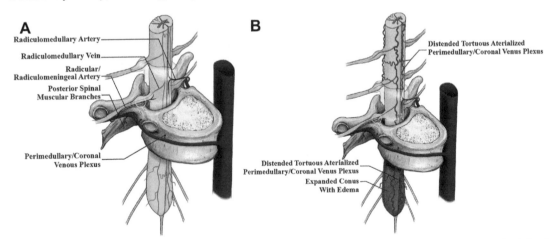

Fig. 1. (A) Normal arterial and venous supply to the spinal cord. (B) Typical location of the fistula in a spinal dural arteriovenous fistula, with consequent venous hypertension.

ischemic strokes of the spinal cord are rare. Venous hypertension is the usual cause of congestive myelopathy in SAVLs, and is the final common pathway that causes neuronal ischemia. The venous system of the spinal cord consists of 3 interconnected venous groups: intradural (extramedullary and intramedullary) veins, extradural/epidural veins, and the intraosseus/paravertebral plexi. In addition, there are longitudinal veins, also called the coronal spinal veins, on the ventral and dorsal aspect of the cord. The intradural (coronal) venous plexi are connected to the epidural venous plexi via the radicular/radiculomedullary veins, also termed the bridging veins (see Fig. 1A),[13] because they do not follow the spinal nerves like the radiculomedullary arteries.[14] There is much more communication between the levels of the venous system than the arterial arcade along the surface and intrinsic/transmedullary pathways of the spinal cord. The transition of a median vein into a radicular vein follows the same characteristic hairpin loop as seen in the radiculomedullary artery. The venous drainage from the spinal cord is centrifugal from the intradural venous plexus into the epidural veins via the radiculomedullary veins, and then ultimately via the azygos and hemiazygos systems into the superior vena cava. The point of dural transgression of the radiculomedullary vein is hypothesized to act as a natural valve that retains the centrifugal venous blood flow of the spinal cord.[15]

CLASSIFICATION

SAVLs are a diverse group of diseases. The traditional classification of SAVLs was purely descriptive and was based on histology, because of a lack of a clear understanding of the pathophysiology of each separate lesion. The evolution of spinal angiography has immensely improved our ability to examine the angioarchitecture of these lesions, which has led to a more accurate classification system based on topographic and anatomic criteria. However, despite these classification refinements an element of subjective judgment persists, because not all lesions conform to the classification system.

The Bicetre group classified SAVLs into 3 main groups. (1) Genetic hereditary lesions are caused by a genetic disorder affecting the vascular germinal cells. The vascular lesions of Hereditary hemorrhagic telangiectasia (HHT) belong to this category.[16] (2) Genetic nonhereditary lesions share metameric links such as Cobb syndrome (or spinal arteriovenous metameric syndrome), which affects the whole myelomere.[17] These patients typically present with multiple shunts of the spinal cord, nerve root, bone, paraspinal muscle, subcutaneous, and skin tissue. Klippel-Trenaunay and Parkes-Weber syndromes are included in this group. (3) Single lesions may reflect incomplete expression of one of the previously mentioned conditions and include spinal cord, nerve root, and filum terminale lesions.[18] The majority of the SAVLs fit this last category.

SAVLs can also be classified into 2 main groups based on hemodynamic criteria: (1) the spinal arteriovenous fistula (AVF) with a direct shunt between the artery and the vein, and (2) an arteriovenous malformation (AVM) with the presence of an intervening nidus of vessels between the artery and the vein (Box 1).[15] Other vascular lesions, such as a capillary telangiectasia and a cavernous hemangioma, do not contain an arteriovenous (AV) shunt and are not amenable to endovascular therapy.[15] The arterial feeders to a spinal dural or pial AV shunt are similar to their cerebral counterparts and are supplied by a radiculomeningeal or a radiculomedullary artery, respectively.

In a recent uniform classification of dural AV shunts, both cerebral and spinal AV shunts were categorized into 3 groups based on the embryologic development of the venous drainage of the surrounding structures: the ventral, dorsal, and lateral epidural groups.[14]

Box 1
Anatomic flow–related classification of spinal arteriovenous lesions

Topographic Classification of Spinal Arteriovenous Lesions

Classification

AVM

1. Intramedullary (also classified as type II glomus-type AVM)

2. Pial

3. Epidural

4. Intramedullary and extramedullary (also known as type III, intradural-extradural, juvenile AVM, or metameric AVM)

AVF

1. Pial AVF (also known as type IV, spinal cord AVF, ventral intradural AVF, or perimedullary AVF)

   a. Small

   b. Large

   c. Giant

2. Dural AVF (also known as type I or a dorsal intradural AVF)

3. Epidural AVF (also known as extradural AVF)

The ventral epidural group consists of shunts into those veins that normally drain structures developed from the notochord (ie, the vertebral body). These veins are known as the basivertebral venous plexus, which subsequently drains into the anterior internal vertebral venous plexus, located at the ventral epidural space of the spinal canal, which joins the basilar venous plexus and cavernous sinus cranially. The previously termed "epidural," "osteodural," or "paravertebral" AV shunts can be categorized in this group. Because the draining veins of these shunts do not drain the spine but the bone, these shunts will not become symptomatic because of venous congestion of the cord. These shunts can become symptomatic as a result of compression of the spinal cord or nerve roots by enlarged epidural venous pouches.[19,20] There are a few case reports describing associated perimedullary reflux causing congestive myelopathy.[21,22]

The dorsal epidural group of AV shunts is related to veins that normally drain the spinous process and lamina at the spinal level. These shunts are related to the major dural venous sinuses (superior sagittal sinus, torcula, and transverse sinuses) at the cranial level; the corresponding veins at the spinal level are poorly developed and consist of a pair of longitudinal channels (ie, the posterior internal venous plexus).[13] Patients with dural AV shunts within this space can present with spontaneous epidural hematomas.[23,24] These shunts are rare.

The most common, classic types of SDAVFs are the lateral epidural AVFs (see **Fig. 1**B). These AV shunts develop in the lateral epidural space at the junction of the bridging (or radicular) veins that connect the spinal cord drainage to the epidural venous system. Outflow obstruction of its adjacent venous outlet, caused either by thrombosis or fibrosis related to aging, will then lead to immediate drainage into the perimedullary veins.[14,25] As a result, patients in this group present with aggressive clinical symptoms related to perimedullary venous congestion.

EPIDEMIOLOGY, CLINICAL PRESENTATION, AND NATURAL HISTORY IN THE ADULT POPULATION
Spinal Cord Arteriovenous Malformation

Spinal cord arteriovenous malformations (SCAVMs) represent 20% to 30% of SAVLs.[26] SCAVMs are high-flow lesions supplied by more than 1 branch of the ASA and/or posterior spinal artery (PSA), with a discrete nidus of vessels that drain into the spinal veins (**Fig. 2**). Associated aneurysms of the feeding arteries and the nidus are common.[27]

SCAVMs are evenly distributed along the spinal cord axis, and may be located within the parenchyma (intramedullary) (also known as type II or glomus-type AVM), the surface of the spinal cord (pial), or the epidural space (epidural), or they may have a complex anatomy with both intramedullary and extramedullary components (also known as type III, intradural-extradural, juvenile AVM, or metameric AVM). The conus medullaris AVM represents a distinct type located on the conus medullaris or cauda equina, and can extend along the filum terminale.[28]

SCAVMs typically appear in childhood or early adulthood, with sudden onset of symptoms attributable to hemorrhage or compression-induced myelopathy. Patients may present with motor and/or sensory deficits, bladder and bowel disturbances, and pain. Most patients have partial improvement after the initial event, but new events are likely and result in progressive deterioration of spinal cord function. Arterial steal and venous hypertension may occur, and can result in progressive myelopathy. Conus medullaris AVMs frequently produce radiculopathy and myelopathy at the same time.[28]

The prognosis for untreated SCAVMs is poor, with 36% of patients younger than 40 years developing severe impairment 3 years after diagnosis.[2] In a report by Hurth and colleagues[29] 13%, 20%, and 57% of patients had severe clinical deterioration 5, 10, and 20 years after diagnosis, respectively.

Pial Arteriovenous Fistula

Pial AVF is characterized by a single or a few intradural direct AV shunts without an intervening nidus. It is usually located on the pial surface of the cord. Arterial supply originates from 1 or more arterial feeders from the ASA or PSA, and the shunt drains into the spinal cord veins (**Fig. 3**).

The pial AVFs are subdivided into small (type I), large (type II), and giant (type III), according to the size and flow of the direct shunt. Small AVFs correspond to a single slow-flow shunt between a nondilated ASA and a slightly dilated spinal vein, and are located in the anterior aspect of the conus medullaris or the filum terminale. Small spinal cord AVFs of the conus medullaris can be easily confused with dural arteriovenous fistulas (DAVFs).

Large AVFs correspond to a single or a few shunts, with greater flow than the small AVFs and moderate dilation of the draining vein. Large AVFs are usually located in the posterolateral aspect of the conus medullaris and are supplied by 1 or more mildly dilated arterial feeders from the PSA. Large AVFs can also occur anteriorly, in

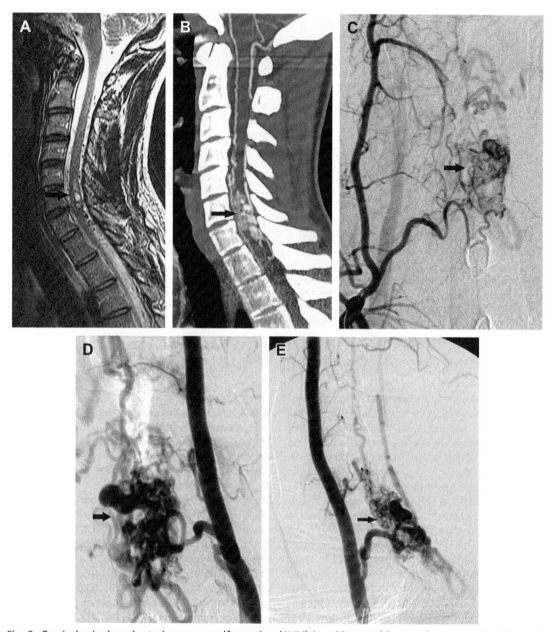

Fig. 2. Cervical spinal cord arteriovenous malformation (AVM) in a 28-year-old man who presented with weakness in his arms and legs. (A) Sagittal T2-weighted MR image of the cervical spine demonstrates flow voids on the surface and within the cord at C6 and C7, with an area of subacute hemorrhage (arrow). (B) Sagittal computed tomography (CT) angiogram of the cervical spine shows a nidus of vessels at the C6 and C7 levels within the spinal cord (arrow) with engorgement of the perimedullary venous plexus. (C) Frontal right thyrocervical trunk angiogram shows indirect arterial supply to this spinal cord AVM (arrow). (D, E) Frontal (D) and lateral (E) left vertebral angiograms show filling of the nidus of vessels at C6 and C7 (arrow) from prominent radicular medullary arteries at C5 and C6, with engorgement of the perimedullary venous plexus from the high-flow shunt.

which case the feeder is a branch of the ASA. Regardless of the location, large AVFs have many arterial feeders, in contrast to 1 or a few shunts.

Giant AVFs have a single or a few high-flow shunts with 1 or more dilated arterial feeders from the ASA and the PSA. The arterial feeders converge to a single shunt, draining into massively dilated arterialized draining veins. Giant AVFs are more common in the conus medullaris region and can be associated with complex vascular malformation syndromes.[30] Giant AVFs can also be seen in the cervical and thoracic levels of the spinal cord.

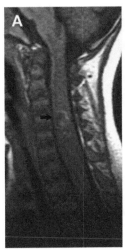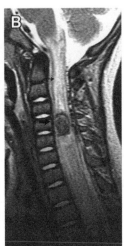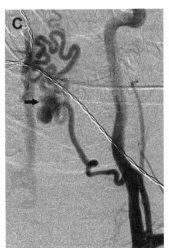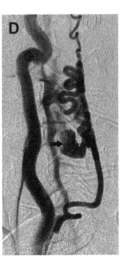

Fig. 3. Cervical spinal cord large pial arteriovenous fistula (AVF) in an 8-year-old boy who presented with quad-riplegia. (*A*) Sagittal T1-weighted MR image of the cervical spine shows expansion of the spinal cord with an area of acute hemorrhage at C4 (*arrow*). (*B*) Sagittal T2-weighted MR image of the cervical spine shows expansion of the cord with diffuse abnormal high signal extending from the medulla inferiorly to involve the entire cervical cord (*thin arrow*). There is an area of acute hemorrhage at C4 within the spinal cord (*thick arrow*). (*C, D*) Left sub-clavian angiogram (*C* frontal, *D* lateral) shows a large pial AVF supplied from the left thyrocervical trunk filling an arterial aneurysm (*arrow*), corresponding to the area of acute hemorrhage of the MR image. There is filling of the perimedullary venous plexus with decompression into the right epidural venous system.

Small spinal cord AVFs present later in life, with progressive neurologic deficits related to venous hypertension, subarachnoid hemorrhage (SAH) being rare. Hematomyelia has also been observed after rupture of the anterior spinal vein, which is subpial in location.[18]

The large and giant spinal cord AVFs usually present in childhood and adolescence with a variety of clinical scenarios. Acute onset of symptoms can occur secondary to SAH, whereas progressive motor and sensory deterioration and sphincter disturbance usually result from vascular steal, venous hypertension, or mass effect on the spinal cord and/or nerve roots from the dilated veins. SAHs usually occur as a result of venous rupture.[31] The mass effect on the cord or nerve roots from dilated veins explains the occasional asymmetric nature of deficits.

Spinal Dural Arteriovenous Fistula

SDAVFs are the most frequent vascular malformation of the spine, and account for approximately 70% of all SAVLs (**Fig. 4**).[32,33] SDAVFs have a male predominance,[34] and diagnosis is most frequent in the sixth decade.[25,35–40] The incidence of SDAVF in the younger population is very rare, especially when compared with other SAVLs. Most fistulas are solitary lesions. The most common location of SDAVFs is in the thoracic region, followed by the lumbar region. Cervical location

of a fistula is rare; however, some patients can have a fistula in the cervical region below C2 that may present with arm weakness.[41] This presentation is only encountered in a cervical SDAVF, and when present has a localizing value.[37] Sacral lesions occur in approximately 4% of patients.[42]

Initial symptoms of venous congestion are nonspecific and include difficulty in climbing stairs, gait disturbances, paresthesias, diffuse or patchy sensory loss, and radicular pain that may affect both of the lower limbs or initially only one limb.[37] Lower back pain without radicular distribution is also frequently encountered. The neurologic symptoms are progressive with time and are often ascending.[39] Bowel and bladder incontinence, erectile dysfunction, and urinary retention are more often seen late in the course of the disease. SDAVFs may mimic more benign conditions such as lumbar spinal canal stenosis, which may lead to a delay in diagnosis or an inappropriate surgery. Leg claudication with exertion tends to be more common in patients with thoracic fistulas.

Spinal cord hemorrhage from an SDAVF is rare, and points toward the presence of a perimedullary (ie, pial) shunt rather than a true SDAVF.[26] Rarely an SDAVF at the level of the foramen magnum with cranial reflux can present with subarachnoid hemorrhage.[43] Two-thirds of the patients at the time of presentation show a combination of gait difficulty, sensory disturbance, fecal or urine in-continence, and sexual dysfunction.[25] In addition,

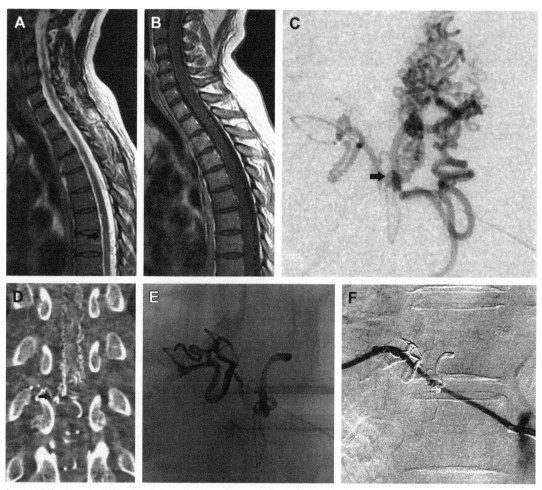

Fig. 4. Right T7 spinal dural AVF in a 58-year-old man who presented with bilateral lower extremity sensory and motor changes along with urinary retention. (*A*) Sagittal T2-weighted MR image of the thoracic spine shows flow voids along the mid-thoracic spinal cord with abnormal intramedullary high signal (*arrow*). (*B*) Sagittal contrast-enhanced T1-weighted MR image shows abnormal enhancement along with surface of the spinal cord. (*C*) T7 intercostal microcatheter angiogram shows fillings of a dural fistula within the right T7 nerve root (*arrow*) with filling of an engorged perimedullary venous plexus. (*D*) Coronal dynamic CT with contrast injected in the right T7 intercostal artery elegantly shows the site of the fistula (*arrow*). (*E*) Spot fluoroscopic image shows the Onyx cast at the site of the fistula and within a portion of the outflow vein. (*F*) Postembolization right T7 intercostal angiogram shows occlusion of the dural fistula.

upper and lower motor neuron involvement can coexist in the same patient, as originally observed by Foix and Alajouanine.[41,44] Hence, physical examination cannot localize the level of the fistula nor does it narrow the differential diagnosis. Confirmation of an SDAVF is based on the findings seen on magnetic resonance (MR) imaging and a spinal angiogram.

Epidural Arteriovenous Fistula

The epidural AVF is a rare lesion associated with significant neurologic morbidity, representing an abnormal shunt between an artery and an epidural vein/venous plexus (**Fig. 5**). Neurologic symptoms

occur by mass effect on the spinal cord and/or nerve roots from the enlarged draining veins, arterial steal, or venous hypertension. Epidural AVFs are primarily described in case reports and small case series, with the cervical spine the most common location.[45–48]

PATHOPHYSIOLOGY

SAVLs may be associated with myelopathy (sensory and motor deficits, bladder and bowel dysfunction), radicular pain or deficit, back pain, or spinal column deformity. Hemorrhage, venous hypertension, arterial steal, and mass effect are

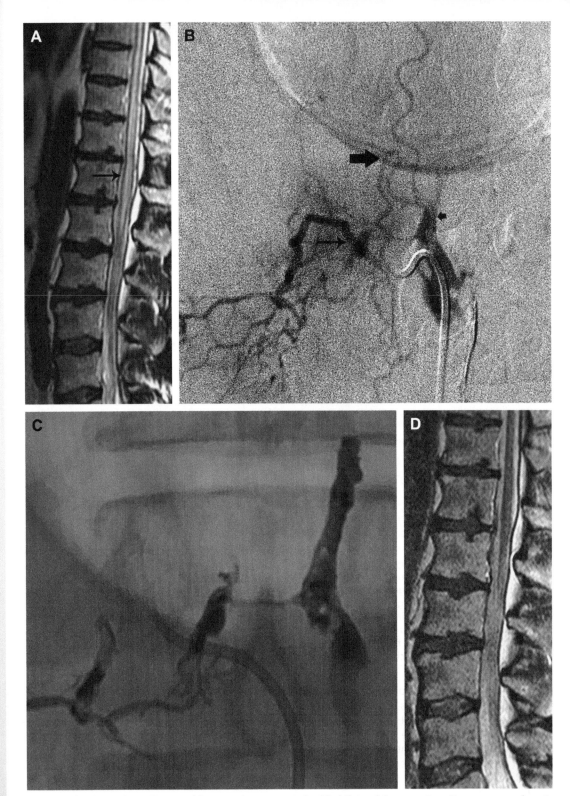

Fig. 5. Epidural AVF in a 62-year-old man who presented with bilateral lower extremity sensory and motor changes, bowel incontinence, and urinary retention. (*A*) Sagittal T2-weighted MR image of the thoracic/lumbar spine shows abnormal high signal (*arrow*) within the conus medullaris extending superior into the thoracic cord. (*B*) Frontal right L2 lumbar angiogram shows an epidural AVF (*thin arrow*) with filling of the epidural venous system within the right L2 nerve root crossing the midline through a bridging vein filling the left epidural venous system (*small thick arrow*), decompressing into perimedullary veins on the left (*large thick arrow*). (*C*) Spot frontal fluoroscopic image shows the Onyx cast filling the site of the fistula and right epidural venous system crossing the midline through a bridging vein and then filling the left epidural venous system. (*D*) Six months after embolization, sagittal T2-weighted MR image shows resolution of the abnormal high signal within the spinal cord.

the possible mechanisms for spinal cord damage, and their importance varies for each type of lesion. Hemorrhage can occur in the cord parenchyma and/or subarachnoid space, leading to acute onset of neurologic deficits.

The risk of hemorrhage is greater in SCAVMs. Large and giant spinal cord AVFs and cervical DAVFs may also present with hemorrhage, whereas small spinal cord AVFs and thoracic and lumbar DAVFs are less likely to bleed.[49,50] Spinal artery and intranidal aneurysms are associated with a high risk for hemorrhage.[27] Rarely, SCAVMs with intracranial venous drainage may lead to intracranial hemorrhage.[51] Venous hypertension is typically associated with SAVLs with perimedullary venous drainage.

The classic lesion associated with venous hypertension is the SDAVF, but this phenomenon can be seen with any lesion that has perimedullary venous drainage, such as the pial AVF. The pressure in the perimedullary veins is abnormally increased by the direct AV shunt, and this increased pressure is transmitted to the intrinsic veins of the cord owing to the lack of valves, resulting in "arterialization" of these veins, with thickened and tortuous walls, decreased intramedullary AV pressure gradient, decreased tissue perfusion, and hypoxia of the spinal cord.[52] In addition, loss of autoregulation of the intrinsic cord vessels leads to cord edema and disruption of the blood-cord barrier.[25] Because the conus medullaris is the lowest part of the spine in the upright position, venous hypertension usually predominates there, aided by the valveless venous system. The pressure in the draining veins varies with arterial pressure, resulting in exacerbated symptoms during exercise. Venous hypertension can be confirmed with angiography of the artery of Adamkiewicz by demonstrating severe prolongation of the venous phase.[33] Lesions with high-flow AV shunts may lead to steal of arterial blood from adjacent normal spinal cord tissue.[53] Lesions in the dorsal aspect of the cord that are fed by the ASA are also prone to arterial steal because of the low potential for collateral arterial supply to the normal cord tissue. Mass effect is a rare mechanism for myelopathy. Large aneurysms and large dilated veins/varices like the ones seen with giant spinal cord AVFs may compress the spinal cord or nerve roots.[54]

IMAGING FINDINGS
Spinal Cord Arteriovenous Malformation

Myelography, which was historically performed before the availability of MR imaging, typically reveals a "bag of worms" appearance and widening of the spinal cord.

Postmyelography computed tomography (CT) is valuable for localizing the lesion inside or outside the spinal cord and for evaluating the local bony changes associated with prolonged pressure by the large tangle of dilated vessels.

In making the diagnosis, contrast-enhanced MR imaging is currently the noninvasive imaging modality of choice. It offers an accurate diagnosis of the AVM and evaluation of the cord surrounding the lesions. Moreover, it may identify an area of acute or chronic hematomyelia. Spinal angiography gives exquisite detail of the arterial feeders, angioarchitecture of the AVM nidus, and venous drainage.

Pial Arteriovenous Fistula

Plain films of the spine are unremarkable except in the case of a giant AVF, which may produce bone erosion. MR imaging may show vascular dilation on the surface of the cord. Arteriography is indispensable not only for precise diagnosis but also to differentiate between the different types of pial AVFs.

Spinal Dural Arteriovenous Fistula

An MR image of the entire spine, with contrast, should be the diagnostic imaging modality of choice to evaluate a patient with a suspected SDAVF. In a recently published large series of 153 patients with an SDAVF, T2 signal hyperintensity on MR imaging was demonstrated in the conus medullaris in 95% of cases.[34] None of the patients in the series had isolated cervical or thoracic T2 signal involvement within the cord, even when the fistula was located at the cervical levels. The findings typically seen on MR imaging are the presence of edema at the conus medullaris, with variable cranial extension and distended tortuous flow voids in the coronal venous plexus. On the T1-weighted sequence, the spinal cord is hypointense and swollen. Following the administration of contrast, there is diffuse enhancement within the spinal cord secondary to chronic venous congestion and breakdown of the blood–spinal cord barrier.[55,56] Identification of a tortuous coronal venous plexus along the spinal cord on the MR image confirms the diagnosis, and should prompt a spinal angiogram to identify the level of the fistula. The presence of diffuse hyperintense T2 signal in the spinal cord in the absence of a mass lesion or diffuse enhancement following contrast administration, with or without a distended tortuous coronal venous plexus, still warrants a spinal angiogram to exclude an SDAVF.

Sometimes flow voids can be subtle and difficult to identify. A steady-state high-resolution MR sequence can sometimes demonstrate the distended coronal venous plexus, which may not be seen on a standard MR imaging sequence of the spine. A steady-state sequence is a heavily weighted T2 sequence. The sequence makes the flow voids in the distended coronal venous plexus more apparent and conspicuous against the bright signal from the cerebrospinal fluid (CSF).[9] This sequence may be useful to confirm an SDAVF when there is a lack of flow voids on a standard MR image of the spine, or when it is difficult to distinguish between pulsation artifact in CSF and distended venous flow voids.

A small group of patients with an SDAVF may not demonstrate T2 signal abnormality within the spinal cord in the presence of a distended coronal venous plexus. In 2 reports, a small group of patients had a negative spinal angiogram and absence of hyperintense T2 signal within the spinal cord, but still harbored an SDAVF.[34,57] The investigators claim the SDAVF was not identified on the initial angiogram, because a selective injection of contrast was not administered at the site of the fistula. An SDAVF also may not be seen on a spinal angiography if it has undergone spontaneous thrombosis. These 2 groups of patients typically present with mild clinical symptoms that do not become worse on exertion. A recent article reported that hyperintense T2 signal involving the entire spinal cord was associated with clinical symptoms that became worse on exertion.[35] Moreover, the extent of T2 signal abnormality did not correlate with the severity of disability on presentation, although it did correlate with the presence of the pinprick level. Sato and colleagues,[58] in their retrospective review of SDAVFs, demonstrated that lack of cord edema correlated with the absence of medullary dysfunction. The spinal angiograms of the asymptomatic patients in this report distinctively demonstrated early radicular venous outflow from affected perimedullary veins to the extradural venous plexus as a potential alternative route for the venous hypertension to be released.

Once the diagnosis of an SDAVF is confirmed on noninvasive imaging, the next step is to identify the level of the fistula and to plan for treatment. The location of pathologic vessels or the extent of intramedullary findings on MR imaging does not correlate with the level of the fistula.[59] The fistula location can be at any level from the foramen magnum to the sacrum. Locating of the fistula can be difficult and challenging, especially when the cord edema is distant from the fistula site. The search for the optimal noninvasive imaging modality with which to identify the fistula and guide spinal angiography is still a work in progress.[60] A

few reports document the value of first-pass gadolinium-enhanced MR spinal angiography for determining the level of the fistula.[61–64] This technique can consistently identify early filling of the coronal venous plexus; however, its ability to accurately identify the level of the fistula remains limited. CT angiography of the spine also has been used to tin an attempt to identify the level of the fistula[65]; however, given that the location of the fistula can be anywhere from the foramen magnum to the sacrum, the radiation and contrast burden to the patient is significant, so this is not a practical approach.[35] The authors consider that the level of the fistula is best determined by a spinal angiogram.

Epidural Arteriovenous Fistula

Contrast CT of the spine demonstrates a tangle of vessels that show enhancement. MR imaging can confirm the diagnosis, and identifies the location and extent of the lesion. Spinal angiography accurately identifies the site of the fistula usually fed by branches of the costocervical and thyrocervical trunk; the vertebral, intercostal, and lumbar arteries; and arteries that supply the sacrum and the pelvis. Venous drainage is usually into an epidural vein, although drainage into the perimedullary venous plexus is possible if there is thrombosis of the epidural venous system.

Diagnostic Spinal Angiography: Technique and Findings

At the authors' institution, all spinal angiograms are performed under general endotracheal anesthesia to minimize motion artifact, given the length of the procedure. The angiographic suite is composed of a biplane angiographic unit with conebeam CT capability (Axiom Artis; Siemens, Munich, Germany). The patient is placed supine on the angiographic table, and access is obtained by puncturing the right common femoral artery using ultrasound guidance and a micropuncture kit. The initial diagnostic portion of the procedure is typically performed with various 5F catheters, depending on the patient's anatomy. A complete spinal angiogram is performed, which includes selective bilateral injections of the internal carotid arteries, external carotid arteries, vertebral arteries, thyrocervical trunks, costocervical trunks, segmental arteries from T1 to L5, and the posterior division of the internal iliac arteries. The median sacral artery is also selectively injected with contrast. In cases with a high clinical suspicion for an SDAVF, a microcatheter angiogram at selective levels based on noninvasive MR imaging is recommended before the diagnosis can be excluded. The typical findings on a spinal angiogram of an SDAVF is a medially directed branch of a segmental artery filling a fistula within the neuroforamen at the site of dural nerve root entry, with early filling of a radicular vein and subsequent opacification of a distended tortuous coronal venous plexus. If the angiogram is performed into the late venous phase, decompression of the radicular veins into the epidural venous system can be identified, usually at a distance from the level of the fistula.[66]

Optimal opacification of the vessel in question with contrast and a selective catheter location in the segmental vessel is critical in visualizing the SDAVF. A small number of patients have a compelling MR imaging appearance of SDAVF, but are occult on selective spinal angiography. Killory and colleagues[67] reported 3 patients who were successfully treated after an occult SDAVF was identified with near-infrared indocyanine green intraoperative spinal angiography. A total of 8 other patients with angiographically occult SDAVF have been described in the literature.[65,68–70]

TREATMENT
Spinal Cord Arteriovenous Malformation

Treatment of an SCAVM aims to decrease the risk of hemorrhage and arrest the progression of neurologic deficits.[71,72] Reduction of the arterial steal within an SCAVM may reverse a neurologic deficit. SCAVMs are supplied by a single or a few arterial feeders; however, the exact supply to the lesion is often difficult to discern because of the high-flow shunts. Several of arterial feeders may have an indirect supply to the AVM. Proximal occlusion of the arterial feeders from a surgical or an endovascular approach will not cure the lesion, but make treatment more difficult because this will not occlude the AVM nidus. Surgical treatment of an intramedullary AVM is accompanied by significant major complications. A large series reported the risk of embolization was 3 to 5 times lower than that of surgery (5.7% irreversible deficit after embolization vs 15%–28% after surgery).[71] The authors are of the opinion that endovascular treatment should be the first method of choice for SCAVMs, even if the lesion is suitable for surgical resection.[73]

Embolization plays an important role in the management of intramedullary SCAVMs, both as primary treatment and as an adjunct to surgical excision. Partial embolization can improve the natural history of these lesions.[74,75] Liquid embolic agents are preferred for endovascular treatment.

Particle embolization is easier to perform, but has serious disadvantages owing to recanalization requiring repeat embolization. A series of thoracic SCAVMs embolized with particles demonstrated an 80% recanalization rate.[71] Clinical improvement was seen in 57% of the patients after the first embolization and in 63% after the last embolization. Treatment with particulate material is not definitive; however, it may be considered palliative treatment because it improves the natural history and can provide a good clinical outcome.

Liquid embolic agents such as cyanoacrylate and Onyx achieve a more permanent occlusion with a very low recanalization rate, but carry a concurrent risk of inadvertent embolization of the perforating branches that are not visualized on angiography. In a large series of SCAVM and AVF embolization with cyanoacrylate, good clinical outcome was observed in 83% of patients.[76] Permanent morbidity related to embolization was seen in 13% of patients with only 4% deemed to have severe deficits, which all were the result of embolization through the ASA. A reduction in lesion size of more than 50% was achieved in 86% of the patients, with no recanalization, during a mean follow-up period of 5.6 years. Recurrent hemorrhage was seen in 4% of patients. All of these cases were cervical SCAVMs in which less than 50% of the lesion was obliterated. Onyx (ev3, Irvine, CA) has also been used to treat SCAVMs. In a series of 17 patients with symptomatic intramedullary AVMs treated with Onyx, total obliteration was achieved in 6 patients, subtotal obliteration in 5, and partial obliteration in 5.[77] The procedure was aborted in 1 patient. Clinical improvement during follow-up (mean 24.3 months) was noted in 14 patients and clinical deterioration in 3 patients, including the 1 treated surgically. There were 3 intraprocedural complications (2 extradural hematomas and 1 SAH), without neurologic consequences.

Pial Arteriovenous Fistula

Pial AVFs represent a heterogeneous group of lesions. The therapeutic approach depends on the angioarchitecture of the lesion. Treatment must be performed early with surgical or endovascular obliteration of the fistula at the point of the AV connection. Embolization can also be used as an adjunct to surgery.[78] Regardless of the treatment approach, complete permanent occlusion of the fistula is the only way to prevent long-term recurrence. Therefore liquid embolic agents are the material of choice, and polyvinyl alcohol (PVA) particles should be used only for embolization before surgical resection.

If a small (type 1) or large (type 2) pial AVF is located posterior or lateral to the spinal cord, surgery may be indicated.[72,79] If the lesion is located anterior to the spinal cord, surgical resection may be associated with a high risk of damage to the spinal cord. For giant (type 3) AVFs, surgery is indicated if endovascular treatment fails.

When treating small AVFs, microcatheter placement at the site of the AV shunt is difficult because this is usually supplied from a distal branch of the ASA.[80] For large AVFs, embolization is rarely successful because of the multiple feeding arteries. Safe microcatheter placement at the AV shunt in a large AVF can be difficult because the arterial feeders are usually from transmedullary or perimedullary branches supplying the spinal cord. Embolization has been reported in select cases. Oran and colleagues[81] reported successful glue embolization in 4 of 5 patients with small AVFs, followed by clinical improvement in 3 patients. Cho and colleagues[82] reported successful complete embolization in 3 of 5 patients (partial embolization in 1 patient) with small AVFs and 0 of 2 patients (partial embolization in 2 patients) with large AVFs. Clinical improvement or stability was seen in 2 of 4 patients with small AVFs (1 worsened) and in one-half of patients with large AVF (1 worsened). One patient treated with PVA demonstrated recurrent fistula 3 months after the embolization.

The goal of surgical treatment is to interrupt the connection between the arterial and the venous system while preserving the ASA branches. Superselective catheterization of the arterial feeder is more feasible in giant AVFs, owing to their increased diameter and the high flow through the shunt. The massively dilated draining veins increase the risk of intraoperative hemorrhage and the difficulty of surgical treatment. An endovascular approach is therefore recommended for these lesions. The major challenge of an endovascular approach is placing the embolization material in the proper position without venous migration. Ricolfi and colleagues[31] reported their results of endovascular treatment of 12 patients with giant AVFs of the spinal cord using balloons or particles. Treatment with nondetachable balloons was curative in 5 of 6 patients; embolization failed secondary to spasm in 1 patient. Treatment with detachable balloons was curative in 3 patients; partial embolization was achieved in 1 patient. In 1 patient who was treated with a detachable balloon, the balloon migrated into the venous site, causing clinical deterioration. The fistula was completely occluded in 2 patients treated with gelatin sponge particles. Clinical improvement was seen in 6 of 10 patients with complete occlusion of the fistula. In a series of 35 patients with pial AVFs, Mourier and colleagues[50] reported their results in 22 giant AVFs treated with detachable balloons. Complete occlusion of the fistula was achieved in 15 patients, all with clinical improvement following treatment. Of 6 patients with partial occlusion, 4 remained unchanged and 2 worsened clinically after treatment. There was 1 periprocedural death.

Detachable balloons are not available in the United States today, and the use of particles alone is not indicated because the particles may pass through the shunt into the venous circulation, where they may cause an inadvertent paradoxic embolus or pulmonary embolism. Instead coils, alone or combined with liquid embolic agents, should be the materials of choice. In giant AVFs, coils can be placed in the fistula to act as a frame for the liquid embolic agent to prevent migration through the high-flow shunt into the venous side. The embolization should occur at the fistula and proximal draining veins to prevent development of inaccessible collateral arterial feeders and recanalization of the fistula. Progressive retrograde thrombosis of the veins draining the fistula may result in transient worsening of symptoms.

Spinal Dural Arteriovenous Fistula

The traditional treatment of an SDAVF consists of a laminectomy with surgical exclusion of the fistula. A meta-analysis of the literature revealed a complete obliteration rate of 98% by surgical exclusion of the fistula.[83] **Table 1** summarizes the reports of surgical treatment for SDAVFs with long-term follow-up. Surgical exclusion is a durable, simple procedure, which can achieve a very high obliteration rate. There are only a few complications associated with surgery, the first of which is the potential for spine instability after a laminectomy; this can be prevented by a limited facet removal during the fistula exposure. Spine instability was not reported in a large meta-analysis of the surgical literature.[83] The second possible complication is development of a pseudomeningocele, which can be minimized by a meticulous dural, muscle, and skin closure. Surgery also continues to evolve with minimally invasive surgical techniques for excision of an SDAVF becoming available, which may limit complications.[84,85]

Although surgical treatment of SDAVFs demonstrates an initial success rate approaching 100% with minimal morbidity, only a few studies have evaluated the long-term outcome following surgical treatment. The majority of surgical series with at least 12 months of follow-up demonstrate either an improvement or stabilization of symptoms after treatment.[86–92] Behrens and Thron,[87] in a review of 21 patients 50 months after surgery, demonstrated improvement in motor activity in 67% of patients, resolution or stabilization in preoperative pain in

Table 1
Reports of surgical treatment for SDAVFs with long-term follow-up

Series,[Ref.] Year	No. of Patients	Treatment Type	Long-Term Outcome	Objective Grading Scheme
Steinmetz et al,[83] 2004	18	Surgery	Yes	Yes
Eskandar et al,[108] 2002	26	Combined	Yes	Yes
Van Dijk et al,[95] 2002	47	Combined	Yes	Yes
Song et al,[91] 2001	32	Combined	Yes	Yes
Behrens and Thron,[87] 1999	21	Surgery	Yes	Yes
Ushikoshi et al,[109] 1999	13	Combined	No	Yes
Westphal & Koch,[110] 1999	47	Combined	Yes	Yes
Lee et al,[88] 1998	9	Surgery	Yes	No
Tacconi et al,[93] 1997	25	Surgery	Yes	Yes
Afshar et al,[86] 1995	19	Surgery	Yes	Yes
Huffmann et al,[111] 1995	21	Surgery	No	
Morgan & Marsh,[112] 1989	17	Combined	No	
Mourier et al,[90] 1989	70	Surgery	Yes	No
Symon et al,[92] 1984	50	Surgery	Yes	Yes
Oldfield et al,[113] 1983	6	Surgery	No	
Merland et al,[33] 1980	13	Combined	No	
Logue,[89] 1979	24	Surgery	Yes	Yes

All studies with surgery or surgery combined with embolization are included. Long-term outcome is period >12 months.

71%, and a reduction in potency in 28% of male patients. One study by Tacconi and colleagues[93] is an exception to the other outcomes reports in the literature. These investigators showed that at a mean follow-up of 147 months, 25% of patients had arrest in progression of disease and 10% had improvement in symptoms. Sixty-three percent of patients showed deterioration in gait and/or micturition. Additional prospective long-term follow-up studies are needed to establish durability of outcome after surgical treatment, and to compare surgery with endovascular treatment.

Endovascular treatment of an SDAVF dates back to 1968, when Doppman and colleagues[75] first performed the procedure with metal pellets. Several reports demonstrating the efficacy of endovascular treatment of SDAVFs have subsequently been published (Table 2). The success rate of endovascular treatment varies from 25% to 75%.[94,95] For the treatment to be effective, the embolic agent has to occlude the fistula site, including the proximal portion of the draining vein, to prevent subsequent intradural collateral filling of the fistula. Therefore, proximal arterial occlusion with coils or Gelfoam is contraindicated. In the 1990s, embolization with particulate material (PVA) led to early recanalization of the fistula, and thus should not be used.[96] Endovascular treatment of the fistula is considered first at the

authors' institution. If there is poor penetration of the liquid embolic agent into the draining vein, persistence of the fistula after embolization, or the fistula cannot be safely embolized owing to the close proximity of an anterior spinal artery, surgical excision is chosen. The level of the fistula is marked by coil deployment into the distal segmental/intercostal artery to aid surgical localization of the level of laminectomy and fistula.[97] If endovascular treatment fails, prompt surgical resection of the fistula is recommended, as a recent study demonstrated poor clinical outcome in the event of delay in secondary intervention.[98]

Table 2 shows the published reports of SDAVFs treated with cyanoacrylate and PVA.[99] Successful endovascular treatment of SDAVFs was reported in 70% to 90% of cases.[36,91,94,100,101] Retrospective studies with significant long-term follow-up following endovascular treatment have recently been reported in the literature.[36,100] Published reports have highlighted a mean reduction for gait of 1 grade on the Aminoff-Logue scale after endovascular or surgical treatment.[91,95,102] In particular, gait disturbances were more likely to improve following endovascular or surgical treatment, whereas micturition disturbances were less likely to improve.[91] Outcomes in the literature following endovascular treatment with limited follow-up times have reported gait improvement in 40% to

Table 2
Studies reporting endovascular treatment of SDAVFs

Series,[Ref.] Year	No. of Patients	Embolization Technique	No. of Successful Embolizations (%)	No. Requiring Surgery (%)	No. of Repeat Embolizations (%)
Criscuolo et al,[114] 1989	1	PVA	0	1 (100)	0
Hall et al,[115] 1989	3	PVA	1 (33)	2 (67)	0
Hasuo et al,[116] 1996	2	PVA	2 (100)	0	0
Morgan & Marsh,[112] 1989	14	PVA	2 (14)	5 (36)	NA
Nichols et al,[96] 1992	14	PVA	3 (21)	NA	NA
Schaat et al,[42] 2002	1	PVA/Tornado coil	1 (100)	0	0
Mourier et al,[50] 1993	22	Latex detachable balloons	15 (68)	NA	NA
Rodiek,[117] 2002	1	TGMs	1 (100)	0	0
Hayashi et al,[118] 2001	1	Histoacryl + lipiodol	1 (100)	0	0
Warakaulle et al,[105] 2003	2	Onyx	1 (50)	1?	0
Jellema et al,[119] 2005	24	Histoacryl + lipiodol	12 (50)	4 (17)	5 (21)
Eskander et al,[108] 2002	21	Liquid acrylic	9 (43)	9 (43)	0
Cenzato et al,[102] 2004	10	Cyanoacrylic glue	NA	NA	NA
Birchall et al,[120] 2000	1	NBCA	0	1 (100)	0
Cognard et al,[121] 1996	7	NBCA	6 (86)	0	0
Guillevin et al,[100] 2005	26	NBCA	21 (81)	5 (19)	0
Mascalchi et al,[122] 2001	18	NBCA	11 (61)	NA	NA
Matsubara et al, 2004	2	NBCA	2 (100)	0	0
Rodesch et al,[123] 2005	18	NBCA	13 (72)	3 (17)	0
Song et al,[91] 2001	20	NBCA	14 (70)	5 (25)	0
Ushikoshi et al,[109] 1999	6	NBCA	4 (67)	2 (33)	0
Van Dijk et al,[95] 2002	44	NBCA	11 (25)	31 (70)	0
Lundqvist et al,[101] 1990	10	NBCA or PVA	9 (90)	1 (10)	0
Narvid et al,[36] 2008	39	NBCA or PVA	27 (69)	12 (31)	0
Niimi et al,[94] 1997	47	NBCA	39 (83)	0	NA
Westphal & Koch,[110] 1999	35	NBCA, embospheres, PVA, fiber coils	13 (37)	20 (57)	2 (6)

Abbreviations: CAP, cellulose acetate polymer; NA, not available; NBCA, *n*-butyl cyanoacrylate; PVA, polyvinyl alcohol; TGMs, trisacryl gelatin microspheres.

100% of patients.[91,94,100,102,103] Niimi and colleagues[94] reported that 25 (71%) of 35 patients who underwent embolization were free of symptomatic recurrence after 12 months. In another study of 44 patients primarily treated with endovascular therapy, Jellema and colleagues[104] found an improvement in motor function in 56% of patients and gait improvement in 64% of patients at 6 years after their procedure. Other symptoms such as pain and urinary symptoms are less likely to significantly improve following treatment.[91,100]

A few reports have documented the use of Onyx for the endovascular treatment of SDAVFs.[105,106] Nogueira and colleagues,[106] in a recent series of SDAVFs treated with Onyx, showed no recurrence on angiography at 12 months. However, another series of SDAVFs treated with Onyx reported by Adamczyk and colleagues[107] showed fistula recurrence even after an initial angiographic cure. The long-term durability of endovascular treatment for SDAVFs is lacking in comparison with surgery.

Epidural Arteriovenous Fistula

A large, high-flow epidural AVF is usually treated by placement of a detachable balloon or coils with a liquid embolic agent at the site of the fistula. If the epidural AVF is small, it can be definitively treated with a liquid embolic agent or with particulate embolization before surgical resection. Surgical resection is another option, but this can be very technically demanding. Endovascular embolization is the first line of treatment, followed by surgery; this can reduce the blood flow through the shunt considerably. Complete surgical exclusion includes the actual fistulous site with a small length of the affected artery and vein.

SUMMARY

This article is an overview of SAVLs, describing the classification, pathophysiology, epidemiology, clinical presentation, natural history, and pathophysiology of SAVLs in adults along with a discussion of the treatment of each lesion. MR imaging is useful as a noninvasive imaging modality to characterize all SAVLs. Spinal angiography remains the gold standard for complete evaluation of SAVLs. Endovascular and surgical techniques both have a role in the treatment of these lesions.

REFERENCES

1. Veznedaroglu E, Nelson PK, Jabbour PM, et al. Endovascular treatment of spinal cord arteriovenous malformations. Neurosurgery 2006;59:S202–9 [discussion: S3–13].
2. Aminoff MJ, Logue V. The prognosis of patients with spinal vascular malformations. Brain 1974;97:211–8.
3. Elsberg CA. Diagnosis and treatment of diseases of the spinal cord and its membranes. Philadelphia: WB Saunders Co; 1916. p. 194–204.
4. Di Chiro G, Doppman J, Ommaya AK. Selective arteriography of arteriovenous aneurysms of the spinal cord. Radiology 1967;88:1065–77.
5. Djindjian R. Embolization of angiomas of the spinal cord. Surg Neurol 1975;4:411–20.
6. Fleming A, Keynes RJ, Tannahill D. The role of the notochord in vertebral column formation. J Anat 2001;199:177–80.
7. Zawilinski J, Litwin JA, Nowogrodzka-Zagorska M, et al. Vascular system of the human spinal cord in the prenatal period: a dye injection and corrosion casting study. Ann Anat 2001;183:331–40.
8. O'Rahilly R, Muller F. Neurulation in the normal human embryo. Ciba Found Symp 1994;181:70–82 [discussion: 89].
9. Krings T, Lasjaunias PL, Hans FJ, et al. Imaging in spinal vascular disease. Neuroimaging Clin N Am 2007;17:57–72.
10. Lasjaunias P, Berenstein A, TerBrugge K. Surgical neuroangiography: clinical vascular anatomy and variations, vol. 1. Berlin: Springer-Verlag; 2001.
11. Krings T, Geibprasert S, Thron A. Spinal vascular anatomy. In: Naidich T, Castillo M, Cha S, editors. Imaging of the spine. New York: Elsevier; 2011. p. 185–200.
12. Thron A. Vascular anatomy of the spinal cord: neuroradiological investigation and clinical syndromes. Berlin: Springer-Verlag; 1988.
13. Groen RJ, Grobbelaar M, Muller CJ, et al. Morphology of the human internal vertebral venous plexus: a cadaver study after latex injection in the 21-25-week fetus. Clin Anat 2005;18:397–403.
14. Geibprasert S, Pereira V, Krings T, et al. Dural arteriovenous shunts: a new classification of craniospinal epidural venous anatomical bases and clinical correlations. Stroke 2008;39:2783–94.
15. Patsalides A, Knopman J, Santillan A, et al. Endovascular treatment of spinal arteriovenous lesions: beyond the dural fistula. AJNR Am J Neuroradiol 2011;32:798–808.
16. Krings T, Ozanne A, Chng SM, et al. Neurovascular phenotypes in hereditary haemorrhagic telangiectasia patients according to age. Review of 50 consecutive patients aged 1 day-60 years. Neuroradiology 2005;47:711–20.
17. Barnwell SL, Dowd CF, Davis RL, et al. Cryptic vascular malformations of the spinal cord: diagnosis by magnetic resonance imaging and outcome of surgery. J Neurosurg 1990;72:403–7.
18. Rodesch G, Hurth M, Alvarez H, et al. Angio-architecture of spinal cord arteriovenous shunts at presentation. Clinical correlations in adults and children. The Bicetre experience on 155 consecutive patients seen between 1981-1999. Acta Neurochir (Wien) 2004;146:217–26 [discussion: 226–7].
19. Alexander MJ, Grossi PM, Spetzler RF, et al. Extradural thoracic arteriovenous malformation in a patient with Klippel-Trenaunay-Weber syndrome: case report. Neurosurgery 2002;51:1275–8 [discussion: 1278–9].
20. Kahara V, Lehto U, Sajanti J. Presacral arteriovenous fistula: case report. Neurosurgery 2003;53:774–6 [discussion: 776–7].
21. Krings T, Mull M, Bostroem A, et al. Spinal epidural arteriovenous fistula with perimedullary drainage. Case report and pathomechanical considerations. J Neurosurg Spine 2006;5:353–8.
22. Silva N Jr, Januel AC, Tall P, et al. Spinal epidural arteriovenous fistulas associated with progressive myelopathy. Report of four cases. J Neurosurg Spine 2007;6:552–8.
23. Asai J, Hayashi T, Fujimoto T, et al. Exclusively epidural arteriovenous fistula in the cervical spine

with spinal cord symptoms: case report. Neurosurgery 2001;48:1372–5 [discussion: 1375–6].

24. Chuang NA, Shroff MM, Willinsky RA, et al. Slow-flow spinal epidural AVF with venous ectasias: two pediatric case reports. AJNR Am J Neuroradiol 2003;24:1901–5.

25. Jellema K, Tijssen CC, van Gijn J. Spinal dural arteriovenous fistulas: a congestive myelopathy that initially mimics a peripheral nerve disorder. Brain 2006;129:3150–64.

26. Krings T, Mull M, Gilsbach JM, et al. Spinal vascular malformations. Eur Radiol 2005;15:267–78.

27. Biondi A, Merland JJ, Hodes JE, et al. Aneurysms of spinal arteries associated with intramedullary arteriovenous malformations. II. Results of AVM endovascular treatment and hemodynamic considerations. AJNR Am J Neuroradiol 1992;13:923–31.

28. Spetzler RF, Detwiler PW, Riina HA, et al. Modified classification of spinal cord vascular lesions. J Neurosurg 2002;96:145–56.

29. Rodesch G, Hurth M, Alvarez H, et al. Classification of spinal cord arteriovenous shunts: proposal for a reappraisel–the Bicetre experience with 155 consecutive patients treated between 1981 and 1999. Neurosurgery 2002;51(2):374–9 [discussion: 379-80].

30. Nakstad PH, Hald JK, Bakke SJ. Multiple spinal arteriovenous fistulas in Klippel-Trenaunay-Weber syndrome treated with platinum fibre coils. Neuroradiology 1993;35:163–5.

31. Ricolfi F, Gobin PY, Aymard A, et al. Giant perimedullary arteriovenous fistulas of the spine: clinical and radiologic features and endovascular treatment. AJNR Am J Neuroradiol 1997;18:677–87.

32. Kendall BE, Logue V. Spinal epidural angiomatous malformations draining into intrathecal veins. Neuroradiology 1977;13:181–9.

33. Merland JJ, Riche MC, Chiras J. Intraspinal extramedullary arteriovenous fistulae draining into the medullary veins. J Neuroradiol 1980;7:271–320.

34. Muralidharan R, Saladino A, Lanzino G, et al. The clinical and radiological presentation of spinal dural arteriovenous fistula. Spine (Phila Pa 1976) 2011;36:E1641–7.

35. Krings T, Geibprasert S. Spinal dural arteriovenous fistulas. AJNR Am J Neuroradiol 2009;30:639–48.

36. Narvid J, Hetts SW, Larsen D, et al. Spinal dural arteriovenous fistulae: clinical features and long-term results. Neurosurgery 2008;62:159–66 [discussion: 166–7].

37. Jellema K, Canta LR, Tijssen CC, et al. Spinal dural arteriovenous fistulas: clinical features in 80 patients. J Neurol Neurosurg Psychiatry 2003;74:1438–40.

38. Hessler C, Regelsberger J, Grzyska U, et al. Therapeutic clues in spinal dural arteriovenous fistulas—a 30 year experience of 156 cases. Cent Eur Neurosurg 2010;71:8–12.

39. Koenig E, Thron A, Schrader V, et al. Spinal arteriovenous malformations and fistulae: clinical, neuroradiological and neurophysiological findings. J Neurol 1989;236:260–6.

40. Aminoff MJ, Barnard RO, Logue V. The pathophysiology of spinal vascular malformations. J Neurol Sci 1974;23:255–63.

41. Schrader V, Koenig E, Thron A, et al. Neurophysiological characteristics of spinal arteriovenous malformations. Electromyogr Clin Neurophysiol 1989;29:169–77.

42. Schaat TJ, Salzman KL, Stevens EA. Sacral origin of a spinal dural arteriovenous fistula: case report and review. Spine (Phila Pa 1976) 2002;27:893–7.

43. Kai Y, Hamada J, Morioka M, et al. Arteriovenous fistulas at the cervicomedullary junction presenting with subarachnoid hemorrhage: six case reports with special reference to the angiographic pattern of venous drainage. AJNR Am J Neuroradiol 2005;26:1949–54.

44. Foix CH, Alajouanine T. La myelite necrotique subaigue. Rev Neurol 1926;46:1–42.

45. Arnaud O, Bille F, Pouget J, et al. Epidural arteriovenous fistula with perimedullary venous drainage: case report. Neuroradiology 1994;36:490–1.

46. Clarke MJ, Patrick TA, White JB, et al. Spinal extradural arteriovenous malformations with parenchymal drainage: venous drainage variability and implications in clinical manifestations. Neurosurg Focus 2009;26:E5.

47. Weingrad DN, Doppman JL, Chretien PB, et al. Paraplegia due to posttraumatic pelvic arteriovenous fistula treated by surgery and embolization. Case report. J Neurosurg 1979;50:805–10.

48. Kawabori M, Hida K, Yano S, et al. Cervical epidural arteriovenous fistula with radiculopathy mimicking cervical spondylosis. Neurol Med Chir (Tokyo) 2009;49:108–13.

49. Rosenblum B, Oldfield EH, Doppman JL, et al. Spinal arteriovenous malformations: a comparison of dural arteriovenous fistulas and intradural AVM's in 81 patients. J Neurosurg 1987;67:795–802.

50. Mourier KL, Gobin YP, George B, et al. Intradural perimedullary arteriovenous fistulae: results of surgical and endovascular treatment in a series of 35 cases. Neurosurgery 1993;32:885–91 [discussion: 891].

51. Di Chiro G, Doppman JL. Endocranial drainage of spinal cord veins. Radiology 1970;95:555–60.

52. Hurst RW, Kenyon LC, Lavi E, et al. Spinal dural arteriovenous fistula: the pathology of venous hypertensive myelopathy. Neurology 1995;45:1309–13.

53. Djindjian M, Djindjian R, Hurth M, et al. Steal phenomena in spinal arteriovenous malformations. J Neuroradiol 1978;5:187–201.

54. el Mahdi MA, Rudwan MA, Khaffaji SM, et al. A giant spinal aneurysm with cord and root compression. J Neurol Neurosurg Psychiatry 1989;52:532–5.

55. Chen CJ, Chen CM, Lin TK. Enhanced cervical MRI in identifying intracranial dural arteriovenous fistulae with spinal perimedullary venous drainage. Neuroradiology 1998;40:393–7.

56. Terwey B, Becker H, Thron AK, et al. Gadolinium-DTPA enhanced MR imaging of spinal dural arteriovenous fistulas. J Comput Assist Tomogr 1989;13: 30–7.

57. Gilbertson JR, Miller GM, Goldman MS, et al. Spinal dural arteriovenous fistulas: MR and myelographic findings. AJNR Am J Neuroradiol 1995; 16:2049–57.

58. Sato K, Terbrugge KG, Krings T. Asymptomatic spinal dural arteriovenous fistulas: pathomechanical considerations. J Neurosurg Spine 2012;16:441–6.

59. Geibprasert S, Pongpech S, Jiarakongmun P, et al. Cervical spine dural arteriovenous fistula presenting with congestive myelopathy of the conus. J Neurosurg Spine 2009;11:427–31.

60. Bowen BC, Fraser K, Kochan JP, et al. Spinal dural arteriovenous fistulas: evaluation with MR angiography. AJNR Am J Neuroradiol 1995;16:2029–43.

61. Farb RI, Kim JK, Willinsky RA, et al. Spinal dural arteriovenous fistula localization with a technique of first-pass gadolinium-enhanced MR angiography: initial experience. Radiology 2002;222: 843–50.

62. Bowen BC, Pattany PM. Contrast-enhanced MR angiography of spinal vessels. Magn Reson Imaging Clin N Am 2000;8:597–614.

63. Mull M, Nijenhuis RJ, Backes WH, et al. Value and limitations of contrast-enhanced MR angiography in spinal arteriovenous malformations and dural arteriovenous fistulas. AJNR Am J Neuroradiol 2007;28:1249–58.

64. Bowen BC, Saraf-Lavi E, Pattany PM. MR angiography of the spine: update. Magn Reson Imaging Clin N Am 2003;11:559–84.

65. Yamaguchi S, Eguchi K, Kiura Y, et al. Multi-detector-row CT angiography as a preoperative evaluation for spinal arteriovenous fistulae. Neurosurg Rev 2007;30:321–6 [discussion: 327].

66. Hetts SW, Moftakhar P, English JD, et al. Spinal dural arteriovenous fistulas and intrathecal venous drainage: correlation between digital subtraction angiography, magnetic resonance imaging, and clinical findings. J Neurosurg Spine 2012;16: 433–40.

67. Killory BD, Nakaji P, Maughan PH, et al. Evaluation of angiographically occult spinal dural arteriovenous fistulae with surgical microscope-integrated intraoperative near-infrared indocyanine green angiography: report of 3 cases. Neurosurgery 2011;68:781–7 [discussion: 787].

68. Alleyne CH Jr, Barrow DL, Joseph G. Surgical management of angiographically occult spinal dural arteriovenous fistulae (type I spinal arteriovenous malformations): three technical case reports. Neurosurgery 1999;44:891–4 [discussion:894–5].

69. Oldfield EH, Bennett A 3rd, Chen MY, et al. Successful management of spinal dural arteriovenous fistulas undetected by arteriography. Report of three cases. J Neurosurg 2002;96:220–9.

70. Sugawara T, Hirano Y, Itoh Y, et al. Angiographically occult spinal dural arteriovenous fistula located using selective computed tomography angiography. Case report. J Neurosurg Spine 2007;7:215–20.

71. Biondi A, Merland JJ, Reizine D, et al. Embolization with particles in thoracic intramedullary arteriovenous malformations: long-term angiographic and clinical results. Radiology 1990;177:651–8.

72. Anson J, Khayata M, Merland J. Spinal arteriovenous malformations. Intravascular techniques. In: Carter LP, Spetzler RF, Hamilton MG, editors. Neurovascular surgery. New York: McGraw-Hill; 1995.

73. Merland J, Reizine D, Laurent A, et al. Embolization of spinal cord vascular lesions. In: Vinuela F, Halbach VV, Dion JE, editors. Interventional neuroradiology: endovascular therapy of the central nervous system. New York: Raven Press; 1992.

74. Djindjian R, Cophignon J, Rey Theron J, et al. Superselective arteriographic embolization by the femoral route in neuroradiology. Study of 50 cases. 3. Embolization in craniocerebral pathology. Neuroradiology 1973;6:143–52.

75. Doppman JL, Di Chiro G, Ommaya A. Obliteration of spinal-cord arteriovenous malformation by percutaneous embolisation. Lancet 1968;1:477.

76. Rodesch G, Hurth M, Alvarez H, et al. Embolization of spinal cord arteriovenous shunts: morphological and clinical follow-up and results—review of 69 consecutive cases. Neurosurgery 2003;53:40–9 [discussion: 49–50].

77. Corkill RA, Mitsos AP, Molyneux AJ. Embolization of spinal intramedullary arteriovenous malformations using the liquid embolic agent, Onyx: a single-center experience in a series of 17 patients. J Neurosurg Spine 2007;7:478–85.

78. Hida K, Iwasaki Y, Goto K, et al. Results of the surgical treatment of perimedullary arteriovenous fistulas with special reference to embolization. J Neurosurg 1999;90:198–205.

79. Hodes JE, Merland JJ, Casasco A, et al. Spinal vascular malformations: endovascular therapy. Neurosurg Clin N Am 1994;5:497–509.

80. Riche MC, Melki JP, Merland JJ. Embolization of spinal cord vascular malformations via the anterior spinal artery. AJNR Am J Neuroradiol 1983;4: 378–81.

81. Oran I, Parildar M, Derbent A. Treatment of slow-flow (type I) perimedullary spinal arteriovenous

fistulas with special reference to embolization. AJNR Am J Neuroradiol 2005;26:2582–6.

82. Cho KT, Lee DY, Chung CK, et al. Treatment of spinal cord perimedullary arteriovenous fistula: embolization versus surgery. Neurosurgery 2005;56:232–41 [discussion: 241].

83. Steinmetz MP, Chow MM, Krishnaney AA, et al. Outcome after the treatment of spinal dural arteriovenous fistulae: a contemporary single-institution series and meta-analysis. Neurosurgery 2004;55:77–87 [discussion: 88].

84. Desai A, Bekelis K, Erkmen K. Minimally invasive tubular retractor system for adequate exposure during surgical obliteration of spinal dural arteriovenous fistulas with the aid of indocyanine green intraoperative angiography. J Neurosurg Spine 2012;17:160–3.

85. Patel NP, Birch BD, Lyons MK, et al. Minimally invasive intradural spinal dural arteriovenous fistula ligation. World Neurosurg 2012. [Epub ahead of print].

86. Afshar JK, Doppman JL, Oldfield EH. Surgical interruption of intradural draining vein as curative treatment of spinal dural arteriovenous fistulas. J Neurosurg 1995;82:196–200.

87. Behrens S, Thron A. Long-term follow-up and outcome in patients treated for spinal dural arteriovenous fistula. J Neurol 1999;246:181–5.

88. Lee TT, Gromelski EB, Bowen BC, et al. Diagnostic and surgical management of spinal dural arteriovenous fistulas. Neurosurgery 1998;43:242–6 [discussion: 246–7].

89. Logue V. Angiomas of the spinal cord: review of the pathogenesis, clinical features, and results of surgery. J Neurol Neurosurg Psychiatry 1979;42:1–11.

90. Mourier KL, Gelbert F, Rey A, et al. Spinal dural arteriovenous malformations with perimedullary drainage. Indications and results of surgery in 30 cases. Acta Neurochir (Wien) 1989;100:136–41.

91. Song JK, Vinuela F, Gobin YP, et al. Surgical and endovascular treatment of spinal dural arteriovenous fistulas: long-term disability assessment and prognostic factors. J Neurosurg 2001;94:199–204.

92. Symon L, Kuyama H, Kendall B. Dural arteriovenous malformations of the spine. Clinical features and surgical results in 55 cases. J Neurosurg 1984;60:238–47.

93. Tacconi L, Lopez Izquierdo BC, Symon L. Outcome and prognostic factors in the surgical treatment of spinal dural arteriovenous fistulas. A long-term study. Br J Neurosurg 1997;11:298–305.

94. Niimi Y, Berenstein A, Setton A, et al. Embolization of spinal dural arteriovenous fistulae: results and follow-up. Neurosurgery 1997;40:675–82 [discussion: 682–3].

95. Van Dijk JM, TerBrugge KG, Willinsky RA, et al. Multidisciplinary management of spinal dural arteriovenous fistulas: clinical presentation and long-

term follow-up in 49 patients. Stroke 2002;33:1578–83.

96. Nichols DA, Rufenacht DA, Jack CR Jr, et al. Embolization of spinal dural arteriovenous fistula with polyvinyl alcohol particles: experience in 14 patients. AJNR Am J Neuroradiol 1992;13:933–40.

97. Marquardt G, Berkefeld J, Seifert V, et al. Preoperative coil marking to facilitate intraoperative localization of spinal dural arteriovenous fistulas. Eur Spine J 2009;18:1117–20.

98. Andres RH, Barth A, Guzman R, et al. Endovascular and surgical treatment of spinal dural arteriovenous fistulas. Neuroradiology 2008;50:869–76.

99. Sivakumar W, Zada G, Yashar P, et al. Endovascular management of spinal dural arteriovenous fistulas. A review. Neurosurg Focus 2009;26:E15.

100. Guillevin R, Vallee JN, Cormier E, et al. N-butyl 2-cyanoacrylate embolization of spinal dural arteriovenous fistulae: CT evaluation, technical features, and outcome prognosis in 26 cases. AJNR Am J Neuroradiol 2005;26:929–35.

101. Lundqvist C, Berthelsen B, Sullivan M, et al. Spinal arteriovenous malformations: neurological aspects and results of embolization. Acta Neurol Scand 1990;82:51–8.

102. Cenzato M, Versari P, Righi C, et al. Spinal dural arteriovenous fistulae: analysis of outcome in relation to pretreatment indicators. Neurosurgery 2004;55:815–22 [discussion: 822–3].

103. Atkinson RP, Awad IA, Batjer HH, et al. Reporting terminology for brain arteriovenous malformation clinical and radiographic features for use in clinical trials. Stroke 2001;32:1430–42.

104. Jellema K, Tijssen CC, van Rooij WJ, et al. Spinal dural arteriovenous fistulas: long-term follow-up of 44 treated patients. Neurology 2004;62:1839–41.

105. Warakaulle DR, Aviv RI, Niemann D, et al. Embolisation of spinal dural arteriovenous fistulae with Onyx. Neuroradiology 2003;45:110–2.

106. Nogueira RG, Dabus G, Rabinov JD, et al. Onyx embolization for the treatment of spinal dural arteriovenous fistulae: initial experience with long-term follow-up. Technical case report. Neurosurgery 2009;64:E197–8 [discussion: E198].

107. Adamczyk P, Amar AP, Mack WJ, et al. Recurrence of "cured" dural arteriovenous fistulas after Onyx embolization. Neurosurg Focus 2012;32:E12.

108. Eskandar EN, Borges LF, Budzik RF, et al. Spinal dural arteriovenous fistulas: experience with endovascular and surgical therapy. J Neurosurg 2002;96:162–7.

109. Ushikoshi S, Hida K, Kikuchi Y, et al. Functional prognosis after treatment of spinal dural arteriovenous fistulas. Neurol Med Chir (Tokyo) 1999;39:206–12 [discussion 12–3].

110. Westphal M, Koch C. Management of spinal dural arteriovenous fistulae using an interdisciplinary neuroradiological/neurosurgical approach: experience with 47 cases. Neurosurgery 1999;45:451–7 [discussion 7–8].

111. Huffmann BC, Gilsbach JM, Thron A. Spinal dural arteriovenous fistulas: a plea for neurosurgical treatment. Acta Neurochir (Wien) 1995; 135:44–51.

112. Morgan MK, Marsh WR. Management of spinal dural arteriovenous malformations. J Neurosurg 1989; 70:832–6.

113. Oldfield EH, Di Chiro G, Quindlen EA, et al. Successful treatment of a group of spinal cord arteriovenous malformations by interruption of dural fistula. J Neurosurg 1983;59:1019–30.

114. Criscuolo GR, Oldfield EH, Doppman JL. Reversible acute and subacute myelopathy in patients with dural arteriovenous fistulas. Foix-Alajouanine syndrome reconsidered. J Neurosurg 1989;70: 354–9.

115. Hall WA, Oldfield EH, Doppman JL. Recanalization of spinal arteriovenous malformations following embolization. J Neurosurg 1989;70:714–20.

116. Hasuo K, Mizushima A, Mihara F, et al. Contrast-enhanced MRI in spinal arteriovenous malformations and fistulae before and after embolisation therapy. Neuroradiology 1996;38:609–14.

117. Rodiek SO. Successful endovascular treatment of a spinal dural arteriovenous fistula with trisacryl gelatin microspheres. Minim Invasive Neurosurg 2002;45:173–6.

118. Hayashi K, Kitagawa N, Takahata H, et al. A case of spinal dural AVF treated by endovascular embolization. No To Shinkei 2001;53:381–5.

119. Jellema K, Sluzewski M, van Rooij WJ, et al. Embolization of spinal dural arteriovenous fistulas: importance of occlusion of the draining vein. J Neurosurg Spine 2005;2:580–3.

120. Birchall D, Hughes DG, West CG. Recanalisation of spinal dural arteriovenous fistula after successful embolisation. J Neurol Neurosurg Psychiatry 2000;68:792–3.

121. Cognard C, Miaux Y, Pierot L, et al. The role of CT in evaluation of the effectiveness of embolisation of spinal dural arteriovenous fistulae with N-butyl cyanoacrylate. Neuroradiology 1996;38:603–8.

122. Mascalchi M, Ferrito G, Quilici N, et al. Spinal vascular malformations: MR angiography after treatment. Radiology 2001;219:346–53.

123. Rodesch G, Hurth M, Alvarez H, et al. Spinal cord intradural arteriovenous fistulae: anatomic, clinical, and therapeutic considerations in a series of 32 consecutive patients seen between 1981 and 2000 with emphasis on endovascular therapy. Neurosurgery 2005;57:973–83 [discussion 83].

Spinal Arteriovenous Shunts in Children

Indran Davagnanam, MD, MB BCh, BAO, BMedSci, FRCR[a,b,*],
Ahmed K. Toma, MD, FRCS (Neurosurg)[c],
Stefan Brew, MBBS, MHB, MSc, FRANZCR, FRCR[a,d]

KEYWORDS

- Spinal arteriovenous shunt • Congenital condition • Pediatrics • Arteriovenous malformation

KEY POINTS

- Spinal arteriovenous shunts are rare.
- Many spinal arteriovenous shunts are associated with congenital conditions (eg, Cobb syndrome).
- Only symptomatic lesions should be treated.
- Spinal arteriovenous shunts are difficult to treat.

INTRODUCTION

Pediatric spinal arteriovenous shunts (PSAVS) are rare and, in contrast to those in adults, are often congenital or associated with underlying genetic disorders.[1] They are thought to represent a more severe and complete phenotypic spectrum of all spinal arteriovenous shunts seen in the overall spinal shunt population. The pediatric presentation thus accounts for its association with significant morbidity and, in general, a more challenging treatment process compared with the adult presentation.[2]

Approximately 10% of all central nervous system arteriovenous shunts are spinal, but of those, a much smaller proportion is thought to present in the pediatric age group.[3–5] The proportion of pediatric patients presenting with this disease seems to vary widely in the published literature, and the incidence is generally underestimated because of the variable clinical presentation and difficulty in establishing the diagnosis. In one series of spinal arteriovenous shunts, pediatric patients accounted for approximately 20% of the population.[6]

CLASSIFICATION OF PSAVS

Several classification systems have been used historically, which were largely inconsistent and imprecise, focusing primarily on being descriptive.[7–12] Mulliken and Glowacki[13] proposed the first classification system for vascular malformations based on endothelial cell characteristics and thus the vascular biology of these lesions. Since then, more recent classification systems have attempted to incorporate the vascular biology of these malformations, because it leads to a better understanding of the character and natural history of these lesions. This classification ultimately aids the neurovascular interventionalist in determining endovascular management.

One of the more recently proposed classification systems, based on 25-year experience at the Bicêtre Hospital,[2] begins with considering underlying hereditary conditions, which provide some evidence for a genetic role in the development of PSAVS. In a series of patients younger than 2 years, 62% with PSAVS demonstrated either hereditary hemorrhagic telangiectasia (HHT) or a

[a] Lysholm Department of Neuroradiology, National Hospital for Neurology & Neurosurgery, Queen Square, London WC1N 3BG, UK; [b] Brain Repair & Rehabilitation Unit, Institute of Neurology, University College London, London WC1N 3BG, UK; [c] Victor Horsley Department of Neurosurgery, National Hospital for Neurology & Neurosurgery, Queen Square, London WC1N 3BG, UK; [d] Department of Neuroradiology, Great Ormond Street Hospital for Children, Great Ormond Street, London WC1N 3JH, UK
* Corresponding author. Lysholm Department of Neuroradiology, National Hospital for Neurology & Neurosurgery, Queen Square, London WC1N 3BG, UK.
E-mail address: indran.davagnanam@uclh.nhs.uk

Neuroimag Clin N Am 23 (2013) 749–756
http://dx.doi.org/10.1016/j.nic.2013.04.002
1052-5149/13/$ – see front matter © 2013 Elsevier Inc. All rights reserved.

somatic nonheritable mutation/spinal arteriovenous metameric syndrome (SAMS).[14] HHT is an autosomal dominant disease with identified mutations in 3 genes, 2 of which are members of the transforming growth factor β (TGF-β) pathway, which plays an important role during the embryologic development of vascular assembly and angiogenesis.[15] Genetic nonhereditary conditions, such as Klippel-Trenaunay syndrome, Parkes Weber syndrome, neurofibromatosis I, and Ehlers-Danlos syndrome type IV, have also been associated with PSAVS.[5,16]

The morphology of the shunt is then determined and classified into either a fistula, consisting of a single direct point of arteriovenous shunting, or a nidus, whereby the arteriovenous shunt occurs through a network of vessels. Fistulas are further classified into either microfistulas or macrofistulas. Micro–arteriovenous fistulas are small-size lesions fed by one or multiple arteries of different caliber, which drain into moderately enlarged veins, whereas macro–arteriovenous fistulas are high-flow shunts supplied by large arteries, which drain directly into a giant varix with secondary congestion of spinal cord veins.

The distinction between a fistula and nidus can be difficult to determine even if characterization via catheter angiography is performed, because arteriovenous shunts can induce progressive vascular changes over time with more prominent venous ectasia and recruitment of further arterial supply. Thus a single fistulous point may appear as a multiply shunting process resembling a nidus with time because of the pattern of pial reflex and congestion.[2]

The compartmentalization of the shunt is the final consideration; this is classified into pial (intradural), dural (epidural), or paraspinal (parachordal). The pediatric dural shunts described here are not to be confused with and are distinct from the adult spinal dural arteriovenous fistulas, which are acquired lesions.[17]

In using this classification system, it becomes apparent that the character of the shunt and its location are the most important factors in determining the management options and thus the likely outcome of subsequent endovascular treatment.

CLINICAL PRESENTATION

Although the angioarchitecture of PSAVS is an important determinant of treatment and its outcome, no definite evidence suggests that it determines clinical presentation, particularly hemorrhage, in these patients. Similarly, considering the strong association with hereditary conditions such as HHT and SAMS, very few patients presenting with PSAVS fulfill the clinical diagnostic criteria for HHT or have stigmata of a metameric syndrome.

A series of patients with intradural PSAVS showed that 19% presented at age 15 years and younger, with a high male predominance in contrast to the gender parity in the adult population.[6] Most of the shunts in this series were in the cervical and thoracic spinal regions, with twice as many nidal-type shunts than fistulas. Hemorrhage at presentation was seen in 21 of the 30 patients: 11 with hematomyelia and 10 with subarachnoid hemorrhage. Patients with hematomyelia had severe deficits at presentation compared with their counterparts with subarachnoid hemorrhage. The remainder of the patients who presented without hemorrhage had acute symptoms attributable to venous congestion with or without venous thrombosis.

In another series in patients younger than 2 years, the proportion presenting with hemorrhage was much smaller, approximately 23% overall, but around 20% of those with intradural PSAVS. The mean age of presentation in that series was 7 months, with a similar male predominance to that seen in older children.[14]

DIAGNOSTIC IMAGING
Magnetic Resonance Imaging

Magnetic resonance imaging (MRI) is the preferred modality for screening for PSAVS, and often requires imaging of the entire spinal axis. Computed tomography (CT) and conventional/CT myelography have little role to play the diagnosis and premanagement evaluation of spinal arteriovenous shunts.

Conspicuous and tortuous flow voids representing congested dilated veins are detectable on standard spin-echo, high-resolution steady-state Constructive Interference in Steady State (CISS)/Fast Imaging Employing Steady State Acquisition (FIESTA), and high-resolution 3-dimensional fast spin-echo with variable excitation pulse Sampling Perfection with Application optimized Contrasts using different flip angle Evolution (SPACE) sequences. The venous dilatation can often elude the site of the shunt in relation to the dura. Current contrast-enhanced time-resolved magnetic resonance angiography techniques are similarly useful in detecting the presence of a shunt, but currently little evidence shows its role in reliably identifying the site of arteriovenous shunting,[18] although it can often visualize the location of an arteriovenous malformation (AVM) and the approximate location of its implied arterial feeders.

MRI is also useful in visualizing flow-related aneurysms, associated compression, edema, and hemorrhage affecting the spinal cord. Gadolinium contrast enhancement is sometimes seen, attributed to venous stasis, ischemia, or infarction of the spinal cord. In cases of SAMS, lesions of the associated metamere can often be seen. The utility of MRI is limited, however, in distinguishing between a nidus and an arteriovenous fistula and detecting small ventral shunts with draining veins within the ventral sulcus of the spinal cord.[19]

Spinal Angiography

Currently, spinal angiography is considered the gold standard imaging modality for PSAVS. It is an invasive procedure performed with the patient under general anesthesia, requiring experienced neurointerventional expertise. Selective injections of all feeding pedicles and analysis of the draining veins is essential in the assessment and understanding of the angioarchitecture of PSAVS. This procedure also includes the assessment of the vascularity of adjacent spinal cord, which is crucial for preembolization treatment planning.

However, the intradural spinal arteries in neonates and infants are proportionately larger and more tortuous than in the normal adult, and therefore should not be misinterpreted as a pathologic finding.

Three-dimensional rotational spinal digital subtraction angiography (DSA) can be helpful in characterizing the PSAVS, particularly in identifying intranidal pseudoaneurysms and evaluating the feasibility of embolization.

THERAPEUTIC STRATEGY

The therapeutic strategy is determined on an individual basis relating to the expected clinical objective, be it preventive, corrective, or palliative. The choice of either primary neurosurgical treatment, with or without preembolization, or primary endovascular treatment will differ depending on the individual case and the institution. The results of either vary accordingly in the published literature.[3,20–24]

The treatment approach and likely outcome is dependent on the angioarchitecture of the PSAVS. Fistulas have a greater likelihood of complete cure than AVMs, because the latter has a more complex anatomy. In AVMs this often precludes complete embolization, which, if attempted, may raise the risk of permanent neurologic deficit; partial targeted embolization of AVMs thus offers an improvement without unduly increasing this risk.

Treatment of PSAVS should almost never be on an emergent basis. Careful diagnostic angiographic assessment of the angioarchitecture of

the shunt and determination of a preembolization strategy should be advocated before embarking on treatment.

Patients presenting with hemorrhage are supportively managed initially to allow recovery before any intervention is performed with embolization, usually 6 to 8 weeks after the initial event. Early or frequent rehemorrhage is not a typical feature in PSAVS, although differences may exist in extremely young patients.[2] If an arterial pseudoaneurysm is identified in association with a ruptured PSAVS, partial targeted embolization may be considered, similar to the approach for ruptured brain AVMs.

The choice of delivery catheters and embolic material, and the choice of arterial, venous, or combination approaches can be variable. The methods outlined in the following sections reflect the treatment choice and strategy developed at the authors' institution, elements of which are common to other institutions but not prescriptive.

PIAL AVMS

Pial AVMs of the spinal cord rarely present in children, and are seldom seen in neonates, casting doubt on the widely held assumption that they are congenital. Their natural history is poorly characterized, and the risks of treatment are often high. Decision making is therefore difficult. In general, only symptomatic lesions should be treated, and treatment should be targeted at specific angioarchitectural features, such as rapidly shunting components or aneurysms.[14,25] Treatment may be surgical, endovascular, or a combination of these. Although cure is occasionally achieved, often partial treatment aiming for a reduction in shunt volume or the exclusion of aneurysms believed to be the site of hemorrhage is all that can be achieved.

Imaging should include MRI of the brain and spine (which will allow assessment of the cord parenchyma and determination of the presence or absence of blood) and catheter angiography. For a pial AVM, the anterior spinal axis above and below the lesion must be identified on catheter angiography, and all segmental arteries to the region must be injected. Meticulous analysis of the angiographic study is mandatory, because the distinction between anterior and posterior spinal arterial supply is critical in determining the least risky route for embolization.

Endovascular treatment is technically demanding and carries significant risk. In the spinal cord, the operator must be mindful that the best position that can be obtained for embolization is still within millimeters of the anterior spinal and its branches. Inadvertent occlusion of these arteries can result in, at best, a hemicord syndrome, and potentially cord transection. Communication between feeding pedicles to the AVM should be anticipated, even if not visible. The technique used at the authors' institution involves catheterization of the appropriate segmental artery with a 4-Fr Catheter, and subsequent catheterization of the targeted feeding pedicle with a Magic microcatheter. The appropriate component of the AVM is then closed using cyanoacrylate glue rendered radio-opaque with Lipiodol.

PIAL ARTERIOVENOUS FISTULAS

Pail arteriovenous fistulas (**Fig. 1**) usually present with progressive neurologic deficit caused by either mechanical deformation of the cord or cord edema from venous hypertension. Spinal subarachnoid hemorrhage is surprisingly rare. It often presents in children, and is clearly associated with HHT.[26] This finding does not necessarily imply that they are congenital (ie, present at birth), and the authors have never seen a pial arteriovenous fistula of the spinal cord present in the neonatal or infant period.

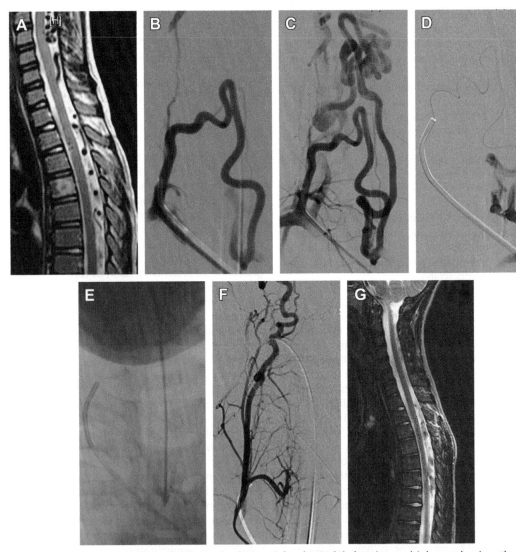

Fig. 1. Spinal cord arteriovenous fistula. Sagittal T2-weighted MRI (*A*) showing multiple, predominantly dorsal, dilated, and tortuous pial veins. Arterial (*B*) and venous (*C*) phases of a right costocervical artery angiogram showing the fistula and the prominent draining veins. Superselective microcatheterization of the feeding artery and angiography shows the point of fistulation (*D*) from which glue embolization was undertaken (*E*). The post-embolization follow-up angiogram through the costocervical artery (*F*) reveals no residual arteriovenous shunting and a perceptible absence of prominent pial veins on the sagittal T2-weighted MRI of the spinal cord (*G*).

Although the natural history is poorly character-ized, almost all present with progressive neuro-logic deficit, and treatment is therefore clearly indicated. The goal should be cure. Imaging should include MRI of the brain and spine (which will allow assessment of the cord parenchyma and determi-nation of the presence or absence of any other le-sions) and catheter angiography. As for pial AVMs, spinal angiography can be technically demanding, again requiring the anterior spinal axis above and below the lesion to be identified, and all segmental arteries to the region should be injected. Often massively distended pial arteries supply the fistula from remote segmental arteries, and extensive angiography may be necessary.

Treatment is usually endovascular, and usually cure can be achieved. The same issues outlined earlier for pial AVM apply: inadvertent occlusion of the intrinsic blood supply to the spinal cord re-sults in, at best, a hemicord syndrome, and poten-tially functional cord transection. As with the pial AVMs, the preceding diagnostic angiogram must be meticulously conducted and analyzed, be-cause distinction between anterior and posterior spinal arterial supply is critical in determining the least risky route for embolization. In pial AVF, the anatomy is often grossly distorted, and it may be difficult to judge the point at which the fistula lies or to precisely identify the artery that enters the fistula.

A similar technique of catheterizing the appro-priate segmental artery with a 4-Fr catheter is per-formed, followed by microcatheterization of the targeted feeding pedicle with a Magic microcath-eter. The microcatheter is passed through the fis-tula to the venous side, and then withdrawn to lie at the arteriovenous junction. Very concentrated Histoacryl, rendered radio-opaque with Tantalum powder to minimize delay in polymerization from Lipiodol, is then injected in free flow, forming a localized plug at the arteriovenous junction. If the initial embolization does not result in cure, but a significant reduction in the arteriovenous shunt has been achieved, it is often much easier to un-derstand the anatomy after an interval of several months, when the arteries and veins have reduced in caliber.

Coil embolization is technically easier, and prob-ably safer, although in the authors' experience, when used in this situation often does not result in cure and may make definitive treatment more difficult by blocking access to the feeding pedicles.

DURAL ARTERIOVENOUS FISTULAS

Dural arteriovenous fistulas are extremely rare, and usually have different morphology to the corresponding lesions in adults, with a more diffuse zone of arteriovenous shunting and much more prominent congestion of the pial plexus of the cord. Many are associated with Cobb syn-drome, a spinal metameric vascular malformation characterized by a pial AVM, dural arteriovenous fistula, paraspinal AVM, and cutaneous lesion, all at the same metameric level.[27,28]

PARASPINAL ARTERIOVENOUS FISTULAS

Paraspinal arteriovenous fistulas are referred to as parachordal arteriovenous fistulas by Rodesch and Lasjaunias (Fig. 2), and when present raise the possibility of associated genetic conditions, particularly HHT or SAMS.[5,14,29–32] These are rapidly shunting direct arteriovenous fistulas that may present with heart failure,[33] or drain into the intradural venous system and produce pial congestion and cord symptoms such as cord dysfunction as a result of mass effect or edema, hematomyelia, or subarachnoid hemorrhage.[14,34] The most common site is the cervicothoracic junc-tion. Paraspinal arteriovenous fistulas are often mistaken for vertebro-vertebral fistulas when in the cervical region, because they generally drain into the vertebral venous plexus. When angio-graphically analyzed, they are always supplied by a segmental artery rather than directly off the vertebral artery. The distinction is important, because closing the vertebral artery itself will not result in cure and will risk neurologic deficit from cord ischemia.

In the head and neck region, the brachial arte-riovenous shunts also include maxillary and pharyngeal arteriovenous fistulas. Children with this condition may present with a bruit or a slowly enlarging pulsatile mass.[35] Thoracolumbar arte-riovenous shunts are extremely rare in children with minimal clinical symptoms, which may re-main indolent until venous drainage is rerouted centripetally.

The authors' preferred approach to these le-sions is balloon occlusion using a detachable balloon. The balloon is positioned and inflated, closing the fistula, but not detached. Catheter angiography of the artery supplying the fistula, and all surrounding segmental arteries, is per-formed before detachment (via the contralateral femoral artery) to confirm exclusion of the fistula and preservation of blood supply to the spinal cord. Although coils are technically simpler, the irreversible deployment and inadvertent exclusion of a significant radicular artery, which may arise from an occluded segmental artery, may have disastrous consequences.

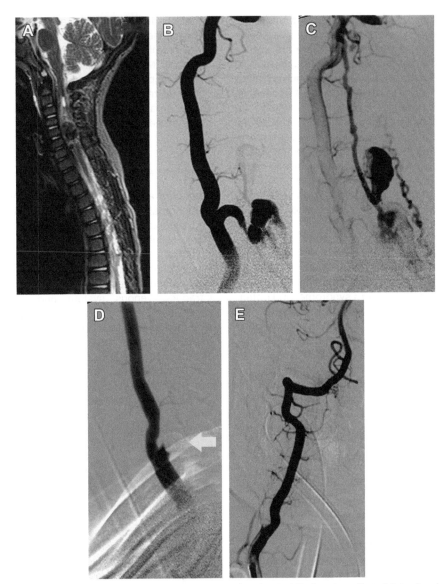

Fig. 2. Parachordal arteriovenous fistula. Sagittal T2-weighted MRI (*A*) showing dilated intradural vessels and myelopathic spinal cord changes. Arterial (*B*) and venous (*C*) phases of a selective right vertebral artery angiogram showing a parachordal arteriovenous fistula filling via a segmental artery shunting into marked distended intradural veins. A balloon is inflated (*white arrow*) with exclusion of the fistula (*D*). The 6-month follow-up of right subclavian angiogram (*E*) shows no arteriovenous shunt post-balloon occlusion.

SUMMARY

Spinal arteriovenous shunts that are diagnosed in the neonates, infants, and children are not anatomically different from those in adults. They have a high association with genetic abnormalities, including HHT and SAMS in children versus adults. Evaluation for these syndromes should be sought when a child presents with a spinal arteriovenous shunt. These lesions tend to affect male pediatric patients more commonly than adult patients. A hemorrhagic presentation is much more frequent in children than adults, except in very young children. Many spinal arteriovenous shunts are amendable to endovascular therapy; however, this group of lesions can cause significant morbidity.

REFERENCES

1. Rodesch G, Lasjaunias P. Spinal cord arteriovenous shunts: from imaging to management. Eur J Radiol 2003;46(3):221–32.

2. Cullen S, Krings T, Ozanne A, et al. Diagnosis and endovascular treatment of pediatric spinal arteriovenous shunts. Neuroimaging Clin N Am 2007;17(2): 207–21.

3. Cogen P, Stein BM. Spinal cord arteriovenous malformations with significant intramedullary components. J Neurosurg 1983;59:471–8.

4. Stapf C, Mast H, Sciacca RR, et al. The New York Islands AVM study: design, study progress and initial results. Stroke 2003;34:29–33.

5. Rodesch G, Hurth M, Alvarez H, et al. Classification of spinal cord arteriovenous shunts: proposal for a reappraisal—the Bicetre experience with 155 consecutive patients treated between 1981 and 1999. Neurosurgery 2002;51:374–80.

6. Rodesch G, Hurth M, Alvarez H, et al. Angio-architecture of spinal cord arteriovenous shunts at presentation. Clinical correlations in adults and children. Acta Neurochir (Wien) 2004;146:217–27.

7. Anson JA, Spetzler RF. Classification of spinal arteriovenous malformations and implications for treatment. BNI Q 1992;8:2.

8. Bao YH, Ling F. Classification and therapeutic modalities of spinal vascular malformations in 80 patients. Neurosurgery 1997;40:75–81.

9. Heros R, Debrun G, Ojemann RG, et al. Direct spinal arteriovenous fistula: a new type of spinal AVM. J Neurosurg 1986;64:134–9.

10. Marsh WR. Vascular lesions of the spinal cord: history and classification. Neurosurg Clin N Am 1999;10:1–8.

11. Merland JJ, Reizine D, Laurent A, et al. Embolization of spinal cord vascular lesions. In: Vinuela F, Halbach VV, Dion J, editors. Interventional neuroradiology: endovascular therapy of the central nervous system. New York: Raven Press; 1992. p. 153–65.

12. Spetzler RF, Detwiler PW, Riina HA, et al. Modified classification of spinal cord vascular lesions. J Neurosurg 2002;96:145–56.

13. Mulliken JB, Glowacki J. Hemangiomas and vascular malformations in infants and children: a classification based on endothelial characteristics. Plast Reconstr Surg 1982;69:412–22.

14. Cullen S, Alvarez H, Rodesch G, et al. Spinal arteriovenous shunts presenting before 2 years of age: analysis of 13 cases. Childs Nerv Syst 2006;22(9): 1103–10.

15. Fernandez-Lopez A, Sanz-Rodriguez F, Blanco FJ, et al. Hereditary hemorrhagic telangiectasia a vascular dysplasia affecting the TGF-B signalling pathway. Clin Med Res 2006;4:66–78.

16. Deans W, Bloch S, Leibrock L, et al. Arteriovenous fistula in patients with neurofibromatosis. Radiology 1982;144:103–7.

17. Berenstein A, Lasjaunias P, ter Brugge KG. Spinal arteriovenous malformations. In: Berenstein A, Lasjaunias P, editors. Surgical neuroangiography, clinical and endovascular treatment aspects in adults, vol. 22. Berlin: Springer Verlag; 2004. p. 738–847.

18. Meckel S, Maier M, Ruiz DS, et al. MR angiography of dural arteriovenous fistulas: diagnosis and follow-up after treatment using a time-resolved 3D contrast-enhanced technique. AJNR Am J Neuroradiol 2007;28(5):877–84.

19. Lasjaunias P, Maillot C, Terbrugge K. Pial relations with spinal cord veins explain MRI occult spinal AV shunts. Interv Neuroradiol 2000;6:333–6.

20. Rodesch G, Hurth M, Ducot B, et al. Embolization of spinal cord arteriovenous shunts: morphological and clinical follow-up and results—review of 69 consecutive cases. Neurosurgery 2003;53:40–50.

21. Krayenbuehl H, Yasargil MG, McClintock HG. Treatment of spinal cord vascular malformations by surgical excision. J Neurosurg 1969;30:427–35.

22. Rosenblum B, Oldfield EH, Doppman JL, et al. Spinal arteriovenous malformations: a comparison of dural arteriovenous fistulas and intradural AVMs in 81 patients. J Neurosurg 1987;67:795–802.

23. Spetzler RF, Zabramski JM, Flom RA. Management of juvenile spinal AVMs by embolization and surgical excision. J Neurosurg 1989;70:628–32.

24. Connolly ES, Zubay GP, McCormick PC, et al. The posterior approach to a series of glomus (type II) intramedullary spinal cord arteriovenous malformations. Neurosurgery 1998;42:774–86.

25. Berenstein A, Lasjaunias P. Spinal cord arteriovenous malformations. In: Berenstein A, Lasjaunias P, editors. Surgical neuroangiography: endovascular treatment of spine and spinal cord lesions, vol. 5. New York: Springer Verlag; 1992. p. 24–109.

26. Rodesch G, Hurth M, Alvarez H, et al. Spinal cord intradural arteriovenous fistulae: anatomic, clinical, and therapeutic considerations in a series of 32 consecutive patients seen between 1981 and 2000 with emphasis on endovascular therapy. Neurosurgery 2005;57(5):973–83.

27. Ling J, Agid R, Nakano S, et al. Metachronous multiplicity of spinal cord arteriovenous fistula and spinal dural AVF in a patient with hereditary haemorrhagic telangiectasia. Interv Neuroradiol 2005; 11(1):79.

28. Tubridy Clark M, Brooks EL, Chong W, et al. Cobb syndrome: a case report and systematic review of the literature. Pediatr Neurol 2008;39(6): 423–5.

29. Alexander MJ, Grossi PM, Spetzler RF, et al. Extradural thoracic arteriovenous malformation in a patient with Klippel-Trenaunay-Weber syndrome. Case report. Neurosurgery 2002;51:1275–8.

30. Kahara V, Lehto U, Ryymin P, et al. Vertebral epidural arteriovenous fistula and radicular pain in neurofibromatosis type 1. Acta Neurochir (Wien) 2002; 144:493–6.

31. Rodesch G, Alvarez H, Chaskkis C, et al. Clinical manifestations in paraspinal arteriovenous malformations. Spinal cord symptoms, pathophysiology and treatment objectives. Intern J Neuroradiol 1996;2:430–6.

32. Goyal M, Willinsky R, Montanera W, et al. Paravertebral arteriovenous malformations with epidural drainage: clinical spectrum, imaging features, and results of treatment. AJNR Am J Neuroradiol 1999; 20:749–55.

33. Lasjaunias P. A revised concept of the congenital nature of cerebral arteriovenous malformations. Interv Neuroradiol 1997;3:275–81.

34. Kominami S, Liu Y, Alvarez H, et al. A case of VVF presenting with a subarachnoid hemorrhage. Interv Neuroradiol 1996;2:229–33.

35. Waitzman AA, Anderson J, Willinsky RA. Endovascular management of vertebral arteriovenous fistulas: the Toronto experience. J Otolaryngol 1996; 25:322–8.

Cerebral Arteriovenous Shunts in Children

Ahmed K. Toma, MD, FRCS (Neurosurg)[a],
Indran Davagnanam, MD, MB BCh, BAO, BMedSci, FRCR[b,c,*],
Vijeya Ganesan, MD, FRCP[d],
Stefan Brew, MBBS, MHB, MSc, FRANZCR, FRCR[b,e]

KEYWORDS

• Arteriovenous malformations • Children • Vein of Galen • Shunt

KEY POINTS

• Divided into arteriovenous malformations and arteriovenous fistulae.
• Presentation is different from adults: eg, heart failure in neonates.
• Commonest cause of haemorrhagic stroke in children.
• Digital subtraction angiography is the gold standard method of investigation.
• High projected life-time risk of haemorrhage warrant more aggressive treatment strategy.

INTRODUCTION

Intracranial arteriovenous shunts (AVSs) in children can be divided into pial arteriovenous malformations (AVMs), vein of Galen malformations (VGAMs), and arteriovenous fistulae (AVF), including single-hole fistulae. Dural AVF and dural sinus malformations (DSMs) are rare entities within this group.

The relative immaturity of the anatomy and physiology of the neonatal and infant brain results in the inability of the hydrovenous system to compensate in the face of such disorders.[1] The AVSs in this population are of a distinct angioarchitecture often containing fistulous components with direct arteriovenous (AV) connections. AVMs can be multifocal and also often exhibit a complex pattern of venous drainage that can affect the entire venous system, often associated with venous malformations.

Thus, the clinical presentation reflects this difference in the underlying anatomy, physiology, and disorder between children and adults.[2] Most intracranial AVSs in adults are pial AVMs or dural AVFs. The clinical presentation of heart failure is rare in adults; however, pediatric AVSs often present with heart failure in the neonatal period. Other differences in children include their association with other vascular abnormalities and genetic influences.[3]

PIAL AVMS
Cause

Pial AVMs (Fig. 1) are the commonest cerebrovascular lesion in children. The lesion is thought to develop between the third and eighth week of fetal life.[4,5] They are usually congenital lesions that arise from the abnormal development of the arteriolar-capillary network that exists between the arterial

[a] Victor Horsley Department of Neurosurgery, National Hospital for Neurology & Neurosurgery, Queen Square, London WC1N 3BG, UK; [b] Lysholm Department of Neuroradiology, National Hospital for Neurology & Neurosurgery, Queen Square, London WC1N 3BG, UK; [c] Brain Repair & Rehabilitation Unit, Institute of Neurology, University College London, London WC1N 3BG, UK; [d] Department of Pediatric Neurology, Great Ormond Street Hospital for Children, Great Ormond Street, London WC1N 3JH, UK; [e] Department of Neuroradiology, Great Ormond Street Hospital for Children, Great Ormond Street, London WC1N 3JH, UK
* Corresponding author. Lysholm Department of Neuroradiology, National Hospital for Neurology & Neurosurgery, Queen Square, London WC1N 3BG, UK.
E-mail address: indrandavagnanam@gmail.com

Neuroimag Clin N Am 23 (2013) 757–770
http://dx.doi.org/10.1016/j.nic.2013.05.001

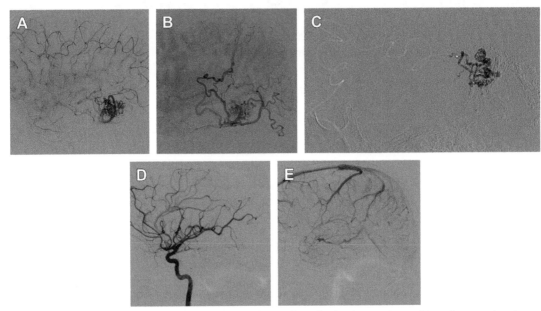

Fig. 1. Pial AVM. (*A*) A late arterial/early capillary phase of a selective internal carotid angiogram showing an AVM nidus of the posterior temporal area. (*B*) Capillary phase of the angiogram shows multiple congested draining veins. (*C*) Histoacryl glue embolization through microcatheter with good penetration of the nidus. (*D*) Final angiogram (arterial phase) and (*E*) (venous phase) shows complete exclusion of the AVM with no AV shunt.

and venous circulations with an organ. Only 18% of AVMs that become symptomatic do so before the age of 15 years. The mortality from hemorrhage in a child is 25%. Intracranial pial AVMs may be associated with facial AVMs or cerebrofacial metameric syndromes (CAMS; or Bonnet-Dechaume-Blanc or Wyburn-Mason syndrome) as well as genetic conditions such as hemorrhagic hereditary telangiectasia (HHT; or Osler-Weber-Rendu syndrome) and neurofibromatosis type I.[6–8] Single-hole AVFs, once considered a subset of AVMs, are thought to be a distinct vascular entity according to their angioarchitecture[9] and thus are discussed separately in this article.

Presentation

Pial AVMs are rarely seen in the first year of life. They may present in infancy, but most present in the second and third decade of life up to the age of 15 years.[2] If the contention that they are congenital is correct, this pattern implies that they undergo postnatal angioarchitecture evolution leading to presentation when the child is older.

Although presentation in the newborn is infrequent, AVMs may manifest as congestive heart failure (50%), followed by hemorrhage (37.5%). In infants, hemorrhage (30%) and macrocrania (27%) are more common than heart failure (23%).[1] The commonest presentation of an AVM in childhood is hemorrhage (75%), either intraparenchymal or intraventricular, followed by seizures,

which constitute approximately 15% of the presenting population. AVMs are the commonest cause of hemorrhagic stroke in children (30%–55%) and, as such, any child with spontaneous intracranial hemorrhage should be presumed to have an AVM until proved otherwise.[10,11] Associated aneurysms are found in about 16% of children with AVMs.[12]

Natural History

Enlargement of an AVM in children occurs with growth as a result of increased flow through poorly differentiated vessels and the potential recruitment of new arterial supply.[13,14] Children have a higher rate of hemorrhage from an AVM at initial presentation compared with adults, which may reflect the underlying angioarchitectural differences in the age groups but equally may reflect the lower frequency of intracranial imaging for pediatric nonhemorrhagic symptoms.

The annual risk and rate of hemorrhage of a previously nonruptured AVM is probably similar to that of adults, ranging between 2% and 4%.[15,16] Although children are more likely to present with hemorrhage, similar to adults, the rate of subsequent hemorrhage in children with AVM is approximately 90% lower than in adults with AVM. However, despite the annualized risk of hemorrhage being similar to that of adults, the cumulative risk is greater in children given the greater number of years left to live.[17]

Diagnosis

Computed tomography (CT) is useful in the context of a ruptured AVM to assess the location and size of the hematoma, the presence of hydrocephalus, and mass effect. However, CT scan often fails to identify the precise source of bleeding. Magnetic resonance (MR) imaging is useful for localization of the AVM, its size, presence of hematoma, or posthemorrhagic changes. Functional MR imaging and MR tractography may be useful in an AVM located in an eloquent part of the brain, particularly in preparation for treatment.[18,19] CT and MR angiography are useful to determine the afferent vessels of the AVM and the venous outflow of the malformation.[20,21]

Digital subtraction angiography is the gold standard for the diagnosis of a cerebral AVM; no imaging modality other than digital subtraction angiography can exclude the presence of an intracranial AVS. It has a vital role in determining the angioarchitecture and hemodynamic features of the AVM and is essential to plan treatment. Angiography may be used during surgery to localize the lesion, distinguish arteries from veins, and ensure complete removal.

Treatment

The main goal of AVM treatment is to prevent intracranial hemorrhage and, to achieve this, the AVM must be completely obliterated. Although complete cure is desirable, it should be considered in the context of the anticipated natural history of the AVM in any particular child versus the risk of treatment. Clear indications for treatment of an AVM include hemorrhage, rapid neurologic deterioration, or the presence of an intranidal or feeding artery aneurysm. In children, consideration should be given to treatment of an asymptomatic AVM, because lifelong risk of hemorrhage is high.

Different therapeutic approaches include surgical resection, endovascular embolization, gamma knife radiosurgery, and proton beam therapy. These approaches are used as single treatment modalities or in combination, determined by the size, location, and vascular anatomy of the lesion.[22–25] The treatment approach should be determined by factors that include the age of the patient, the clinical presentation, and the angioarchitecture of the AVM.[26] Management is guided by a multidisciplinary team with experience in the treatment of neonates, infants, and children with intracranial AVMs. Grading systems have been used to guide treatment and assess outcome. The most widely used is the Spetzler-Martin classification, which is a surgical grading system. The Spetzler-Martin grade is determined by the size of the AVM, eloquence of the involved brain, and pattern of venous drainage.[27]

Transarterial endovascular embolization with liquid embolic agents (see **Fig. 1**) has gained popularity in the last 2 decades, largely as a result of improvements in angiographic image quality, endovascular access products, and embolic materials, becoming a favored method in children in many centers. The choice of embolic material depends on the angioarchitecture of the AVM and operator expertise and preference. Each material has advantages and disadvantages. Liquid embolic agents are of 2 main types:

- Cyanoacrylate (glue)-based materials that polymerize on contacting hydroxyl ions in blood. Commonly used preparations include Histoacryl (n-butyl-2 cyanoacrylate [NBCA]), and TRUFILL NBCA liquid embolic system. Polymerization time can be modified by the addition of oil-based contrast agents like Lipiodol (labeled Ethiodol in the United States), which also confers radiopacity to the embolic to allow fluoroscopic visualization. Lipiodol is an ethyl ester of iodized fatty acids of poppy seed oil. GLUBRAN 2 (General Enterprise Marketing, Viareggio, Lucca, Italy) is comonomer of NBCA and metachryloxysulfolan monomer. The longer radical chain allows a lower temperature of polymerization and slightly slower polymerization than Histoacryl, which may result in lower toxicity and less inflammatory reaction. Glubran is approved for use in Europe and carries the CE mark.[28]
- Precipitated polymers: Onyx is a nonadhesive liquid embolic agent composed of ethylene vinyl alcohol (EVOH) copolymer dissolved in dimethyl sulfoxide (DMSO), and suspended micronized tantalum powder to provide contrast for visualization under fluoroscopy. Onyx is available in 2 product formulations: Onyx 18 (6% EVOH) and Onyx 34 (8% EVOH). Onyx 18 travels more distally and penetrates deeper into the nidus because of its lower viscosity compared with Onyx 34. Onyx is delivered by slow controlled injection through a microcatheter into the brain AVM under fluoroscopic control. The DMSO solvent dissipates into the blood, causing the EVOH copolymer and suspended tantalum to precipitate in situ into a spongy, coherent embolus. Onyx immediately forms a skin as the polymeric embolus solidifies from the outside to the inside, while traveling more distally in the lesion.[29]

Glue can be useful in direct AVF, where flow is rapid and high-concentration embolic polymerizes rapidly at the AV junction without escape into the venous system. Glue may be superior in occlusion of intranidal aneurysms and may be delivered through smaller flow-direct catheters in more remote locations. Small glue volumes can be injected because of rapid polymerization with limited nidal penetration, usually requiring repeated pedicle catheterizations, which may result in lower cure rates in larger nidal AVMs compared with Onyx. Glue injections unfold over seconds and are more difficult to control compared with Onyx injections, which unfold over minutes with time to pause, repeat angiography, and reflect. Onyx generally achieves better nidal penetration with larger volume of nidus occluded on each injection.[30] Onyx offers potential complete cure of even large brain AVMs and has a higher rate of occlusion, but postprocedural hemorrhage rates may be higher.[31] Onyx delivery requires DMSO-compatible microcatheters that generally are more rigid compared with the best glue-delivery microcatheters, thus making catheterization of tortuous small arterial pedicles more difficult. DMSO is toxic, and injection of large volumes should be avoided in small, sick children.

Outcome

Children in general have high compensatory capacity with good outcome compared with adults. Outcome following hemorrhage depends on the location and size of hemorrhage, with mortalities in hospital series around 8% to 50% and moderate to severe cognitive deficits at around 23%.[10,11] Overall AVM obliteration has been reported in up to 40% of patients undergoing endovascular embolization, often taking multiple procedures.[2,3,32] Embolization cure rates are better in small malformations (<1 cm) and those with single pedicles, including the fistula-type lesions, than in large lesions with more pedicles.

AVFS OF CHILDHOOD

Pediatric AVFs are characterized by a direct AV connection with no intervening network of vessels, and therefore typically exhibit rapid flow, often causing high-output cardiac failure. The pediatric AVFs include VGAM, pial AVF, DSM, and infantile high-flow dural fistula (Figs. 2–7).

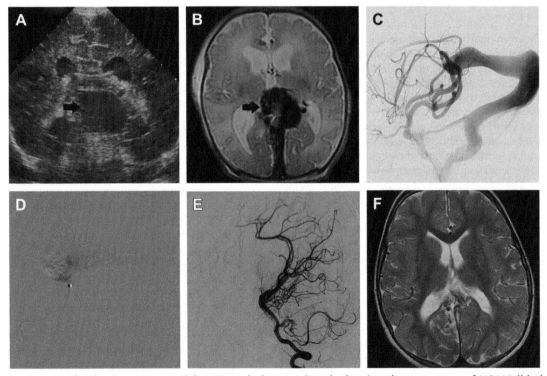

Fig. 2. Vein of Galen in a neonate. (A) Antenatal ultrasound study showing the venous sac of VGAM (black arrow). (B) Axial T2-weighted MR imaging in a neonate with VGAM (black arrow). (C) Left internal carotid artery (ICA) angiogram in a neonate with VGAM showing a profuse shunting through multiple feeders into a large venous sac. (D) Concentrated Histoacryl microcatheter embolization. (E) Six-month follow-up left vertebral artery angiogram showing no evidence of AV shunt. (F) Follow-up axial T2-weighted MR imaging.

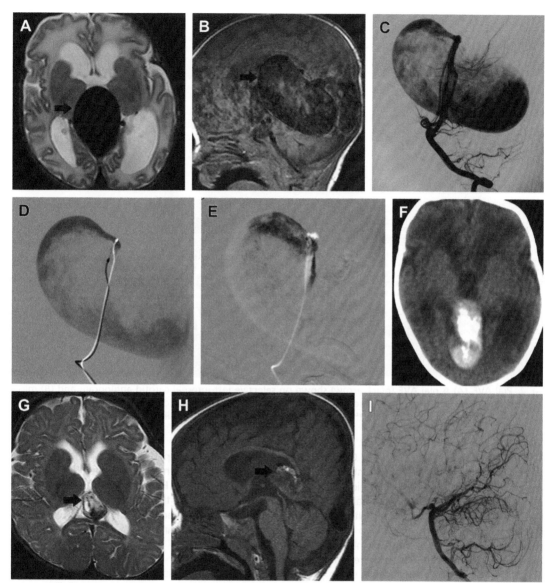

Fig. 3. Vein of Galen in a child. (*A*) Axial T2-weighted and (*B*) sagittal T2-weighted MR imaging of the brain in a child with VGAM showing a large venous sac (*black arrow*). (*C*) Left vertebral artery angiogram showing a large venous sac draining multiple feeders. (*D*) Microcatheter angiogram. (*E*) Concentrated Histoacryl embolization of the fistulous points. (*F*) Postoperative CT scan of the brain. (*G*) Early follow-up T2-weighted axial and (*H*) T1-weighted sagittal MR imaging shows occlusion of the VGAM (*black arrows*). (*I*) Follow-up left vertebral angiogram showing no evidence of AV shunt. Note the improved brain perfusion.

VGAM

Definition and cause

VGAM (see **Figs. 2** and **3**) can be defined as a congenital AV shunt, centered on the tela choroidea of the third ventricle, supplied predominantly by choroidal arteries, and usually draining into an aberrant falcine sinus. In VGAMs, the thalamostriate and internal cerebral veins do not communicate with the vein of Galen but instead drain into the posterior and inferior thalamic veins, and either join a subtemporal vein or, more commonly, the lateral mesencephalic vein to open into the superior petrosal sinuses, which gives the characteristic angiographic epsilon shape or epsilon vein on the lateral angiogram. The straight sinus is usually absent, with a falcine sinus draining the malformation to the superior sagittal sinus.

In some instances it may be difficult to distinguish between a VGAM and a thalamic or tectal

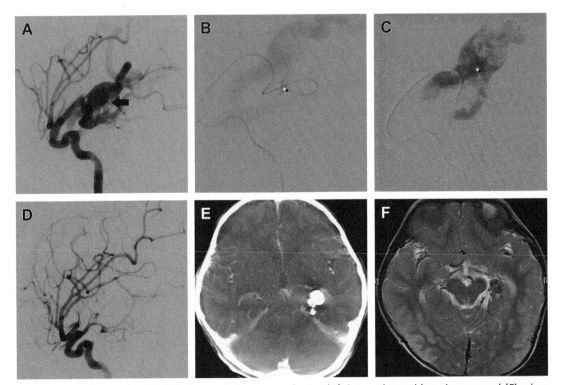

Fig. 4. Pial AVF. (*A*) A pial AVF (*black arrow*) shown on selective left internal carotid angiogram and (*B*) microcatheter angiogram. (*C*) Histoacryl glue embolization. (*D*) Final left ICA angiogram arterial phase. (*E*) DynaCT at the end of the procedure showing the glue cast. (*F*) T2-weighted MR imaging follow-up scan.

AVM draining into a dilated vein of Galen, and a medially located pial AVF draining into the vein of Galen. In general, 2 types of angioarchitecture are described in VGAMs: choroidal and mural. The former corresponds with a primitive condition involving all of the choroidal arteries and an interposed network before opening into the large venous pouch. The latter type corresponds with direct AVF within the wall of the median vein of the prosencephalon. The fistulas may be single but are often multiple, converging into a single venous chamber or into multiple venous chambers located along the anterior aspect of a venous pouch or along 1 dilated choroidal vein before reaching the venous pouch.

VGAM is rare, but is the most common intracranial AV shunt presenting in the neonatal period. Our institution receives around 1 to 2 new VGAM referrals per month, but it is difficult to be certain what catchment population this comes from, or what proportion reaches us. Disproportionate attention is given to VGAM, because the logic for treatment of all other high-flow AVSs of the neonatal period is based largely on our experience with VGAMs.

Paget first explicitly dealt with the embryology of this condition, referring to the possibility of an early embryonic AV shunt developing in the tela choroidea of the third ventricle, and postulating as to its consequences.[33] Raybaud and colleagues[34] in 1989 stated that the ectatic vein in VGAM was the embryonic precursor, the median vein of the prosencephalon, and not the vein of Galen itself.

Presentation

Antenatal diagnosis of VGAM is increasingly made using ultrasound and MR imaging. It is puzzling that it has never been shown on a 20-week gestational age antenatal scan, because the embryology suggests that it must be present at this stage. Antenatal diagnosis of VGAM raises some difficult considerations; some develop in utero parenchymal brain damage, and have a poor prognosis. Most have normal brain in utero, and present with either antenatal or perinatal heart failure.[35,36]

Gold[37] in 1964 described the following clinical stages in patients with VGAMs: (1) neonates with cardiac insufficiency, (2) infants and young children with hydrocephalus and seizures, and (3) older children or adults with headaches and subarachnoid hemorrhage. Amacher[38] later added a further clinical group that included neonates and infants with macrocephaly and minimal cardiac

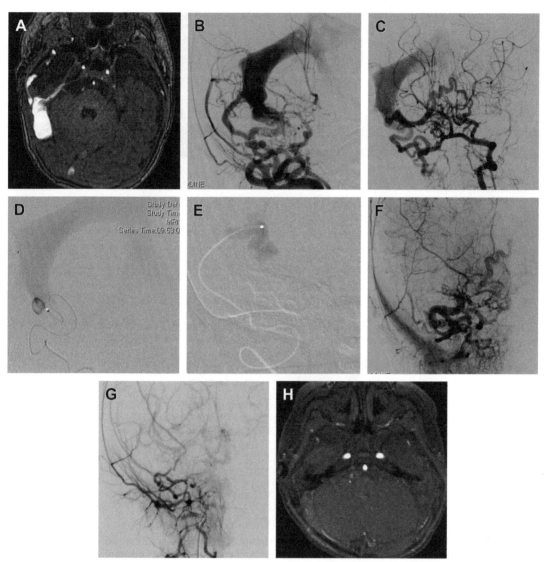

Fig. 5. Dural AVF. (*A*) MR angiogram of a child with dural AVF. (*B*) Anteroposterior (AP) projection of right common carotid artery angiogram before embolization. (*C*) AP projection of left vertebral artery before embolization. (*D*) AP projection of microcatheter angiogram at fistulous point. (*E*) AP projection of first glue embolization. (*F*) AP projection of final angiogram. (*G*) AP projection of 6-month angiogram. (*H*) MR angiography follow-up.

symptoms. The most common mode of presentation in a neonate is heart failure caused by extremely low-resistance flow through the AV shunt. These children are often gravely ill, and may progress to multiorgan failure and ischemic brain damage within hours to days, despite optimal support in an intensive care unit. Infants and children may also present with hydrocephalus or macrocephaly, often associated with the development of jugular bulb stenosis and venous hypertension.

Ventricular drainage in VGAM should be avoided if possible. Johnston and colleagues,[39] in a

literature review, noted that of 11 shunted infants 7 died and only 1 had no deficit. In an additional group of 6 shunted children, only 2 had no deficit. In the series by Zerah and colleagues,[40] only 1 of 17 infants had an uneventful shunting procedure. Wherever possible in this group, we advocate embolization, aiming to cure the AV shunt, and deferral of ventricular drainage wherever possible. Third ventriculostomy has been used successfully in this setting, although preferably after embolization to reduce the rate of the AV shunt.

Older children or adults sometimes present with previously undiagnosed (or untreated or partially

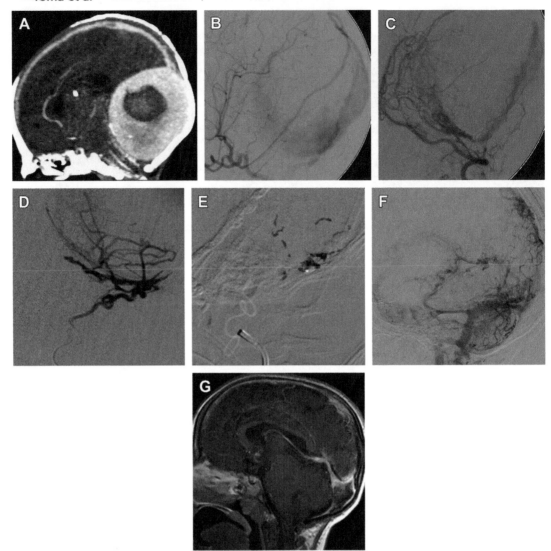

Fig. 6. DSM. (*A*) CT head of a child with DSM. (*B*) Left vertebral and (*C*) left internal carotid selective angiograms showing a DSM. (*D*) Microcatheter angiogram. (*E*) Glue embolization. (*F*) After glue embolization, left vertebral angiogram showing no AV shunt. (*G*) Sagittal T1 MR imaging follow-up.

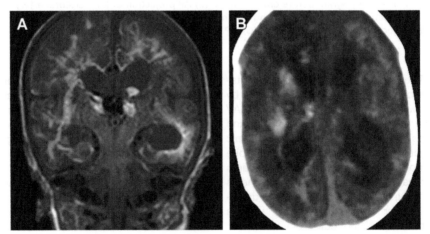

Fig. 7. Not to treat VGM. (*A*) Coronal T1 MR imaging scan of a child with VGAM with extensive parenchymal hemorrhage and volume loss. (*B*) CT showing parenchymal hemorrhage, calcification, and volume loss.

treated) VGAM. Most present with hemorrhage, or signs of increased intracranial pressure caused by venous hypertension. Treatment is technically difficult, and has a higher complication rate than in children.

Natural history

The natural history data are not robust; the diagnosis is often never made, and the literature confuses VGAMs with other disorders. Most neonates in heart failure die untreated. Infants and children presenting with hydrocephalus have a more indolent course, but often evolve toward chronic venous ischemia resulting in developmental delay, seizures, and parenchymal hemorrhage.[35,36] Adults typically present with hemorrhage or signs of increased intracranial pressure. Spontaneous thrombosis of VGAM is probably rare; in the series by Lasjaunias and colleagues,[41] 5 out of 120 patients (4%) developed spontaneous thrombosis, with 2 neurologically normal.

Diagnosis

Antenatal diagnosis is usually by identification of an anechoic structure in the region of the cistern of the vein of Galen with demonstrable flow within it on Doppler ultrasound, although ultrasound is poor at assessing the brain parenchyma. Fetal MR imaging is useful, both to characterize the VGAM and to assess the brain parenchyma. Many neonates are not diagnosed promptly; any neonate with unexplained high-output cardiac failure should have imaging of the head to exclude a VGAM. MR imaging is optimal in this regard, because it allows both diagnosis and assessment of brain parenchyma, although CT and CT angiography (CTA) are more often used in the clinical setting. Older children and adults are best imaged by MR imaging.[39,42]

However, the angioarchitecture of the lesion is best shown and appreciated by catheter angiography. Catheter angiography should only be performed as a prelude to treatment; iliac artery occlusion is common in angiography in neonates, and becomes an issue in subsequent treatment.[43] The dominant arterial supply usually comes from the posterior choroidal arteries, although their morphology is distorted from the usual adult pattern. The pericallosal and anterior choroidal arteries also often contribute. In older children, subependymal vessels passing through the thalamus and midbrain also often contribute to the AV shunt.

Although the distinction in angioarchitecture is well described as choroidal and mural types according to Lasjaunias and colleagues,[41] in our experience there is a spectrum ranging from a single AV shunt to innumerable arterial feeders from

multiple sources. In VGAM, the dilated median vein of the prosencephalon is thought not to communicate with the deep venous system of the brain, although there are reports of thalamic hemorrhage after embolization; in this regard we have observed at least 2 cases in which we performed retrograde catheterization of the thalamic veins off the sac.

Treatment

Neonates

Whether presenting antenatally, or more commonly perinatally, it is not clear when these children are best treated (see Fig. 7); Lasjaunias traditionally decided by a scoring system, aiming to avoid treatment of neonates wherever possible, to allow treatment when the child is larger and it is technically easier and safer.[21] At Great Ormond Street Hospital (GOSH) for Children, our approach has changed over time, influenced by both the death of neonates and infants from heart failure while awaiting treatment, and excellent outcomes in children who were regarded as too systemically unwell to treat by other operators. Our current approach is to perform embolization on any VGAM with cardiac failure as soon as possible after delivery, provided there is no imaging evidence of severe parenchymal damage to the brain.

The initial aim of treatment is to relieve heart failure, rather than cure the malformation. Subsequent staged embolization aims for cure by 6 months. It is self-evident that the very sick children with low scores tend to have worse outcomes, but at GOSH for Children we offer treatment to even very sick children provided there is not evidence of diffuse parenchymal damage. We have seen cured patients growing up as normal children.

The first step is catheter angiography (see Fig. 2). We generally use a femoral approach, using a 4-Fr sheath, and a short Berenstein diagnostic catheter. Bilateral internal carotid and left vertebral high-frame-rate angiography is performed, which consumes most of the available contrast dose in a neonate, and most of the subsequent intervention is performed under fluoroscopy, with occasional microcatheter angiography.

In our practice at GOSH for Children, all neonates are treated by transarterial embolization using concentrated Histoacryl rendered radiopaque with tantalum. This technique is quick, and reliably relieves heart failure in these gravely ill children. All neonates return to the intensive care unit after embolization, and almost all need a combination of positive inotropes and vasodilators, aiming for management of pulmonary arterial hypertension, and careful control of systemic pressure. They are generally kept heavily sedated and intubated in the intensive care unit for 48 hours after embolization.

Although no clear statement can be made, the optimal target is probably around 50% reduction in cardiac output in the first stage of embolization. The fraction of cardiac output passing through the AV shunt in a VGAM has exceeded 90% in all neonates in whom we have measured, a state that is clearly incompatible with life, and for which no animal model exists. Sudden closure of a shunt of this magnitude often precipitates severe left ventricular failure, and occasionally intracranial hemorrhage. Such an abrupt physiologic alteration needs to be carefully managed; before, during and after the procedure, and requires the input of pediatric cardiology, intensive care unit specialists, anesthesia, and experienced pediatric interventional neuroradiologists.

Infants and children

Those children who are not treated in the neonatal period usually present, sometimes repeatedly, with hydrocephalus, macrocephaly, seizures, or developmental delay, probably mediated by increased intracranial venous pressure (**Fig. 3**). The logical approach would be an attempt at reduction of intracranial venous pressure. In contrast, the optimal solution is cure of the AV shunt, although this should probably be staged, and is not always possible because by this age there are often innumerable transthalamic and transtectal arterial feeders. Cerebrospinal fluid diversion should be avoided wherever possible.

Every conceivable approach has been used for VGAM; transarterial occlusion with coils, glue, or Onyx, retrograde transvenous embolization with coils, and, in our center, retrograde embolization using glue and stent placement of stenosis of the jugular bulb. Stereotactic radiosurgery and conventional neurosurgery have also been attempted. It is not clear which of these approaches is best in any set of circumstances and hence a multidisciplinary approach is essential.

Outcomes

The poorer the state of the child at the outset of the disease process, the lower the probability of a good outcome. Our reluctance to use the rigid Lasjaunias clinical criteria for treatment stems from our personal experience. At our institution, we have seen children deemed too sick to treat by these criteria who end up normal, and children deemed too well to treat end up dead. Our approach in VGAM has evolved to mirror that in any other pediatric neurovascular disorder: a multidisciplinary decision involving pediatric neurology, neurosurgery, interventional neuroradiology, and pediatric intensive care specialists is made, taking into account the radiological state of the brain, the clinical state of the child, and the wishes of the parents. The only absolute exclusion to treatment is evidence of severe parenchymal damage to the brain (see **Fig. 7**). Severe physiologic derangement (high shunt volume, renal failure, hepatic failure, heart failure on maximal inotropes, requirement of high-frequency ventilation and so forth) makes periprocedural management more difficult, but tends to polarize outcomes into death or good outcome, provided the brain is intact at the time of embolization. Overall, neonates presenting to GOSH for Children now have around a 60% chance of being neurologically intact, 15% chance of mild disability, 10% chance of severe disability, and 15% chance of death. This probability includes many patients who would be refused treatment by conventional criteria.

High-flow Pial AVF

Definition and cause

Pial AVFs of the brain (see **Fig. 4**) are sometimes termed single-hole AVFs and account for approximately 3.3% to 4.7% of all intracranial AVMs.[9,44] They are characterized by direct connections between arteries and veins with arterial supply derived from cortical or pial arteries, and are frequently associated with large to giant venous pouches, which can occur as a solitary fistulae, but frequently are multiple, which is a characteristic finding of this entity. Most of these are situated in the supratentorial neuroparenchyma and are more common in the frontal and temporal lobes.

Natural history

The exact incidence of a pial AVF in children is not known because of its rarity.[44] Most published papers have included this type of angioarchitecture within the overall population of the cerebral AVMs or even the VGAMs. As within most vascular anomalies in this age group, there is a male predominance and strong genetic association in pediatric cases in which there are multiple intracranial AVFs. Conditions such as HHT[6,7,9,45] and encephalocraniocutaneous lipomatosis[9,46] are well-recognized associations in the literature.

Presentation

Presentation is usually within the first 5 years of life with the mean age in one series at 23 months.[9] Symptoms attributable to pial AVFs are usually the consequence of high-flow AV shunting, leading to cardiac failure, hemorrhage, macrocrania, seizures, focal neurologic deficits, edema, or mass effect from the venous varices.[9] When presenting with hemorrhage, AVF can also be associated with false arterial or venous aneurysms; these should be vigilantly identified, because this is an indication and a focal target for treatment.[47] Venous outflow obstruction in the form of pial venous outflow stenosis, dural sinus stenosis and thrombosis seems to be associated with hemorrhagic presentations, similar to the experience with AVMs.[9,48]

Diagnosis and treatment

The diagnosis follows the imaging algorithm of pial AVM as detailed earlier using CT, CTA, MR imaging, MR angiography, and catheter angiography methods.

The goal of treatment in pial AVFs in young children, even when asymptomatic, is the rapid control of the lesion (AV shunt), because of the worse neurocognitive prognosis and mortality when managed conservatively.[49,50] Surgery has been reported to be successful in a small number of cases of neonates and infants presenting with a symptomatic nongalenic AVF.[51,52] However, our experience is that endovascular embolization is a safe and often curative treatment[53]; the technique used is identically to that described with concentrated glue and coils to occlude the fistula.

DSM and Infantile Dural AVF

Definition and cause

These disorders are collectively rare (see **Figs. 5** and **6**) and the true incidence and prevalence are difficult to quantify accurately. We receive around 1 per year; around 10% of the neonatal VGAM caseload. DSMs are thought to be a consequence of uncontrolled development of the posterior sinuses, including transverse sinus, sigmoid sinus, and/or confluence of sinuses, rather than of embryologic nondevelopment.

Presentation

DSMs generally present in the neonatal and infancy periods, although they usually become symptomatic on the average at 5 month of age. The most frequent clinical presentation is macrocrania followed by seizures, psychomotor delay, and intracranial hemorrhage. The other clinical presentations include congestive cardiac failure, cranial bruit, facial vein dilatation, and intracranial hypertension (intracranial hypertension being associated with macrocrania).[54]

Natural history

Anatomically there are 2 types of DSM[54]:

1. DSM involving the adjacent posterior sinuses, with giant pouches and slow-flow mural AV

shunting. Partial thrombosis of the sinus may occur and can also be observed in utero. The dural sinus pouch at birth communicates with the other sinuses and drains normal cerebral veins.

2. DSM of the jugular bulb malformation with otherwise normal sinuses that appears as a sigmoid sinus-jugular bulb diaphragm and is associated with a petromastoid-sigmoid sinus high-flow AVF, which is usually a single-hole type. DSMs usually have a benign course, remain asymptomatic for a long time, and are incidentally discovered. Their treatment by embolization is technically easy, and the outcome of most patients is complete exclusion of the shunt and favorable neurologic outcome.

Associated multiple slow-flow AV shunts are consistently shown within the dural wall of the DSM contributing to the hydrovenous restriction by venous congestion of the brain. The brain at birth has to drain solely through the diseased sinus before cavernous capture.[55] Early and rapid spontaneous thrombosis of a DSM lake and secondary dysmaturation of the jugular outlets further compromise cerebral venous drainage and can lead to venous infarction and lethal intraparenchymal hemorrhage. Unilateral DSMs, which have lateralized from the torcular, have a more favorable outcome as 1 normal draining venous sinus is maintained. It is important to have the ipsilateral cerebral hemisphere drain via an alternate normal venous pathway, either by cavernous capture or by a persistent medial occipital sinus bypassing the thrombosed sinus into the ipsilateral jugular vein or into the contralateral sinus via the superior sagittal sinus.

Diagnosis and treatment

Diagnosis on antenatal ultrasonography or MR imaging is possible but requires recognition of the disease condition by an experienced sonographer or neuroradiologist. Following antenatal diagnosis, MR imaging of the brain should be performed to determine the location of the DSM and quantify the extent of brain damage. If the DSM is located on the midline and large, early angiography is recommended to assess the anatomy of the cerebral veins. The physiologic issues and decision making are similar to other AVSs but the techniques used are more variable.

The therapeutic options thus depend on the angioarchitecture of each individual case and the state of maturation or dysmaturation of the venous sinuses. When partial or no cavernous capture and no pial reflux are seen, there is an option of treating with heparin and embolization of the shunts with glue, in anticipation of cavernous capture to take place with minimal or no consequences for the hydrovenous equilibrium of the maturing brain. If there is a significant shunt causing pial reflux, embolization is necessary to prevent venous hypertension and cerebral ischemic damage. The goal is to reduce pial reflux by occluding the shunts while maintaining patency of the sinuses. If there is complete occlusion of a mural AVS, this will likely lead to complete sinus thrombosis, resulting in an absence of a venous outlet for the brain and leading to poor outcome.

The prognosis, and specifically the mortality, associated with dural AVSs reported in the literature are extremely high, on the order of 38% in all ages and 67% in the neonatal subgroup.[56] However, the perception of a DSM at the torcular being lethal has not been verified by our experience. Although these lesions are difficult to manage, we have achieved outcomes broadly similar to those of VGAM. Pial AVF and infantile dural AVF have a better prognosis.[54]

Cranial AV shunts key facts:
- Divided into AVM and AVF
- Presentation is different in adults (eg, heart failure in neonates)
- Commonest cause of hemorrhagic stroke in children
- Digital subtraction angiography is the gold standard method of investigation
- High lifetime risk for significant mortality and morbidity warrants more aggressive treatment strategy

REFERENCES

1. Ozanne A, Alvarez H, Krings T, et al. Neurovascular pathology malformation of the child: aneurysmal malformations of the vein of Galen (VGAM), pial arteriovenous malformations (PAVM), dural sinus malformation (DSM). J Neuroradiol 2007;34(3): 145–66.

2. Berenstein A, Ortiz R, Niimi Y, et al. Endovascular management of arteriovenous malformations and other intracranial arteriovenous shunts in neonates, infants, and children. Childs Nerv Syst 2010; 26(10):1345–58.

3. Lasjaunias P, Hui F, Zerah M, et al. Cerebral arteriovenous malformations in children. Management of 179 consecutive cases and review of the literature. Childs Nerv Syst 1995;11(2):66–79.

4. Guidetti B, Delitala A. Intracranial arteriovenous malformations. Conservative and surgical treatment. J Neurosurg 1980;53:149–52.

5. So SC. Cerebral arteriovenous malformations in children. Childs Brain 1978;4:242–50.

6. Bharatha A, Faughnan ME, Kim H, et al. Brain arteriovenous malformation multiplicity predicts the diagnosis of hereditary hemorrhagic telangiectasia: quantitative assessment. Stroke 2012;43(1):72–8.

7. Krings T, Chng SM, Ozanne A, et al. Hereditary haemorrhagic telangiectasia in children. Endovascular treatment of neurovascular malformations. Results in 31 patients. Interv Neuroradiol 2005;11:13–23.

8. Bhattacharya JJ, Luo CB, Suh DC, et al. Wyburn-Mason or Bonnet-Dechaume-Blanc as cerebrofacial arteriovenous metameric syndromes (CAMS). A new concept and a new classification. Interv Neuroradiol 2001;7(1):5–17.

9. Weon YC, Yoshida Y, Sachet M, et al. Supratentorial cerebral arteriovenous fistulas (AVFs) in children: review of 41 boxes with 63 non-single-hole choroidal AVFs. Acta Neurochir (Wien) 2005;147:17–31.

10. Beslow LA, Jordan LC. Pediatric stroke: the importance of cerebral arteriopathy and vascular malformations. Childs Nerv Syst 2010;26(10):1263–73.

11. De Ribaupierre S, Rilliet B, Cotting J, et al. A 10-year experience in paediatric spontaneous cerebral haemorrhage: which children with headache need more than a clinical examination? Swiss Med Wkly 2008;138(5–6):59–69.

12. Anderson RC, McDowell MM, Kellner CP, et al. Arteriovenous malformation-associated aneurysms in the pediatric population. J Neurosurg Pediatr 2012;9(1):11–6.

13. Lasjaunias P, Piske R, Terbrugge K, et al. Cerebral arteriovenous malformations (C. AVM) and associated arterial aneurysms (AA). Acta Neurochir 1988;91(1):29–36.

14. Rubin D, Santillan A, Greenfield JP, et al. Surgical management of pediatric cerebral arteriovenous malformations. Childs Nerv Syst 2010;26(10): 1337–44.

15. Ondra SL, Troupp H, George ED, et al. The natural history of symptomatic arteriovenous malformations of the brain: a 24-year follow-up assessment. J Neurosurg 1990;73:387–91.

16. ApSimon HT, Reef H, Phadke RV, et al. A population-based study of brain arteriovenous malformation: long-term treatment outcomes. Stroke 2002;33:2794–800.

17. Fullerton HJ, Achrol AS, Johnston SC, et al. Long-term hemorrhage risk in children versus adults with brain arteriovenous malformations. Stroke 2005;36(10):2099–104.

18. Lee L, Sitoh YY, Ng I, et al. Cortical reorganization of motor functional areas in cerebral arteriovenous malformations. J Clin Neurosci 2013;20(5):649–53. http://dx.doi.org/10.1016/j.jocn.2012.07.007 [Epub ahead of print].

19. Ellis MJ, Rutka JT, Kulkarni AV, et al. Corticospinal tract mapping in children with ruptured arteriovenous malformations using functionally guided

diffusion-tensor imaging. J Neurosurg Pediatr 2012;9(5):505–10.

20. Nüssel F, Wegmüller H, Huber P. Comparison of magnetic resonance angiography, magnetic resonance imaging and conventional angiography in cerebral arteriovenous malformation. Neuroradiology 1991;33(1):56–61.

21. Ozsarlak O, Van Goethem JW, Maes M, et al. MR angiography of the intracranial vessels: technical aspects and clinical applications. Neuroradiology 2004;46(12):955–72.

22. Hladky J, Lejeune J, Blond S, et al. Cerebral arteriovenous malformations in children: report on 62 cases. Childs Nerv Syst 1994;10:328–33.

23. Pan D, Kuo Y, Guo W, et al. Gamma knife surgery for cerebral arteriovenous malformations in children: a 13-year experience. J Neurosurg Pediatr 2008;2(3):229–304.

24. Shin M, Kawamoto S, Kurita H, et al. Retrospective analysis of a 10-year experience of stereotactic radio surgery for arteriovenous malformations in children and adolescents. J Neurosurg 2002;97: 779–84.

25. Kano H, Kondziolka D, Flickinger JC, et al. Stereotactic radiosurgery for arteriovenous malformations, part 2: management of pediatric patients. J Neurosurg Pediatr 2012;9(1):1–10.

26. Zacharia BE, Vaughan KA, Jacoby A, et al. Management of ruptured brain arteriovenous malformations. Curr Atheroscler Rep 2012;14(4):335–42.

27. Spetzler RF, Martin NA. A proposed grading system for arteriovenous malformations. J Neurosurg 1986;65:476–83.

28. Raffi L, Simonetti L, Cenni P, et al. Use of Glubran 2 acrylic glue in interventional neuroradiology. Neuroradiology 2007;49(10):829–36.

29. Available at: http://www.ev3.net/neuro/us/liquid-embolics/onyx-liquid-embolic-system.htm. Accessed May 6, 2012.

30. Mounayer C, Hammami N, Piotin M, et al. Nidal embolization of brain arteriovenous malformations using Onyx in 94 patients. AJNR Am J Neuroradiol 2007;28(3):518–23.

31. Available at: http://www.cxvascular.com/nn-latest-news/neuro-news--latest-news/onyx-vs-glue-end-the-battle. Accessed May 6, 2012.

32. Valavanis A, Yaşargil MG. The endovascular treatment of brain arteriovenous malformations. Adv Tech Stand Neurosurg 1998;24:131–214.

33. Padget DH. The cranial venous system in man in reference to development, adult configuration, and relation to the arteries. Am J Anat 2005;98(3): 307–55.

34. Raybaud C, Strother C, Hald J. Aneurysms of the vein of Galen: embryonic considerations and anatomical features relating to the pathogenesis of the malformation. Neuroradiology 1989;31(2):109–28.

35. Gupta A, Varma D. Vein of Galen malformations: review. Neurol India 2004;52(1):43.

36. Berenstein A, Fifi JT, Niimi Y, et al. Vein of Galen malformations in neonates: new management paradigms for improving outcomes. Neurosurgery 2012;70(5):1207.

37. Gold AP. Vein of Galen aneurysmal malformation. Acta Neurol Scand 1964;11(40):5–31.

38. Amacher AL. The syndromes and surgical treatment of aneurysms of the great vein of Galen. J Neurosurg 1973;39(1):89–98.

39. Johnston IH, Whittle IR, Besser M, et al. Vein of Galen malformation: diagnosis and management. Neurosurgery 1987;20(5):747.

40. Zerah M, Garcia-Monaco R, Rodesch G, et al. Hydrodynamics in vein of Galen malformations. Childs Nerv Syst 1992;8(3):111–7.

41. Lasjaunias P, Alvarez H, Rodesch G, et al. Aneurysmal malformations of the vein of Galen. Follow-up of 120 children treated between 1984 and 1994. Interv Neuroradiol 1996;2(1):15–26.

42. Campi A, Scotti G, Filippi M, et al. Antenatal diagnosis of vein of Galen aneurysmal malformation: MR study of fetal brain and postnatal follow-up. Neuroradiology 1996;38(1):87–90.

43. Roebuck DJ, Vendhan K, Barnacle AM, et al. Ultrasound-guided transaxillary access for diagnostic and interventional arteriography in children. J Vasc Interv Radiol 2010;21(6):842–7.

44. Tomlison FH, Rufenacht DA, Sundt TM Jr, et al. Arteriovenous fistula of the brain and spinal cord. J Neurosurg 1993;79:16–27.

45. Matsubara S, Mandzia JL, ter Brugge K, et al. Angiographic and clinical characteristics of patients with cerebral arteriovenous malformations associated with hereditary hemorrhagic telangiectasia. AJNR Am J Neuroradiol 2000;21(6): 1016–20.

46. Batista LL, Mahadevan J, Sachet M, et al. Encephalocraniocutaneous lipomatosis syndrome in a child: association with multiple high flow cerebral arteriovenous fistulae: case report and review. Interv Neuroradiol 2002;8: 273–83.

47. Garcia Monaco R, Rodesch G, Alvarez H, et al. Pseudoaneurysms within ruptured intracranial arteriovenous malformations: diagnosis and early endovascular treatment. AJNR Am J Neuroradiol 1993;14(2):315–21.

48. Miyasaka Y, Yaka K, Ohwada T, et al. An analysis of the venous drainage system as a factor in hemorrhage from arteriovenous malformations. J Neurosurg 1992;76:239–43.

49. Lasjaunias P, Ter Brugge K. Pial arteriovenous malformation. Vascular diseases in neonates, infants, and children. Berlin, New York, Tokyo: Springer; 1997. p. 203–19.

50. Nelson PK, Niimi Y, Lasjaunias P, et al. Endovascular embolization of congenital arteriovenous fistulas. In: Vinuela F, editor. Neuroimaging Clinics of North America, vol. 2. Philadelphia: Saunders; 1992. p. 309–31.

51. Aoki N, Sakai T, Oikawa A. Intracranial arteriovenous fistula manifesting as progressive neurological deterioration in an infant: case report. Neurosurgery 1991;28:619–23.

52. Barnwell SL, Ciricillo SF, Halbach VV, et al. Intracranial arteriovenous fistulas associated with intraparenchymal varix in childhood: case reports. Neurosurgery 1990;26:122–5.

53. Newman CB, Hu YC, McDougall CG, et al. Balloon-assisted Onyx embolization of cerebral single-channel pial arteriovenous fistulas. J Neurosurg Pediatr 2011;7(6):637–42.

54. Barbosa M, Mahadevan J, Weon YC, et al. Dural sinus malformations (DSM) with giant lakes, in neonates and infants. Review of 30 consecutive cases. Interv Neuroradiol 2003;9(4):407–24.

55. Lasjaunias P, Magufis G, Goulao A, et al. Anatomoclinical aspects of dural arteriovenous shunts in children: review of 29 cases. Interv Neuroradiol 1996;2: 179–91.

56. Morita A, Meyer FB, Nichols DA, et al. Childhood dural arteriovenous fistulae of the posterior dural sinuses: three case reports and literature review. Neurosurgery 1995;37(6):1193–9.

Pediatric Cerebral Aneurysms

Joseph J. Gemmete, MD, FSIR[a],*,
Ahmed K. Toma, MD, FRCS (Neurosurg)[b],
Indran Davagnanam, MD, MB BCh, BAO, BMedSci, FRCR[c],
Fergus Robertson, MRCP, FRCR[c],
Stefan Brew, MBBS, MHB, MSc, FRANZCR, FRCR[c]

KEYWORDS

• Pediatric aneurysm • SAH • Intracranial cerebral aneurysm • Endovascular treatment

KEY POINTS

- Childhood intracranial aneurysms are rare.
- They are distinct pathologically from adult aneurysms.
- They are associated with other congenital diseases.
- They have a higher incidence of de novo growth and recurrence.
- The endovascular method is the main treatment modality.

INTRODUCTION

Intracranial aneurysms in children are rare. (Table 1) shows the larger series of intracranial pediatric aneurysms to date. Most of the risk factors associated with intracranial aneurysms in adults do not exist in children, therefore the pathogenesis is thought to be different. The location and size of intracranial aneurysms in children differ from those found in adults. Most children with intracranial aneurysms present with subarachnoid hemorrhage (SAH) typically with a good clinical grade. This article reviews the incidence and gender prevalence, cause, location, and different types of intracranial aneurysms in children. The clinical presentation, diagnosis, and treatment of intracranial aneurysms in children are discussed, and data from endovascular treatments are presented.

INCIDENCE AND GENDER PREVALENCE

Intracranial aneurysms in children are rare; 0.5% to 4.6% of intracranial aneurysms occur in patients aged 18 years or younger.[1–4] In a cooperative study reported in 1966, only 41 of 6368 (0.6%) ruptured aneurysms were found in patients younger than 19 years.[5] In children, boys are more likely to harbor aneurysms than are girls.[2,6–8] After puberty, women have a 3 to 5 times higher incidence of aneurysms than men.[9,10] In some reports, a female dominance has been found before the age of 2 years.[11] Other reports that include older children have shown a less evident male dominance.[12]

CAUSES

Cerebral aneurysms are often thought to form as a result of chronic hemodynamic stress at branch points of arteries or areas where arteries abruptly change curvature. The classic risk factors in adults are largely acquired, such as hypertension, obesity, high cholesterol, diabetes, alcohol abuse, and smoking, and are often absent in children. Many pediatric patients have medical comorbidities that may be related to an underlying genetic

Grants: None.
[a] Division of Interventional Neuroradiology and Cranial Base Surgery, Departments of Radiology, Neurosurgery, and Otolaryngology, University of Michigan Health System, UH B1D 328, 1500 East Medical Center Drive, Ann Arbor, MI 48109-5030, USA; [b] Victor Horsley Department of Neurosurgery, National Hospital for Neurology & Neurosurgery, University College London Hospitals, Queen Square, London, UK; [c] Lysholm Department of Neuroradiology, National Hospital for Neurology & Neurosurgery, University College London Hospitals, Queen Square, London, UK
* Corresponding author.
E-mail address: gemmete@med.umich.edu

Table 1
Largest recent series of pediatric aneurysms

	Lasjaunias et al,[11] 2005	Hetts et al,[18] 2009	Koroknay-Pal et al,[20] 2012	Mehrotra et al,[19] 2012
Patients (n)	59	77	114	57
Number of aneurysms	75	103	130	73
Age (range)	7.6 y (8 d–15 y)	12 y (3 mo–18 y)	14.5 y (3 mo–18 y)	12.7 y (4 y–18 y)
Sex	M/F 3:2	F/M 1.1:1	M/F 3:2	M/F 1:1.2
Morphology				
Fusiform (%)	56	31	10	2.7
Saccular (%)	27	46	78	78
Infectious (%)	14	12	0	2.7
Traumatic (%)	3	14	7.6	8
Giant (>25 mm) (%)	1.3	11	12	19
Multiple (%)	15	16	11	11
Anterior Circulation (%)	73	78	89	71.3
Posterior Circulation (%)	27	22	11	28.7
SAH (%)	54	32	78.1	88.7
Mass Effect (%)	—	—	6.1	7
Mortality (%)	10.4	1.3	7.7	8.7

abnormality or developmental defect in the arterial tissue. Such factors might predispose these patients to aneurysm formation at a faster rate than that in patient without these factors, accounting for their earlier clinical presentation. Pediatric aneurysms are associated with conditions such as polycystic kidney disease, fibromuscular dysplasia, Ehlers-Danlos syndrome, Klippel-Trénaunay syndrome, tuberous sclerosis, hereditary hemorrhagic telangiectasia, pseudoxanthoma elasticum, or Marfan disease.[13,14] There is also a higher incidence of traumatic aneurysm.

Aneurysms are called saccular or berry when they have a saccular appearance, and dissecting when the aneurysm has a fusiform appearance and has preaneurysmal or postaneurysmal narrowing.[12] Childhood cerebral aneurysms are morphologically different from their saccular counterparts in adults, including a high number of fusiform shape, giant size, and de novo formation. Dissecting aneurysms are dominant during the first 5 years of life, whereas saccular aneurysms are more common in children older than 6 years.

ANEURYSM FEATURES

The size and location of aneurysms in children are different than those found in the adult population. Aneurysms of the internal carotid artery (ICA) occur with similar frequency in both populations;

however, there is a greater incidence of ICA terminus aneurysms in the pediatric population.[2,7,15–20] Aneurysms of the anterior cerebral artery (ACA) including the anterior communicating artery occur 34% of the time in the adult population, whereas, in children, recent reviews have encountered ACA aneurysms only about 5% to 10% of the time.[9,21] Aneurysms involving the middle cerebral artery occur in a similar distribution in both adults and children. Posterior circulation aneurysms are more common in children, occurring approximately 25% of the time.[6,8,11,12,16,22,23] In contrast, in the adult population they occur in only 8% of patients presenting with an aneurysm. The multiplicity of saccular aneurysms in children is low compared with adults, except in children with aneurysms of infectious origin.[11,12,24,25] In our series, 33% of aneurysms were located in the ICA, 33% in the middle cerebral artery, 17% in the posterior cerebral artery, 8% in the posterior communicating artery, and 8% in the basilar artery.

Traumatic Aneurysms

Traumatic aneurysms account for about 5% to 40% of pediatric aneurysms.[12,18,23,25–27] These aneurysms usually involve the distal ACA adjacent to the falx (40%), involve the major vessels along the skull base (35%), or have a cortical location (25%).[27–29] The child usually presents with a hemorrhagic episode about 4 weeks after the initial injury; however, immediate bleeding has also been reported.[30] Most children have sustained a closed head injury, but other causes include penetrating injuries and surgery.[30,31]

Infectious Aneurysms

Infectious aneurysms account for 5% to 15% of pediatric aneurysms.[11,18,26,32] They are most often of bacterial origin.[33–35] The most common organism is staphylococcus, followed by streptococcus and other gram-negative organisms.[24] Infectious arterial aneurysms are usually caused by bacterial endocarditis in infants with congenital or rheumatic heart disease. Infections involving the sphenoid sinus or mastoid air cells and sinus thrombophlebitis may also involve the adjacent artery causing an infectious aneurysm.[12,36,37] Infectious arterial aneurysms have also been observed in children with chronic mucocutaneous candidiasis and human immunodeficiency virusinfection.[38–43]

Saccular Aneurysms

Saccular aneurysms are the most common type of aneurysm occurring in the pediatric population

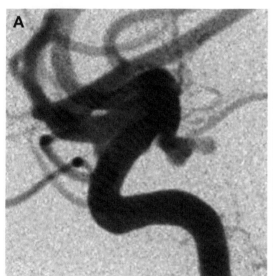
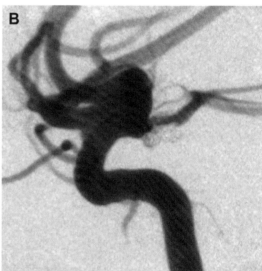
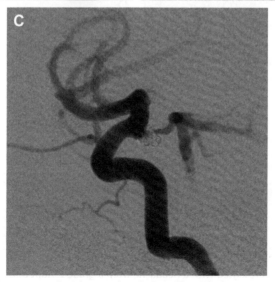

Fig. 1. An 8-year-old girl who presented with worst headache of her life from a grade 3 Hunt and Hess SAH. (A) Lateral view of a selective internal carotid angiogram shows a posterior communicating artery (PCOM) aneurysm. (B) Final angiogram shows the aneurysm coiled to exclusion with preservation of the PCOM artery. (C) A 6-month follow-up angiogram shows persistent exclusion of the aneurysm with patent PCOM artery.

(between 46% and 70%).[11,12,24,26] The cause of saccular aneurysms is unknown. They usually occur at bifurcation points of vessels, suggesting hemodynamic factors.[10,21]

Dissecting Aneurysms (Nontraumatic)

Dissecting aneurysms in the pediatric population occur 4 times more often than in the adult population.[11,12] This type of aneurysm can occur in the anterior or posterior circulation, especially the P1 and P2 segments of the posterior cerebral artery, supraclinoid ICA, and middle cerebral artery. Hetts and colleagues,[18] in the largest reported series, evaluated 77 patients with 103 intracranial aneurysms and showed a greater incidence of dissecting aneurysms in the anterior circulation. Lasjaunias and colleagues,[11] in their series of 59 consecutive children with 79 aneurysms, showed an almost equal distribution between the anterior and posterior circulation. Agid and colleagues,[12] in their series of 33 patients with 37 aneurysms, showed that most dissecting aneurysms involve the posterior circulation. There are reports of dissecting aneurysms in children healing spontaneously with occlusion of the parent artery.[44]

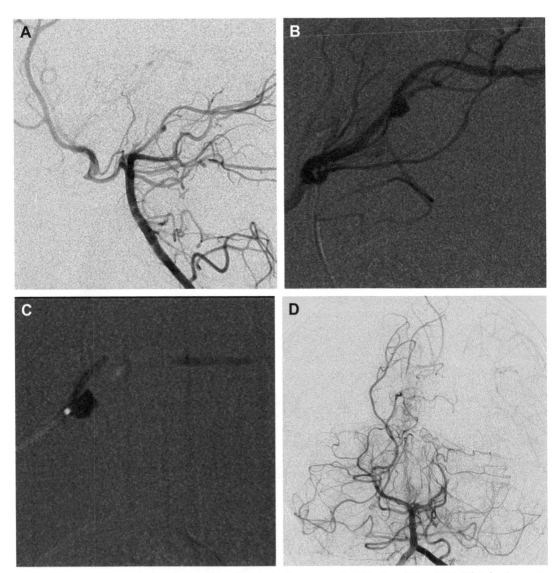

Fig. 2. A 4-year-old boy who presented with a headache from a grade 2 Hunt and Hess SAH. (*A*) Selective vertebral artery angiogram shows a left posterior cerebral artery (PCA) aneurysm. (*B*) Selective PCA angiogram shows the aneurysm at the P2/P3 segment. (*C*) Lateral spot fluoroscopic images shows the Histoacryl glue within the aneurysm and adjacent PCA segment. (*D*) Final vertebral angiogram confirming exclusion of the aneurysm with arterial collaterals supplying left PCA territory.

Giant Aneurysms

Giant aneurysms (>25 mm) in children are about 4 times more common than in adults.[22,25,45–47] Their reported incidence in children is between 25% and 45%.[48] Giant aneurysms should be considered in the dissection category. Children who have giant aneurysms often present with mass effect and only 35% of the time with SAH.[12,18,49]

NATURAL HISTORY

Given the pediatric patient's lifespan, the cumulative risks of aneurysm growth, rupture, recurrence, de novo aneurysm formation, and retreatment are considerable, hence treatment and posttreatment follow-up are mandatory.

CLINICAL PRESENTATION

Children with intracranial aneurysms can present with SAH, headache, direct compressive effects, focal neurologic deficits, or seizures.[19] Sixty percent of children with SAH have a cerebral aneurysm.[50] Fusiform aneurysms tend to present with nonhemorrhagic deficits.[18] Many children with SAH present with a Hunt and Hess grade between 1 and 3.[11,12,47,48,51] The reason for the better clinical grade at presentation is unclear, but this may be related to fewer comorbidities, a superior nitric oxide synthase pathway, or the robustness of the leptomeningeal arterial collaterals.[11,52] In our series, 56% of patients presented with SAH, 33% with mass effect, and 11% after trauma.

DIAGNOSIS

For a child with suspected SAH, the diagnosis begins with a noncontrast computed tomography (CT) scan of the head. If this study is normal and the clinical history is strongly suspicious for SAH, then a lumbar puncture is required. The presence of xanthochromia or blood requires additional imaging in the form of a CT angiogram or a magnetic resonance (MR) angiogram of the circle of Willis. The choice of imaging modality is made on a case-by-case basis with an effort to reduce unnecessary radiation exposure while obtaining the necessary data to plan treatment and postoperative management. Digital subtraction angiography (DSA) is still the gold standard for the diagnosis of cerebral aneurysms. For patients with unruptured aneurysms who may present with headache, seizures, or mass effect, MR imaging of the brain with an MR angiogram of the circle of Willis is valuable to limit radiation exposure because these patients may need long-term follow-up imaging.

TREATMENT

In the past, aneurysms have been treated surgically, with either excision or clipping of the aneurysmal segment. In recent years there has been a shift toward the use of endovascular intervention with a strong desire to avoid open surgery in young children. A multidisciplinary team consisting of stroke neurologists, cerebrovascular neurosurgeons, and neurointerventional radiologists is

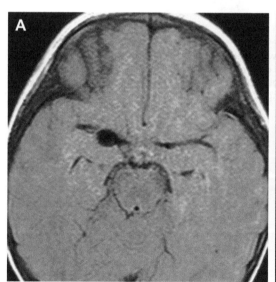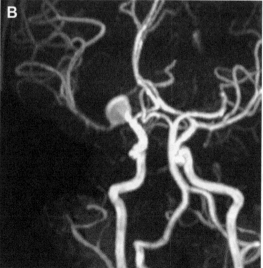

Fig. 3. A 9-month-old boy who presented with left-sided weakness. (*A*) Axial fluid-attenuated inversion recovery MR image of the brain shows a large flow void in the right M1 segment. (*B*) Three-dimensional time of flight MR angiogram shows a wide-necked saccular aneurysm involving the right M1 segment.

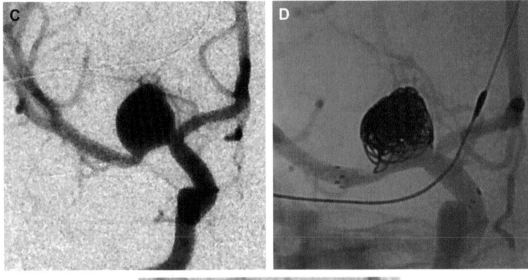

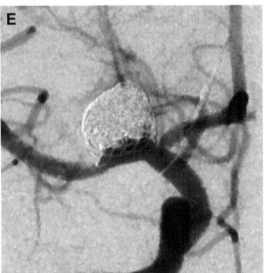

Fig. 3. (*C*) Right internal carotid angiogram shows a wide-necked saccular aneurysm involving the right M1 segment. (*D*) Right internal carotid angiogram shows an enterprise stent from the distal right M1 segment across the neck of the aneurysm extending into the supraclinoid ICA with coils within the aneurysm. (*E*) Final right internal carotid angiogram after embolization shows filling at the base of the aneurysm with a small filling defect within the distal stent.

mandatory to treat complex intracranial aneurysms and achieve excellent results.[53] Treatment options include observation, endovascular therapy, or surgical clipping. The treatment modality depends on location, vascular anatomy, and aneurysm shape. Surgical treatment includes direct clipping, clip reconstruction, and aneurysm trapping with or without bypass procedures.

For endovascular treatment, we generally use a femoral approach, using a 4-Fr to 6-Fr access system. Cerebral angiography and aneurysm catheterization techniques are similar to those used in adults apart from the careful use of contrast according to child size. Other specific issues related to small children include the careful monitoring of blood loss and fluid requirements. Simple coiling with or without adjuvant techniques such as balloon remodeling or stent placement are primarily used for most aneurysms (Fig. 1); however, glue is used for distal fusiform aneurysms (Fig. 2). Stents, including flow-diverting stents, may be necessary for fusiform and giant aneurysms (Fig. 3).

In our series, 8 patients were treated with endovascular techniques, and 1 was managed conservatively, because risk of treatment was considered to outweigh the benefit. Endovascular techniques included coil (n = 5) or glue (n = 1) embolization, stent coiling (n = 1), and balloon occlusion (n = 1).

OUTCOME

In our series, 6 of the patients had an excellent outcome, 1 was left severely disabled, and 2 patients died. Of the 2 patients who died, 1 was managed conservatively, and the other rebled during the occlusion procedure. In the Toronto series, children treated by an endovascular approach had a better clinical outcome than those in the surgically treated group.[12] Seventy-seven percent of the patients who received endovascular treatment made a good recovery (modified Rankin scale 0–1) compared with 44.4% of patients treated with open surgery. Lasjaunias and colleagues[11] also reported good long-term results and outcome in their endovascular-treated aneurysms. Saraf and colleagues,[54] in a study of 23 pediatric patients with intracranial aneurysms, showed an overall favorable outcome in 22 of 23 treated with endovascular techniques. A report from China of 22 patients with intracranial aneurysms treated by endovascular techniques showed a good outcome in 96% of patients with a Glasgow Outcome Scale of 4 or 5.[55]

SUMMARY

Childhood intracranial aneurysms differ from those in the adult population in incidence and gender prevalence, cause, location, and clinical presentation. Endovascular treatment of pediatric aneurysms is the suggested approach because it offers both reconstructive and deconstructive techniques and a better clinical outcome compared with surgery; however, the long-term durability of endovascular treatment is still questionable, therefore long-term clinical and imaging follow-up is necessary.

REFERENCES

1. Locksley HB, Sahs AL, Knowler L. Report on the cooperative study of intracranial aneurysms and subarachnoid hemorrhage. Section II. General survey of cases in the central registry and characteristics of the sample population. J Neurosurg 1966; 24:922–32.

2. Gerosa M, Licata C, Fiore DL, et al. Intracranial aneurysms of childhood. Childs Brain 1980;6: 295–302.

3. Roche JL, Choux M, Czorny A, et al. Intracranial arterial aneurysm in children. A cooperative study. Apropos of 43 cases. Neurochirurgie 1988;34: 243–51 [in French].

4. Sedzimir CB, Robinson J. Intracranial hemorrhage in children and adolescents. J Neurosurg 1973; 38:269–81.

5. Locksley HB. Natural history of subarachnoid hemorrhage, intracranial aneurysms and arteriovenous malformations. Based on 6368 cases in the cooperative study. J Neurosurg 1966;25:219–39.

6. Meyer FB, Sundt TM Jr, Fode NC, et al. Cerebral aneurysms in childhood and adolescence. J Neurosurg 1989;70:420–5.

7. Patel AN, Richardson AE. Ruptured intracranial aneurysms in the first two decades of life. A study of 58 patients. J Neurosurg 1971;35:571–6.

8. Amacher LA, Drake CG. Cerebral artery aneurysms in infancy, childhood and adolescence. Childs Brain 1975;1:72–80.

9. Molyneux A, Kerr R, Stratton I, et al. International Subarachnoid Aneurysm Trial (ISAT) of neurosurgical clipping versus endovascular coiling in 2143 patients with ruptured intracranial aneurysms: a randomised trial. Lancet 2002;360:1267–74.

10. Unruptured intracranial aneurysms–risk of rupture and risks of surgical intervention. International Study of Unruptured Intracranial Aneurysms Investigators. N Engl J Med 1998;339:1725–33.

11. Lasjaunias P, Wuppalapati S, Alvarez H, et al. Intracranial aneurysms in children aged under 15 years: review of 59 consecutive children with 75 aneurysms. Childs Nerv Syst 2005;21:437–50.

12. Agid R, Souza MP, Reintamm G, et al. The role of endovascular treatment for pediatric aneurysms. Childs Nerv Syst 2005;21:1030–6.

13. Pope FM, Kendall BE, Slapak GI, et al. Type III collagen mutations cause fragile cerebral arteries. Br J Neurosurg 1991;5:551–74.

14. Taira T, Tamura Y, Kawamura H. Intracranial aneurysm in a child with Klippel-Trenaunay-Weber syndrome: case report. Surg Neurol 1991;36: 303–6.

15. Pasqualin A, Mazza C, Cavazzani P, et al. Intracranial aneurysms and subarachnoid hemorrhage in children and adolescents. Childs Nerv Syst 1986; 2:185–90.

16. Storrs BB, Humphreys RP, Hendrick EB, et al. Intracranial aneurysms in the pediatric age-group. Childs Brain 1982;9:358–61.

17. Almeida GM, Pindaro J, Plese P, et al. Intracranial arterial aneurysms in infancy and childhood. Childs Brain 1977;3:193–9.

18. Hetts SW, Narvid J, Sanai N, et al. Intracranial aneurysms in childhood: 27-year single-institution experience. AJNR Am J Neuroradiol 2009;30: 1315–24.

19. Mehrotra A, Nair AP, Das KK, et al. Clinical and radiological profiles and outcomes in pediatric patients with intracranial aneurysms. J Neurosurg Pediatr 2012;10:340–6.

20. Koroknay-Pal P, Lehto H, Niemela M, et al. Long-term outcome of 114 children with cerebral aneurysms. J Neurosurg Pediatr 2012;9: 636–45.

21. Wiebers DO, Whisnant JP, Huston J 3rd, et al. Unruptured intracranial aneurysms: natural history, clinical outcome, and risks of surgical and endovascular treatment. Lancet 2003;362:103–10.

22. Allison JW, Davis PC, Sato Y, et al. Intracranial aneurysms in infants and children. Pediatr Radiol 1998;28:223–9.

23. Agid R, Terbrugge K. Pediatric aneurysms. J Neurosurg 2007;106:328 [author reply: 9].

24. Choux M, Lena G, Genitori L. Intracranial aneurysms in children. In: Raimondi A, Choux M, Di Rocco C, editors. Cerebrovascular disease in children. Vienna (Austria): Springer; 1992. p. 123–31.

25. Lasjaunias P, Campi A, Rodesch G, et al. Aneurysmal disease in children: review of 20 cases with intracranial arterial localisations. Interv Neuroradiol 1997;3:215–29.

26. Herman JM, Rekate HL, Spetzler RF. Pediatric intracranial aneurysms: simple and complex cases. Pediatr Neurosurg 1991;17:66–72 [discussion: 3].

27. Yazbak PA, McComb JG, Raffel C. Pediatric traumatic intracranial aneurysms. Pediatr Neurosurg 1995;22:15–9.

28. Ventureyra EC, Higgins MJ. Traumatic intracranial aneurysms in childhood and adolescence. Case reports and review of the literature. Childs Nerv Syst 1994;10:361–79.

29. Nakstad P, Nornes H, Hauge HN. Traumatic aneurysms of the pericallosal arteries. Neuroradiology 1986;28:335–8.

30. Kneyber MC, Rinkel GJ, Ramos LM, et al. Early posttraumatic subarachnoid hemorrhage due to dissecting aneurysms in three children. Neurology 2005;65:1663–5.

31. Sutton LN. Vascular complications of surgery for craniopharyngioma and hypothalamic glioma. Pediatr Neurosurg 1994;21(Suppl 1):124–8.

32. Kanaan I, Lasjaunias P, Coates R. The spectrum of intracranial aneurysms in pediatrics. Minim Invasive Neurosurg 1995;38:1–9.

33. Barrow DL, Prats AR. Infectious intracranial aneurysms: comparison of groups with and without endocarditis. Neurosurgery 1990;27:56–73.

34. Bohmfalk GL, Story JL, Wissinger JP, et al. Bacterial intracranial aneurysm. J Neurosurg 1978;48: 369–82.

35. Horten BC, Abbott GF, Porro RS. Fungal aneurysms of intracranial vessels. Arch Neurol 1976; 33:577–9.

36. Suwanwela C, Suwanwela N, Charuchinda S, et al. Intracranial mycotic aneurysms of extravascular origin. J Neurosurg 1972;36:552–9.

37. Marsot-Dupuch K, Riachi S, Berthet K, et al. Infectious aneurysms of the cavernous carotid artery. J Radiol 2000;81:891–8 [in French].

38. Leroy D, Dompmartin A, Houtteville JP, et al. Aneurysm associated with chronic mucocutaneous candidiasis during long-term therapy with ketoconazole. Dermatologica 1989;178:43–6.

39. Grouhi M, Dalal I, Nisbet-Brown E, et al. Cerebral vasculitis associated with chronic mucocutaneous candidiasis. J Pediatr 1998;133:571–4.

40. Philippet P, Blanche S, Sebag G, et al. Stroke and cerebral infarcts in children infected with human immunodeficiency virus. Arch Pediatr Adolesc Med 1994;148:965–70.

41. Dubrovsky T, Curless R, Scott G, et al. Cerebral aneurysmal arteriopathy in childhood AIDS. Neurology 1998;51:560–5.

42. Shah SS, Zimmerman RA, Rorke LB, et al. Cerebrovascular complications of HIV in children. AJNR Am J Neuroradiol 1996;17:1913–7.

43. Park YD, Belman AL, Kim TS, et al. Stroke in pediatric acquired immunodeficiency syndrome. Ann Neurol 1990;28:303–11.

44. Tanabe M, Inoue Y, Hori T. Spontaneous thrombosis of an aneurysm of the middle cerebral artery with subarachnoid haemorrhage in a 6-year-old child: case report. Neurol Res 1991;13:202–4.

45. Amacher AL, Drake CG, Ferguson GG. Posterior circulation aneurysms in young people. Neurosurgery 1981;8:315–20.

46. Heiskanen O, Vilkki J. Intracranial arterial aneurysms in children and adolescents. Acta Neurochir (Wien) 1981;59:55–63.

47. Proust F, Toussaint P, Garnieri J, et al. Pediatric cerebral aneurysms. J Neurosurg 2001;94:733–9.

48. Huang J, McGirt MJ, Gailloud P, et al. Intracranial aneurysms in the pediatric population: case series and literature review. Surg Neurol 2005;63:424–32 [discussion: 32–3].

49. Peerless SJ, Nemoto S, Drake CG. Giant intracranial aneurysms in children and adolescents. In: Edwards MS, Hoffman HJ, editors. Cerebral vascular disease in children and adolescents. Baltimore (MD): Williams and Wilkins; 1989.

50. Jordan LC. Assessment and treatment of stroke in children. Curr Treat Options Neurol 2008;10: 399–409.

51. Krishna H, Wani AA, Behari S, et al. Intracranial aneurysms in patients 18 years of age or under, are they different from aneurysms in adult population? Acta Neurochir (Wien) 2005;147:469–76 [discussion: 76].

52. Khurana VG, Meissner I, Sohni YR, et al. The presence of tandem endothelial nitric oxide synthase gene polymorphisms identifying brain aneurysms more prone to rupture. J Neurosurg 2005;102: 526–31.

53. Johnston SC. Effect of endovascular services and hospital volume on cerebral aneurysm treatment outcomes. Stroke 2000;31:111–7.

54. Saraf R, Shrivastava M, Siddhartha W, et al. Intracranial pediatric aneurysms: endovascular treatment and its outcome. J Neurosurg Pediatr 2012;10:230–40.

55. Liang JT, Bao YH, Zhang HQ, et al. Intracranial aneurysms in childhood and adolescence. Zhonghua Yi Xue Za Zhi 2011;91:2744–6 [in Chinese].

Arterial Ischemic Stroke in Children

Joseph J. Gemmete, MD, FSIR[a],*,
Indran Davagnanam, MD, MB BCh, BAO, BMedSci, FRCR[b],
Ahmed K. Toma, MD, FRCS (Neurosurg)[c],
Stefan Brew, MBBS, MHB, MSc, FRANZCR, FRCR[b],
Vijeya Ganesan, MD, FRCP[d]

KEYWORDS

- Acute ischemic stroke in children • Vasculitis • Moyamoya • Hyperacute thrombolysis
- Arterial dissection • Sickle cell disease • Congenital heart disease

KEY POINTS

- Nonatheromatous abnormalities of the cerebral and/or cervical arterial circulation are very common in childhood arterial ischemic stroke and are the most important determinants of treatment and prognosis.
- Intracranial disease is far commoner than cervical disease but imaging needs to include the aortic arch to the circle of Willis.
- There are standardized disease definitions that should be used precisely to promote accuracy of diagnosis.
- Key diagnostic dilemmas are the identification of vasculitis and moyamoya.
- Hyperacute thrombolysis is unlikely to be an appropriate treatment for most children with arterial ischemic stroke but may have a role in selected patients.
- As well as medical approaches, including anticoagulation, anti-inflammatories, and antiplatelet therapies, surgical revascularization and endovascular approaches may have a role in the management of these diseases.

INTRODUCTION

Arterial ischemic stroke (AIS) affects 3.3 of 100,000 children per year, with residual morbidity in two-thirds of patients, resulting in significant health care, personal, and social costs.[1–5] The cause of AIS is commonly multifactorial, with one-half of the affected children having a premorbid illness, such as congenital or acquired heart disease, vascular disorders, or an infection.[6,7] With the advent of noninvasive cerebrovascular imaging, especially magnetic resonance angiography (MRA), it has become apparent that most affected children have abnormalities, or arteriopathies, of the cerebral or cervical arterial circulation.[3] This article discusses the clinical presentation, epidemiology, and cause of AIS in children. Then, diagnostic imaging, treatment options, and outcomes as they relate to AIS in children are discussed. Hemorrhagic stroke in children is not included in this article.

[a] Division of Interventional Neuroradiology and Cranial Base Surgery, Departments of Radiology, Neurosurgery, and Otolaryngology, University of Michigan Health System, UH B1D 328, 1500 East Medical Center Drive, Ann Arbor, MI 48109-5030, USA; [b] Lysholm Department of Neuroradiology, National Hospital for Neurology and Neurosurgery, University College London Hospitals, Queen Square, London, UK; [c] Victor Horsley Department of Neurosurgery, National Hospital for Neurology and Neurosurgery, University College London Hospitals, Queen Square, London, UK; [d] Department of Pediatric Neurology, Great Ormond Street Hospital for Children, NHS Trust, London WC1N 3JH, UK
* Corresponding author.
E-mail address: gemmete@med.umich.edu

Neuroimag Clin N Am 23 (2013) 781–798
http://dx.doi.org/10.1016/j.nic.2013.03.019
1052-5149/13/$ – see front matter © 2013 Elsevier Inc. All rights reserved.

CLINICAL PRESENTATION

The clinical presentation of an AIS in children varies according to the age of the child, the cause, and the involved artery.[8] In general, embolic episodes tend to present suddenly, whereas a stenosis or thrombosis may have a more gradual onset.[9] Focal neurologic deficits such as hemiplegia are the most common presentation of AIS in children.[10] Other signs and symptoms, such as headache, language and speech difficulties, mood or behavior disturbances, and seizures, are less specific.[10–12] In children less than 1 year of age, seizures and encephalopathy are more common than focal neurologic signs.[13] Stroke in the posterior circulation can present as vertigo, ataxia, and vomiting. In infancy, a typical presentation includes seizure, lethargy, and/or apnea often without a focal neurologic deficit.[14] Braun and colleagues[15] found that children with nonarteriopathic AIS were significantly more likely than those with arteriopathy to have an abrupt onset of symptoms.

INCIDENCE

The reported incidence of childhood stroke has increased in the last 20 years according to population studies, most likely related to improvements in neuroimaging techniques. Schoenberg and colleagues[16] studied stroke in children in Rochester, MN, from 1965 through 1974. They found an estimated average annual incidence rate of 1.89 of 100,000 and 0.63 of 100,000 per year for hemorrhagic and ischemic strokes, respectively. Their overall average annual incidence rate was 2.52 of 100,000 per year. Broderick and colleagues[17] in the 1990s, studying childhood stroke in metropolitan Cincinnati, found an overall incidence of 2.7 of 100,000 per year. Surprisingly, hemorrhagic stroke (incidence 1.5/100,000/y) was shown to be more frequent than ischemic stroke (incidence 1.2/100,000/y). Updated incidence figures from the Canadian Pediatric Ischemic Stroke Registry showed that ischemic stroke in childhood occurs in 3.3 of 100,000 per year, with 2.6 of 100,000 per year and 0.7 of 100,000 per year as the rates for arterial and sinovenous strokes, respectively.[1,18] When the authors included hemorrhagic strokes, the overall childhood stroke incidence exceeded 6 of 100,000 per year. A retrospective analysis of a California-wide hospital discharge database estimated an incidence of stroke (AIS, cerebral venous thrombosis, and hemorrhagic stroke including subarachnoid hemorrhage) of 2.3 of 100,000 per year and a prospective study across the United Kingdom and Ireland reported an incidence of stroke (AIS, cerebral venous thrombosis, and hemorrhagic stroke including subarachnoid hemorrhage) of 2.3 of 100,000 per year.[19,20] Adverse outcomes include death in 10%, neurologic deficits or seizures in 70%, and recurrent strokes in more than 20% of children affected with a stroke.[2,3] Strokes in children can result from either vascular occlusion (ischemic stroke) or from bleeding caused by a ruptured blood vessel (hemorrhagic stroke). The incidence of ischemic versus hemorrhage stroke is different in children versus adults. Ischemic stroke accounts for 55% of strokes in children, whereas it causes 85% of adult strokes.[11] Boys have a higher risk of pediatric stroke than girls, with the type of stroke varying with age.[21] Infants (30 days to 1 year) have a higher reported rate of ischemic stroke, whereas older children (15–19 years) show a higher incidence of hemorrhagic stroke. Black children have more than twice the risk of stroke of white children. Hispanic children have a lower risk that white children, and Asian children show a roughly equal risk.[19]

ETIOLOGY

There are major differences in the risk factors for stroke in children compared with adults. Compared with adults, children are more likely to have an infectious or inflammatory disorder underlying the stroke.[22] The causes of AIS in childhood are often multifactorial and different than in adults. The most fundamental difference between strokes in children and adults is the wide array of risk factors seen in children versus adults (**Box 1**). The causes of AIS can be broadly divided into the following 6 categories: cardiac disease, sickle cell disease, moyamoya, arterial dissection, other arteriopathy, and other causes.[23] Approximately 24% of the cases are classified as idiopathic.[3]

Cardiac Abnormalities

Cardiac procedures, including catheterization, extracorporeal membrane oxygenation, and surgery, are all considered risk factors for childhood AIS.[24,25] These cardiac procedures are all likely mediated from a heart embolus. Congenital heart disease (**Fig. 1**), valvular heart disease, cardiac arrhythmias, and cardiomyopathy are also risk factors for childhood AIS.[25–28] Abnormalities of the cardiac valves, major vessels, and myocardium may result in turbulent blood flow and the formation of a thrombus that can embolus to the cerebral vessels, which is particularly a problem in children with a right-to-left shunt. In a retrospective national database review of children with AIS, the most frequent comorbidity was noted to be congenital heart disease.[26] Almost 25% of children diagnosed with AIS in the Canadian Registry

Box 1
Causes of pediatric ischemic stroke

Heart disease
Congenital heart disease
Rheumatic heart disease
Cardiomyopathy
Endocarditis/myocarditis
Dysrhythmias

Hematologic disorders
Hemoglobinopathy (sickle cell disease)
Polycythemia
Thrombocytosis
Leukemia/lymphoma

Coagulopathies
Protein C/S deficiency
Antithrombin III deficiency
Antiphospholipid antibody syndrome
Lupus anticoagulant
Factor V Leiden mutation
Disseminated intravascular coagulation

Metabolic
Mitochondrial disorders
Homocystinuria/hyperhomocysteinemia/Fabry disease
Dyslipidemias

Vasculopathy
Moyamoya syndrome
Fibromuscular dysplasia
Neurocutaneous disorders

Vasculitis
Connective tissue diseases
Henoch-Schonlein purpura
Polyarteritis nodosa
Kawasaki disease

Trauma to the head or neck

Infection
  Meningitis
  Varicella
  HIV

Idiopathic

Data from Refs.[10,11,122]

had cardiac disease at presentation.[29] In another childhood AIS cohort study, 28% of the children had cardiac abnormalities.[30]

Hypertension may also be a risk factor for childhood AIS. Ganesan and colleagues[30] showed an association with vasculopathy and systolic hypertension. Lo and colleagues[26] also found that hypertension was a risk factor for pediatric stroke. It is hypothesized that hypertension in children may be related to chronic anemia, comorbid medical conditions, or a systemic response to an acquired vasculopathy.[29]

It is uncertain if a patent foramen ovale (PFO) is a significant risk factor for childhood AIS. In 4 of 6 children with idiopathic AIS, transcranial Doppler with Valsalva suggested a right-to-left shunt.[31] PFO is a known risk factor for AIS in the adult literature; however, the incidence of a PFO in healthy children is unknown.[32]

Sickle Cell Disease

Sickle cell disease (SCD) is one of the most common causes for AIS in childhood, particularly among individuals such as African Americans, of recent historical descent from populations inhabiting malaria-endemic regions. The prevalence of cerebrovascular events in patients with SCD is reported to be 4.0% and the incidence 0.6 per 100 patient-years. The highest risk for stroke is between the ages of 2 and 5 years of age.[33,34] The risk of recurrence is as high as 67%. AIS in SCD is largely related to occlusive disease of in the terminal internal carotid artery (TICA)/proximal middle cerebral artery (MCA)/anterior cerebral artery (ACA), which is caused by endothelial injury from the deformed erythrocytes. Other factors, such as anemia and hypoxemia, may additionally predispose to AIS. Pathologic features of SCD are often associated with thrombotic occlusion and the presence of collateral vessels.[35–37] Blood transfusion, aiming to reduce the circulating level of Hemoglobin S (HbS) and correct anemia sufficiently to suppress bone marrow production of HbS, is extremely effective in both primary and secondary prevention of AIS. The standard of care in many countries is now to institute screening for cerebrovascular disease in children with SCD using transcranial Doppler ultrasound from the age of 2 years, at annual intervals, and instituting blood transfusion for those with abnormally elevated velocity in the middle cerebral arteries. Blood transfusion is also recommended for children who have had clinical AIS, for secondary prevention. Unfortunately, despite its efficacy, blood transfusion places a major burden on the child and family, as well as carrying medical risks such

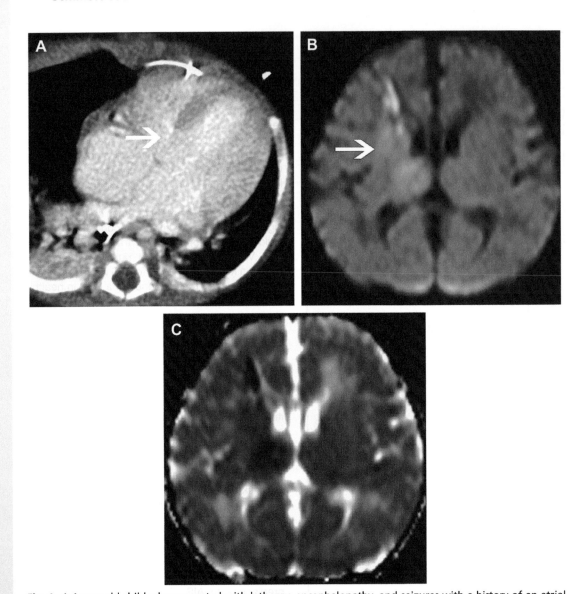

Fig. 1. A 1-year-old child who presented with lethargy, encephalopathy, and seizures with a history of an atrial septal defect, ventricular septal defect, and transposition of great vessels. (*A*) Axial contrast-enhanced CT thorax (*white arrow*) shows a large ventricular septal defect (VSD). (*B*) Axial diffusion-weighted MRI of the brain shows abnormal high signal within the right frontal lobe, basal ganglia, and thalamus (*white arrow*); this is low signal on the corresponding apparent diffusion coefficient (ADC) (*C*).

as blood-borne infection. The logistics of blood transfusion also make it impossible in resource-poor settings. There is ongoing research into the role of other therapies, such as hydroxyurea. Bone marrow transplantation may be considered in children with AIS but the major hurdle with this is identifying a suitable donor. Patients with SCD who have a moyamoya morphology of occlusive disease terminal internal carotid artery (TICA), M1 segment of the middle cerebral artery (M1), A1 segment of the anterior cerebral artery (A1) (TICA/M1/A1 occlusive disease with basal collaterals) are at highest risk of recurrence. Surgical

revascularization may have a role in such individuals but the role of surgery in the context of the overall management of SCD is as yet unclear.

Moyamoya

Moyamoya is a radiological term characterized by bilateral stenosis of the distal internal carotid arteries with lenticulostriate collateralization that results in the pathognomonic "puff of smoke" appearance (**Fig. 2**) on conventional cerebral angiogram and is diagnosed in up to 20% of childhood AIS.[38–41] The condition is common in

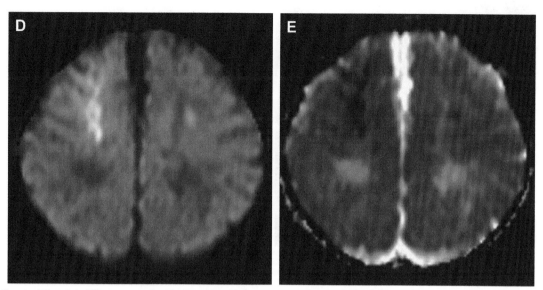

Fig. 1. (*D*) Axial diffusion-weighted MRI image of the brain in same patient shows areas of high signal within both frontal lobes, which is low signal on the corresponding ADC map (*E*). These findings are consistent with embolic AIS in multiple vascular distributions from the patient's congenital heart disease.

Japan and East Asia, where familial cases are also clearly recognized. Currently several genetic loci have been implicated in these.[42] The disease definition relates to Japanese patients and the degree of radiological and phenotypic overlap between them and patients of other ethnicities is not clear. Moyamoya may be apparently idiopathic (moyamoya disease) or secondary to a large variety of other conditions (moyamoya syndrome), including trisomy 21, neurofibromatosis type 1, and cranial irradiation.[43–46] This wide spectrum of associations suggests multiple mechanisms are implicated in the genesis of the arteriopathy. Unfortunately the term is used very loosely in clinical practice and in the literature and is commonly applied in cases of bilateral TICA disease, whether or not the other radiological features are present. The genetics literature describing moyamoya as a feature of many disorders is likely, in fact, to reflect a variety of entities.[42] An example of this is the very distinctive radiological phenotype of cerebral arteriopathy associated with mutations in the alpha-actin-2 (ACTA2) gene, initially described as "moyamoya." In contrast, these patients have several distinctive radiological features, namely proximal ectasia, distal occlusive disease, absence of basal collaterals, and an unusually straight morphology of the intracranial arteries. Because this mutation is dominantly inherited and predisposes to aortic aneurysms, it is an important condition to identify by the radiological signature. There are likely to be further examples of distinctive phenotypes, currently subsumed under imprecise application of the term "moyamoya."

Arterial Dissection

Dissection of the cervical arterial arteries is said to account for 15% to 20% of AIS in children; this is largely seen in older children and adolescents and is usually spontaneous.[47–50] Cases may be attributed to significant or even mild traumatic events, and some to connective tissue disorders, such as Ehlers-Danlos or Marfan syndrome.[51–55] The radiological features required to diagnose dissection can be elusive; absolute evidence comes from visualization of a dissection flap, double vascular lumen, or hematoma within the arterial wall.[56] Indirect evidence includes tapering vascular occlusion (string sign) or irregular caliber change. Vertebral artery (VA) dissection is the most common risk factor for posterior circulation AIS in children and should be actively excluded, by catheter angiography if necessary, unless there is a clear alternative diagnosis (Fig. 3). The V3 loop of the VA is the commonest site of dissection and is often not clearly visualized on MRA. Abnormalities of the cervical spine (eg, calcified arcuate ligament) may be associated with VA dissection and should be excluded by plain radiographs of the neck in flexion and extension. Dissection of the intracranial arteries undoubtedly exists but is difficult to identify and distinguish from other entities, such as focal cerebral arteriopathy (FCA), with confidence.[56] The importance of identifying arterial dissection is that it is one of the diagnoses which,

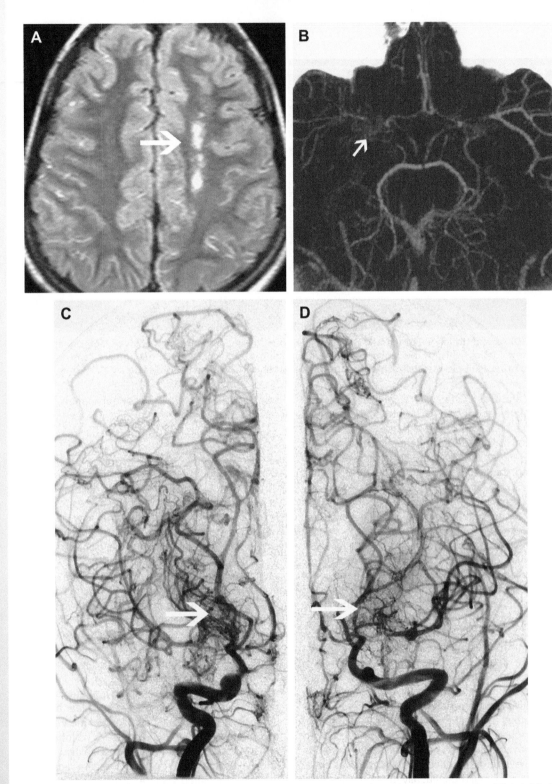

Fig. 2. A 7-year-old boy who presented with headache and weakness in the right upper extremity. (*A*) Axial fluid-attenuated inversion recovery (FLAIR) MRI of the brain shows an area of chronic ischemia with the watershed distribution of the left anterior cerebral artery (ACA) and middle cerebral artery (MCA) (*white arrow*). (*B*) Axial CTA image of the circle of Willis shows a "puff of smoke" in the bilateral basal ganglia (*white arrow*). (*C*) Frontal right internal carotid angiogram shows narrowing of the right supraclinoid, A1, and M1 segments with a "puff of smoke" in the basal ganglia (*white arrow*). (*D*) Frontal left internal carotid angiogram also shows narrowing of the left supraclinoid, A1, and M1 segments with a "puff of smoke" in the basal ganglia (*white arrow*). There is a decreased capillary blush between the left ACA and MCA, consistent with the findings on the MRI shown in (*A*). These findings are consistent with moyamoya and an old watershed infarct between the left ACA and left MCA territory.

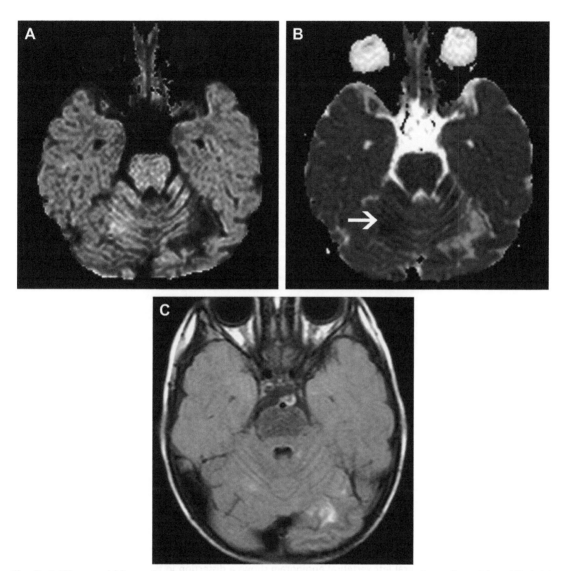

Fig. 3. A 2½-year-old boy who fell from a chair and presented with vertigo, ataxia, and vomiting. (*A*) Axial diffusion-weighted MRI of the brain shows an area of high signal in the right cerebellar hemisphere. (*B*) Axial corresponding ADC map shows an area of restricted diffusion in the right cerebellar hemisphere (*white arrow*). (*C*) Axial FLAIR MRI of the brain, same level as *A* and *B*, shows a majority of these areas of abnormality demonstrate high signal consistent with T2 shine through, or subacute ischemia.

based on current treatment recommendations, alters the treatment approach. Furthermore, the literature suggests that patients with an index event are at increased risk of recurrent dissection in the future. It is likely that affected patients have an underlying genetically determined predisposition, potentially exacerbated by environmental triggers, such as infection or trauma.

Focal Cerebral Arteriopathy of Childhood

To promote consistency, the International Pediatric Stroke Study group has advocated application of standard disease definitions.[57] The most commonly identified cerebral arteriopathy in childhood is focal occlusive disease of the TICA/proximal MCA or ACA; this morphology of disease was originally termed "transient cerebral arteriopathy," a definition that required demonstration of disease stability or regression over time.[41,58] More recently, this term has been superseded by the term "focal cerebral arteriopathy of childhood" (FCA) (**Fig. 4**) to refer to this pattern of focal proximal occlusive disease identified at a single time point. The FCA pattern of arteriopathy is commonly seen in children after varicella

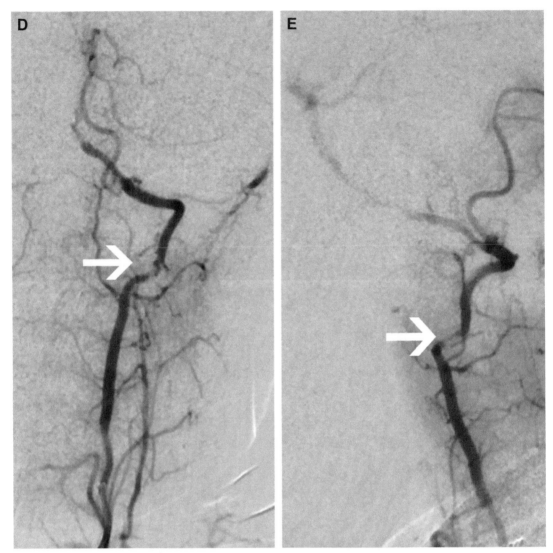

Fig. 3. (*D*) Frontal and (*E*) lateral left vertebral angiogram shows a dissection in the V3 segment (*white arrow*). These findings are consistent with multiple embolic events of different ages from a vertebral artery dissection.

cerebral infarction and in these cases it is hypothesized that the disease represents a focal inflammatory response to the viral infection.[59] The role of infection and vascular inflammation in the genesis of arteriopathy in other cases remains controversial; however, there does seem to be an increased rate of antecedent upper respiratory tract infection in children with FCA. The distinction between FCA and primary angiitis of the central nervous system (PACNS) is controversial. Although vascular inflammation is thought to be a disease mechanism common to both entities, they are distinguished by their clinical course, with PACNS typically having a multifocal and progressive course, in contrast to the monophasic course observed in FCA.[60] Currently there are no

biomarkers that robustly distinguish between FCA and PACNS and there is confusion in the literature, with cases that appear identical in terms of imaging being cited as examples of one or another entity.[61] Catheter angiography may be useful in cases of suspected PACNS if there is multifocal disease affecting smaller arteries. If this is undertaken, it is worth considering systemic angiography, looking for evidence of systemic vascular involvement.

Inflammatory Arteriopathy

Inflammatory arteriopathy of the central nervous system may be part of a systemic vasculitis or isolated PACNS.[30,62] A variety of vessel sizes may be

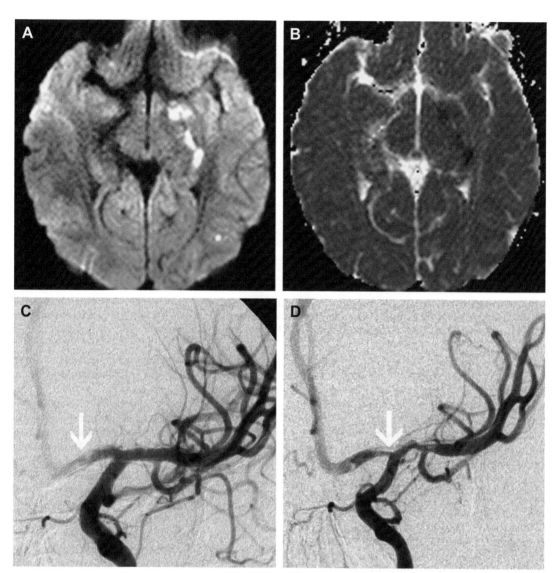

Fig. 4. A 7-year-old girl who presented with headache and right-sided weakness. (*A*) Axial diffusion-weighted MRI of the brain shows an area of high signal in the left mesial temporal lobe, amygdala, and left internal capsule with tiny foci in the left parietal occipital lobe. The corresponding ADC map (*B*) shows low signal in these areas. (*C*) Frontal left internal carotid angiogram at the time of stroke shows a filling defect within the L A1 segment (*white arrow*) with delayed filling of the L ACA; there is also mild narrowing of the L M1 segment. (*D*) Frontal left internal carotid angiogram 1 month after the stroke shows near interval resolution of the filling defect within the L A1 segment; however, there is now narrowing of the left supraclinoid, L A1, and L M1 segments (*white arrow*).

involved; small vessel vasculitis (confirmed histologically) may be associated with normal catheter angiography. Central nervous system vasculitis is notoriously difficult to identify and no investigation, including leptomeningeal biopsy, has a sensitivity of more than 40%. Thus the diagnostic approach has to be broad, including serology and cerebrospinal fluid (CSF) examination, looking for evidence of disease in other organ systems. It is important to have a high level of clinical vigilance, especially in patients with recurrent AIS, multifocal infarction, progressive arteriopathy, or a more diffuse, encephalopathic presentation.[39]

Idiopathic—Other Causes

Although the Sebire classification captures most cerebral arteriopathies seen in association with AIS, it is not entirely comprehensive.[41] In the context of a specialist pediatric neurovascular service, a significant proportion of patients cannot be placed in a category using this scheme; common

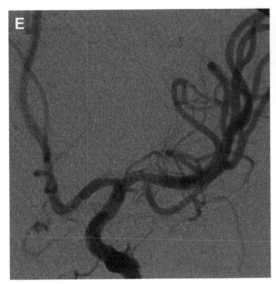
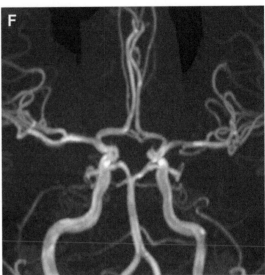

Fig. 4. (*E*) Frontal left internal carotid angiogram 6 months after the stroke shows resolution of the filling defect and areas of narrowing. (*F*) Five-year follow-up MRA shows a normal circle of Willis. These findings are consistent with a stroke related to focal cerebral arteriopathy (FCA) from a varicella infection.

features in them are multifocal arteriopathy (**Fig. 5**), involvement of other organs (especially renal arteries), a genetic or syndrome diagnosis, and the coexistence of occlusive and aneurysmal cerebrovascular disease in the same individual. It is likely that these patients have genetically mediated disease, potentially exacerbated by environmental triggers.

Genetic/Metabolic Conditions

Inherited metabolic disorders are associated with childhood AIS. Some examples include Fabry disease, an X-linked deficiency of α-galactosidase; cerebral autosomal-dominant arteriopathy with subcortical infarcts and leukoencephalopathy; Menkes syndrome, a copper transport disorder; and homocystinuria, a deficiency of cystathionine-β-synthase that results in hyperhomocysteinemia.[63–66]

Sympathomimetic Drugs

Recreational drugs in adolescents is a possible cause of childhood AIS. AIS may be associated with cocaine or amphetamine use related to hypertension and vasospasm.[67,68] It is unclear whether other sympathomimetic agents used in the treatment of migraine headaches or attention deficit disorder are a risk factor for AIS.

Hypercoagulable States

Several prothrombotic conditions seem to contribute to the risk of childhood AIS.[69–74] A meta-analysis of 22 observational cohort studies

showed a significant association between the first AIS and the following prothrombotic conditions: inherited deficiency of protein C, protein S, antithrombin III, factor V Leiden, factor II methylene tetrahydrofolate reductase polymorphism, elevated level of lipoprotein (a), and the presence of antiphospholipid antibodies.[71,72] Thrombophilia may also be an independent risk factor for AIS.[73]

In a study of 50 children with AIS followed for a mean duration of 21 months, elevated D-dimer levels were noted most commonly in children with cardiac disease.[61] D-dimer is a marker of coagulation activation, suggesting an underlying thrombophilia state in cardiac disease, which was also identified in children with AIS and cardiac disease by Strater and colleagues.[70]

Additional hematologic factors that may confer an increased risk of AIS include SCD, iron deficiency anemia, thrombocytosis, and polycythemia.[30,75,76]

DIAGNOSIS

The underlying risk factors of congenital heart disease and SCD are usually known before the AIS. Pertinent history includes head and neck trauma (associated with intracranial hemorrhage and dissection), unexplained fever or infection (particularly varicella), vasculitis, drug ingestion, blood disorders, and an associated headache.[3,21]

Laboratory Testing

Laboratory screening in childhood AIS should include a complete blood cell count, iron studies,

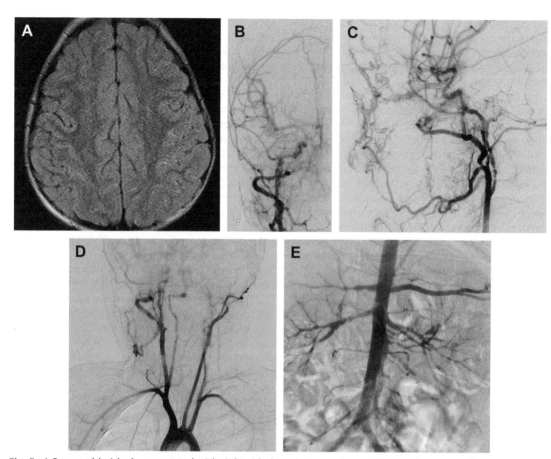

Fig. 5. A 3-year-old girl who presented with right-sided weakness and a systolic blood pressure of 200 mm Hg. (*A*) Axial FLAIR MRI demonstrates no evidence of ischemia with hyperintense cortical vessels. (*B*) Frontal and lateral (*C*) right common carotid angiogram shows severe narrowing and a "string of beads" in the right internal carotid artery. The right external carotid artery is hypertrophied filling collateral vessels to the intracranial circulation. In addition, there is narrowing of the supraclinoid, R A1, and R M1 segments. (*D*) Arch aortogram shows no evidence of narrowing of the great vessels. (*E*) Abdominal aortogram shows severe narrowing and a "string of beads" involving the celiac axis, superior mesenteric artery, and right and left renal arteries. These findings are consistent with moyamoya disease and renal artery stenosis related to fibromuscular dysplasia.

serum electrolytes, C-reactive protein, erythrocyte sedimentation rate, coagulation times, fibrinogen titer, antinuclear antibodies, triglyceride, cholesterol, amino acid chromatography, lactates, protein C, protein S, antithrombin III, antiphospholipid antibodies, urine samples investigation for amino acid, organic acid chromatography, CSF examination for cell count and protein titration, titer of viral antibodies in serum and CSF, and complement and polymerase chain reaction for varicella zoster virus DNA. An echocardiogram, standard electroencephalogram, and a prolonged (24-h) electroencephalogram recording should be obtained.

Imaging Studies

A noncontrast computed tomography (CT) of the head is usually the first imaging modality to rule out an area of acute cerebral infarction or intraparenchymal hemorrhage. In the early stage of ischemia, CT findings can be subtle and a small lesion within the posterior fossa can be missed. Computed tomographic angiography (CTA) can provide further valuable information about the intracranial and extracranial circulation.[77] Arterial dissection, large-vessel occlusion, and stenosis of the circle of Willis can be readily identified on CTA. Disadvantages of CTA include use of IV contrast, radiation exposure, and the difficulty of timing the contrast bolus in small children.

Magnetic resonance imaging (MRI) with diffusion-weighted and perfusion-weighted imaging is optimal for diagnosing stroke. MRA is a noninvasive procedure that can detect large vascular abnormalities similar to cerebral angiography.[14,78] Magnetic resonance spectroscopy and diffusion-weighted imaging with MRA can increase the sensitivity of MRI in detecting ischemia and infarction.[79]

Cerebral angiography should be considered in children when the pathologic abnormalityof a small distal artery is suspected or the cause of an unexplained infarct or hemorrhage cannot be determined by noninvasive imaging.[80] Angiography is also used to diagnose moyamoya disease. At Great Ormond Street Hospital (where there is a large AIS cohort), catheter angiography is performed for any patient when surgery is contemplated, any posterior circulation stroke where the cause is not absolutely determined by noninvasive imaging, and most anterior circulation strokes where the cause is not certain. The yield is very high, especially in the posterior circulation. Great Ormond Street Hospital has never had a diagnostic angiography-related stroke in a child (now over 1000 children).

Transcranial Doppler can identify patients with SCD at high risk for cerebral infarction.[81] In children with SCD with MCA velocities greater than 1.7 m/s (170 cm/s) the risk of stroke increases. A velocity greater than 2 m/s (200 cm/s) in the MCA confers a greater than 10% risk of stroke per year in the next 3 years. Furthermore, a maximum velocity in the ophthalmic artery greater than 0.35 m/s (35 cm/s), a resistance index of the ophthalmic artery less than 0.60 m/s (60 cm/s), and velocity in the ophthalmic artery greater than the ipsilateral MCA have been associated with vascular complications in patients with SCD.[82]

TREATMENT
Acute (Including Hyperacute) Phase

Thrombolysis
A recent review described all of the cases reported in the literature over the last 18 years on the use of endovascular thrombolytic therapies for children with AIS.[83] A total of 34 cases of pediatric AIS treated with endovascular thrombolytic therapies were identified in the literature. This cohort included 18 male and 16 female cases, with a mean age at the time of treatment of 10.9 years (range, 2–18). Systemic risk factors for AIS were identified in 23 of 34 patients (67.6%). Cerebrovascular risk factors were identified in 12 of 34 patients (35.3%). The mean time from the onset of symptoms to endovascular therapy was 14.0 hours (range, 2–72). Only 1 patient underwent treatment with IV tissue plasminogen activator (t-PA) before endovascular therapy. Endovascular therapies included Intraarterial (IA) thrombolysis alone (n = 23), IA thrombolysis + mechanical thrombolysis (n = 9), and mechanical thrombolysis alone (n = 2). One patient underwent definitive treatment of primary vessel pathology using endovascular stent placement.

Recanalization was complete in 12 of 34 cases (35.2%), incomplete in 13 of 34 cases (38.2%), and absent in 3 of 34 cases (8.8%); recanalization status was not reported in 6 of 34 cases (17.6%). Complications (including periprocedural complications and postprocedural hemorrhage) occurred in a total of 10 of 34 cases (29.4%). Postprocedural intracranial hemorrhage occurred in 8 of 34 patients (23.5%), although only 1 of these hemorrhages was symptomatic (2.9% of all cases).

Three studies have suggested that anticoagulation therapy can be given safely in the acute phase of a childhood ischemic stroke.[84–86] The American College of Chest Physicians (ACCP) guidelines recommend initiation of therapy with either unfractionated heparin or low molecular weight heparin (LMWH), given the high frequency of cardioembolism, arterial dissection, and prothrombotic conditions as common causes of childhood AIS.[87] They recommend continuing anticoagulation until cardioembolic sources and extracranial dissection have been excluded. The Royal College of Physicians (RCP) guidelines adopt an approach of using antiplatelet therapy instead of anticoagulation until a cardioembolism or extracranial dissection is diagnosed.[88] The American Heart Association (AHA) guidelines support either approach.[25] Heparin-based anticoagulation is best monitored with antifactor Xa activity U/mL for unfractionated heparin and 0.5 to 1.0 U/mL for LMWH. These recommendations support the use of anticoagulation for cardioembolism and extracranial arterial dissection in the acute and subacute period after a childhood AIS. These recommendations have been called into question based on a recent article of 298 adult patients with carotid dissection, suggesting that aspirin (ASA) may be as effective as anticoagulation in preventing a recurrent stroke.[89] A recent Cochrane Report of nonrandomized studies for carotid artery dissection did not show any evidence of a significant difference between anticoagulants and antiplatelet drugs.[90]

Subacute and Chronic Treatment

Anticoagulation
Secondary prophylaxis with LMWH or Warfarin is recommended by the RCP and ACCP guidelines in children with cardioembolism or extracranial arterial dissection.[87,88] The AHA guidelines also note to consider anticoagulation in children with a high risk of recurrent cardiac embolism and with inherited thrombophilias.[25] In a study focusing on the safety of anticoagulation in

childhood AIS with non-moyamoya arteriopathy, 2 clinical relevant bleeding episodes occurred in 37 patients treated for at least 4 weeks.[86] Cumulative probability of recurrent arterial ischemic stroke at 1 year was 14%. Preliminary clinical studies suggest that anticoagulation may be safe in children with AIS; however, the efficacy and safety of anticoagulation versus antiplatelet therapy has not been evaluated in childhood AIS in the setting of a randomized controlled trial. Antiplatelet therapy is currently recommended by all guidelines for subacute/chronic therapy in childhood AIS without a cardioembolic source or arterial dissection.

Antiplatelet therapy

In children with AIS who do not have SCD, cardioembolic stroke, or arterial dissection, all guidelines (ie, ACCP, RCP, and AHA) recommend secondary prophylaxis with ASA. Dosing recommendations for ASA are 1 to 5 mg/kg/d by ACCP, 1 to 3 mg/kg/d by RCP, and 3 to 5 mg/kg/d by AHA with a reduction to 1 to 3 mg/kg/d if side effects occur.[25,87,88] Duration of treatment remains uncertain; however, many practitioners discontinue treatment after 1 or 2 years.

Other Forms of Treatment

If medical therapy fails to relieve cerebral edema following a stroke, decompressive hemicraniectomy can be of benefit to prevent further ischemia and death.[91]

SECONDARY PREVENTION

There is limited evidence regarding the efficacy of secondary prevention of recurrent AIS in children. ASA is the most common agent prescribed for secondary prevention following an AIS, except in children with SCD or a hypercoagulable condition. The ideal prophylactic dose of ASA in children is unknown; however, a few reports have shown that doses between 1 and 5 mg/kg body weight per day are effective.[87] Antiplatelet therapy is sometimes used in patients with moyamoya disease who are not a surgical candidate or have a mild form of the disease. If ASA is not effective, contraindicated, or not tolerated, other antiplatelets agents can be used; however, the data are limited. ASA should not be combined with other antiplatelet agents with risk factors for intracranial hemorrhage or intracranial vasculopathies.[92]

Long-term anticoagulation with heparin or Warfarin may be indicated for patients with a hypercoagulable condition, an arterial dissection, or an acquired or congenital heart disease. Anticoagulation may also be indicated in patients who have suffered a recurrent AIS on antiplatelet therapy.[93]

Secondary AIS in patients with SCD can be prevented with chronic transfusion therapy every 3 to 4 weeks to maintain an HbS less than 0.3 (30%), which has been shown to decrease the subsequent rate of an AIS by 92%.[94–96] Complications with transfusion therapy include recurrent stroke, iron overload, alloimmunization, autoantibody formation, and noncompliance with transfusions.[95] Iron chelation agents such as deferoxamine are used in cases of iron overload from chronic transfusions.[97–99] The Stroke Prevention in Sickle Cell Disease (STOP) study showed that prophylactic blood transfusion in children with high MCA velocities prevented stroke.[100] The STOP 2 study suggested that transfusions needed to be continued to have a protective effect.[101] Unfortunately, transfusions are expensive and time-consuming; therefore, a search for alternative treatments is warranted.

Hydroxyurea (HU) has also been studied in patients with SCD for AIS prevention.[102,103] HU works by inducing hemoglobin F; this improves red blood cell deformity, reduces the irreversibility of the sickled cell fraction, and is associated with red blood cell survival. However, the maximal benefits of HU are not achieved for 6 months after the initiation of therapy; therefore, patients may require a transfusion overlap period.[104] Iron overload from transfusion is usually treated with blood removal of 10 mL/kg every 2 to 4 weeks to maintain the hemoglobin concentration greater than 8 g/dL.[95,97]

Bone marrow transplant may be curative for patients with SCD and may be an option for stroke prevention.[105] Unfortunately, there is no clear consensus of which SCD patient would most benefit from this form of treatment.[106] There are clinical risks associated with bone marrow transplants, including graft-versus-host disease, seizure, posttransplant hemorrhage, and graft rejection.

Moyamoya disease is usually progressive during childhood and then becomes less progressive when the patient reaches adulthood. Factors related to a poor prognosis include early age at diagnosis, bilateral hemispheric involvement, diffuse angiographic occlusion, and episodes of transient ischemic attack (TIA) followed by stroke.[107] Surgical revascularization has been shown to improve clinical outcome.[108] Revascularization surgery in moyamoya can be either direct such as revascularization superficial temporal-middle cerebral artery bypass or indirect such as encephaloduroarteriosynangiosis, encephalomyosynangiosis, and encephalomyoarteriosynangiosis. Indirect revascularization using an omental flap has been also described.[109,110] Pial synangiosis (**Fig. 6**) is a modification of the encephaloduroarteriosynangiosis procedure and should be considered first-line treatment for

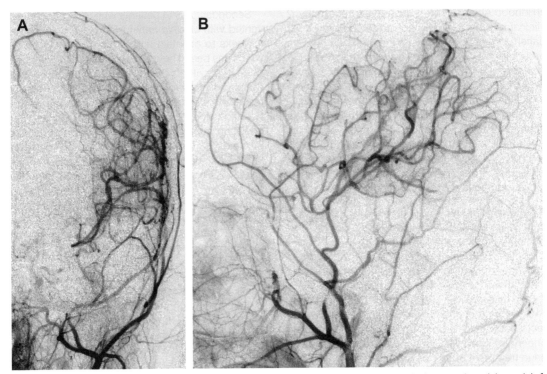

Fig. 6. A patient with moyamoya disease treated with a pial synangiosis. (*A* and *B*) Frontal and lateral left external carotid angiogram shows excellent filling of the left middle cerebral artery branches after treatment.

moyamoya, especially in the pediatric population.[111]

Other risk factors for the prevention of secondary AIS can be modified. For example, patients with hyperhomocysteinemia may respond to supplements of folate, vitamin B12, and vitamin B6. Patients with lipid abnormalities can be treated with exercise, dietary restrictions, and lipid-lowering medications. Inflammatory and autoimmune disorders can be treated with immunosuppressive agents and medications targeting the specific pathways involved.

OUTCOME

The rate of mortality attributable to childhood AIS is 0.09 per 100,000 per year and the case fatality rate is roughly 15%.[4,19] The rate of mortality has fallen since the 1980s.[4] Among survivors there is a high rate of morbidity, with at least two-thirds of children showing neurologic impairment, most commonly sensorimotor.[5,112] Factors associated with an increased risk of death include male gender and preexisting critical illness.[4,19,113] Stroke can also affect other domains, including speech, vision, and cognitive skills; however, these areas have not been studied as well.[114,115] Language difficulties may not present as classical aphasia syndromes but as subcortical aphasia

secondary to involvement of the basal ganglia and internal capsule.[116] In addition, other studies have found impairments in attention, verbal learning, memory, and performance intelligence quotient following an AIS.[117–120] Two-thirds of the children suffering an AIS require help with daily living skills beyond those required by their peers and this has an important impact on quality of life for both the children and their families.[5,119,121]

SUMMARY

AIS affects 3.3 of 100,000 children per year, with residual morbidity in two-thirds, resulting in significant health care, personal, and social costs.[1–5] Focal neurologic deficits, such as hemiplegia, are the most common presentation of AIS in children.[10] The causes of AIS can be broadly divided into the following 6 categories: cardiac disease, SCD, moyamoya, arterial dissection, other arteriopathy, and other causes.[23] Approximately 24% of the cases are classified as idiopathic.[3] Medical approaches, including anticoagulation, antiinflammatory and antiplatelet therapies, surgical revascularization, and endovascular approaches, may have a role in the management of AIS in children. The rate of mortality attributable to childhood AIS is 0.09 per 100,000 per year and the case fatality rate is roughly 15%.[4,19]

REFERENCES

1. DeVeber G. The Canadian Pediatric Ischemic Stroke Study Group: Canadian pediatric ischemic stroke registry: analysis of children with arterial ischemic stroke [abstract]. Ann Neurol 2000;48: 526.

2. Lanska MJ, Lanska DJ, Horwitz SJ, et al. Presentation, clinical course, and outcome of childhood stroke. Pediatr Neurol 1991;7:333–41.

3. Fullerton HJ, Wu YW, Sidney S, et al. Risk of recurrent childhood arterial ischemic stroke in a population-based cohort: the importance of cerebrovascular imaging. Pediatrics 2007;119:495–501.

4. Fullerton HJ, Chetkovich DM, Wu YW, et al. Deaths from stroke in US children, 1979 to 1998. Neurology 2002;59:34–9.

5. Ganesan V, Hogan A, Shack N, et al. Outcome after ischaemic stroke in childhood. Dev Med Child Neurol 2000;42:455–61.

6. Lanthier S, Carmant L, David M, et al. Stroke in children: the coexistence of multiple risk factors predicts poor outcome. Neurology 2000;54:371–8.

7. Mackay MT, Wiznitzer M, Benedict SL, et al. Arterial ischemic stroke risk factors: the International Pediatric Stroke Study. Ann Neurol 2011;69:130–40.

8. Lynch JK. Cerebrovascular disorders in children. Curr Neurol Neurosci Rep 2004;4:129–38.

9. Kirkham FJ. Stroke in childhood. Arch Dis Child 1999;81:85–9.

10. Carlin TM, Chanmugam A. Stroke in children. Emerg Med Clin North Am 2002;20:671–85.

11. Carvalho KS, Garg BP. Arterial strokes in children. Neurol Clin 2002;20:1079–100, vii.

12. Thurman RJ, Jauch EC. Acute ischemic stroke: emergent evaluation and management. Emerg Med Clin North Am 2002;20:609–30, vi.

13. Zimmer JA, Garg BP, Williams LS, et al. Age-related variation in presenting signs of childhood arterial ischemic stroke. Pediatr Neurol 2007;37: 171–5.

14. Nowak-Gottl U, Gunther G, Kurnik K, et al. Arterial ischemic stroke in neonates, infants, and children: an overview of underlying conditions, imaging methods, and treatment modalities. Semin Thromb Hemost 2003;29:405–14.

15. Braun KP, Rafay MF, Uiterwaal CS, et al. Mode of onset predicts etiological diagnosis of arterial ischemic stroke in children. Stroke 2007;38:298–302.

16. Schoenberg BS, Mellinger JF, Schoenberg DG. Cerebrovascular disease in infants and children: a study of incidence, clinical features, and survival. Neurology 1978;28:763–8.

17. Broderick J, Talbot GT, Prenger E, et al. Stroke in children within a major metropolitan area: the surprising importance of intracerebral hemorrhage. J Child Neurol 1993;8:250–5.

18. deVeber G, Andrew M, Adams C, et al. Cerebral sinovenous thrombosis in children. N Engl J Med 2001;345:417–23.

19. Fullerton HJ, Wu YW, Zhao S, et al. Risk of stroke in children: ethnic and gender disparities. Neurology 2003;61:189–94.

20. Williams AN, Eunson PD, McShane MA, et al. Childhood cerebrovascular disease and stroke like illness in the United Kingdom and Eire. A descriptive epidemiological study. Arch Dis Child 2002;86(Suppl 1):A40–1 (G113).

21. Kirkham FJ. Is there a genetic basis for pediatric stroke? Curr Opin Pediatr 2003;15:547–58.

22. Kerr LM, Anderson DM, Thompson JA, et al. Ischemic stroke in the young: evaluation and age comparison of patients six months to thirty-nine years. J Child Neurol 1993;8:266–70.

23. Goldenberg NA, Bernard TJ, Fullerton HJ, et al. Antithrombotic treatments, outcomes, and prognostic factors in acute childhood-onset arterial ischaemic stroke: a multicentre, observational, cohort study. Lancet Neurol 2009;8:1120–7.

24. Billar J. Stroke in children and young adults. 2nd edition. Philadelphia: Saunders/Elsevier; 2009.

25. Roach ES, Golomb MR, Adams R, et al. Management of stroke in infants and children: a scientific statement from a Special Writing Group of the American Heart Association Stroke Council and the Council on Cardiovascular Disease in the Young. Stroke 2008;39:2644–91.

26. Lo W, Stephens J, Fernandez S. Pediatric stroke in the United States and the impact of risk factors. J Child Neurol 2009;24:194–203.

27. Ricci S. Embolism from the heart in the young patient: a short review. Neurol Sci 2003;24(Suppl 1): S13–4.

28. deVeber G. Arterial ischemic strokes in infants and children: an overview of current approaches. Semin Thromb Hemost 2003;29:567–73.

29. DeVeber G. Risk factors for childhood stroke: little folks have different strokes! Ann Neurol 2003;53: 149–50.

30. Ganesan V, Prengler M, McShane MA, et al. Investigation of risk factors in children with arterial ischemic stroke. Ann Neurol 2003;53:167–73.

31. Benedik MP, Zaletel M, Meglic NP, et al. Patent foramen ovale and unexplained ischemic cerebrovascular events in children. Catheter Cardiovasc Interv 2007;70:999–1007.

32. Wu LA, Malouf JF, Dearani JA, et al. Patent foramen ovale in cryptogenic stroke: current understanding and management options. Arch Intern Med 2004; 164:950–6.

33. Prengler M, Pavlakis SG, Prohovnik I, et al. Sickle cell disease: the neurological complications. Ann Neurol 2002;51:543–52.

34. Ohene-Frempong K, Weiner SJ, Sleeper LA, et al. Cerebrovascular accidents in sickle cell disease: rates and risk factors. Blood 1998;91:288–94.

35. Rothman SM, Fulling KH, Nelson JS. Sickle cell anemia and central nervous system infarction: a neuropathological study. Ann Neurol 1986;20: 684–90.

36. Tuohy AM, McKie V, Manci EA, et al. Internal carotid artery occlusion in a child with sickle cell disease: case report and immunohistochemical study. J Pediatr Hematol Oncol 1997;19:455–8.

37. Merkel KH, Ginsberg PL, Parker JC Jr, et al. Cerebrovascular disease in sickle cell anemia: a clinical, pathological and radiological correlation. Stroke 1978;9:45–52.

38. Bernard TJ, Goldenberg NA. Pediatric arterial ischemic stroke. Hematol Oncol Clin North Am 2010;24:167–80.

39. Amlie-Lefond C, Bernard TJ, Sebire G, et al. Predictors of cerebral arteriopathy in children with arterial ischemic stroke: results of the International Pediatric Stroke Study. Circulation 2009;119: 1417–23.

40. Manceau E, Giroud M, Dumas R. Moyamoya disease in children. A review of the clinical and radiological features and current treatment. Childs Nerv Syst 1997;13:595–600.

41. Sebire G, Fullerton H, Riou E, et al. Toward the definition of cerebral arteriopathies of childhood. Curr Opin Pediatr 2004;16:617–22.

42. Roder C, Nayak NR, Khan N, et al. Genetics of Moyamoya disease. J Hum Genet 2010;55:711–6.

43. Rosser TL, Vezina G, Packer RJ. Cerebrovascular abnormalities in a population of children with neurofibromatosis type 1. Neurology 2005;64: 553–5.

44. Kirkham FJ, DeBaun MR. Stroke in children with sickle cell disease. Curr Treat Options Neurol 2004;6:357–75.

45. Jea A, Smith ER, Robertson R, et al. Moyamoya syndrome associated with Down syndrome: outcome after surgical revascularization. Pediatrics 2005;116:e694–701.

46. Morris B, Partap S, Yeom K, et al. Cerebrovascular disease in childhood cancer survivors: a Children's Oncology Group Report. Neurology 2009; 73:1906–13.

47. Chabrier S, Husson B, Lasjaunias P, et al. Stroke in childhood: outcome and recurrence risk by mechanism in 59 patients. J Child Neurol 2000;15:290–4.

48. Chabrier S, Lasjaunias P, Husson B, et al. Ischaemic stroke from dissection of the craniocervical arteries in childhood: report of 12 patients. Eur J Paediatr Neurol 2003;7:39–42.

49. Brandt T, Grond-Ginsbach C. Spontaneous cervical artery dissection: from risk factors toward pathogenesis. Stroke 2002;33:657–8.

50. Patel H, Smith RR, Garg BP. Spontaneous extracranial carotid artery dissection in children. Pediatr Neurol 1995;13:55–60.

51. Sepelyak K, Gailloud P, Jordan LC. Athletics, minor trauma, and pediatric arterial ischemic stroke. Eur J Pediatr 2010;169:557–62.

52. Shaffer L, Rich PM, Pohl KR, et al. Can mild head injury cause ischaemic stroke? Arch Dis Child 2003;88:267–9.

53. Wraige E, Ganesan V, Pohl KR. Arterial dissection complicating tonsillectomy. Dev Med Child Neurol 2003;45:638–9.

54. Kieslich M, Fiedler A, Heller C, et al. Minor head injury as cause and co-factor in the aetiology of stroke in childhood: a report of eight cases. J Neurol Neurosurg Psychiatry 2002;73:13–6.

55. Fullerton HJ, Johnston SC, Smith WS. Arterial dissection and stroke in children. Neurology 2001;57:1155–60.

56. Rafay MF, Armstrong D, Deveber G, et al. Craniocervical arterial dissection in children: clinical and radiographic presentation and outcome. J Child Neurol 2006;21:8–16.

57. DeVeber G. In pursuit of evidence-based treatments for paediatric stroke: the UK and Chest guidelines. Lancet Neurol 2005;4:432–6.

58. Kirkham F, Sebire G, Steinlin M, et al. Arterial ischaemic stroke in children. Review of the literature and strategies for future stroke studies. Thromb Haemost 2004;92:697–706.

59. Askalan R, Laughlin S, Mayank S, et al. Chickenpox and stroke in childhood: a study of frequency and causation. Stroke 2001;32:1257–62.

60. Lanthier S, Armstrong D, Domi T, et al. Post-varicella arteriopathy of childhood: natural history of vascular stenosis. Neurology 2005;64:660–3.

61. Bernard TJ, Fenton LZ, Apkon SD, et al. Biomarkers of hypercoagulability and inflammation in childhood-onset arterial ischemic stroke. J Pediatr 2010;156:651–6.

62. Danchaivijitr N, Cox TC, Saunders DE, et al. Evolution of cerebral arteriopathies in childhood arterial ischemic stroke. Ann Neurol 2006;59:620–6.

63. Rolfs A, Bottcher T, Zschiesche M, et al. Prevalence of Fabry disease in patients with cryptogenic stroke: a prospective study. Lancet 2005;366:1794–6.

64. Granild-Jensen J, Jensen UB, Schwartz M, et al. Cerebral autosomal dominant arteriopathy with subcortical infarcts and leukoencephalopathy resulting in stroke in an 11-year-old male. Dev Med Child Neurol 2009;51:754–7.

65. Hsich GE, Robertson RL, Irons M, et al. Cerebral infarction in Menkes' disease. Pediatr Neurol 2000;23:425–8.

66. Alehan F, Saygi S, Gedik S, et al. Stroke in early childhood due to homocystinuria. Pediatr Neurol 2010;43:294–6.

67. Kaku DA, Lowenstein DH. Emergence of recreational drug abuse as a major risk factor for stroke in young adults. Ann Intern Med 1990;113:821–7.

68. Westover AN, McBride S, Haley RW. Stroke in young adults who abuse amphetamines or cocaine: a population-based study of hospitalized patients. Arch Gen Psychiatry 2007;64:495–502.

69. Kenet G, Sadetzki S, Murad H, et al. Factor V Leiden and antiphospholipid antibodies are significant risk factors for ischemic stroke in children. Stroke 2000;31:1283–8.

70. Strater R, Vielhaber H, Kassenbohmer R, et al. Genetic risk factors of thrombophilia in ischaemic childhood stroke of cardiac origin. A prospective ESPED survey. Eur J Pediatr 1999;158(Suppl 3): S122–5.

71. Kenet G, Lutkhoff LK, Albisetti M, et al. Impact of thrombophilia on risk of arterial ischemic stroke or cerebral sinovenous thrombosis in neonates and children: a systematic review and meta-analysis of observational studies. Circulation 2010;121: 1838–47.

72. Haywood S, Liesner R, Pindora S, et al. Thrombophilia and first arterial ischaemic stroke: a systematic review. Arch Dis Child 2005;90:402–5.

73. Nowak-Gottl U, Strater R, Heinecke A, et al. Lipoprotein (a) and genetic polymorphisms of clotting factor V, prothrombin, and methylenetetrahydrofolate reductase are risk factors of spontaneous ischemic stroke in childhood. Blood 1999;94: 3678–82.

74. Nowak-Gottl U, Junker R, Hartmeier M, et al. Increased lipoprotein(a) is an important risk factor for venous thromboembolism in childhood. Circulation 1999;100:743–8.

75. Maguire JL, deVeber G, Parkin PC. Association between iron-deficiency anemia and stroke in young children. Pediatrics 2007;120:1053–7.

76. Alvarez-Larran A, Cervantes F, Bellosillo B, et al. Essential thrombocythemia in young individuals: frequency and risk factors for vascular events and evolution to myelofibrosis in 126 patients. Leukemia 2007;21:1218–23.

77. Atkinson DS Jr. Computed tomography of pediatric stroke. Semin Ultrasound CT MR 2006;27: 207–18.

78. Husson B, Rodesch G, Lasjaunias P, et al. Magnetic resonance angiography in childhood arterial brain infarcts: a comparative study with contrast angiography. Stroke 2002;33:1280–5.

79. Venkataraman A, Kingsley PB, Kalina P, et al. Newborn brain infarction: clinical aspects and magnetic resonance imaging. CNS Spectr 2004; 9:436–44.

80. Ganesan V, Savvy L, Chong WK, et al. Conventional cerebral angiography in children with ischemic stroke. Pediatr Neurol 1999;20:38–42.

81. Riebel T, Kebelmann-Betzing C, Gotze R, et al. Transcranial Doppler ultrasonography in neurologically asymptomatic children and young adults with sickle cell disease. Eur Radiol 2003;13:563–70.

82. Seibert JJ, Glasier CM, Kirby RS, et al. Transcranial Doppler, MRA, and MRI as a screening examination for cerebrovascular disease in patients with sickle cell anemia: an 8-year study. Pediatr Radiol 1998;28:138–42.

83. Ellis MJ, Amlie-Lefond C, Orbach DB. Endovascular therapy in children with acute ischemic stroke: review and recommendations. Neurology 2012; 79:S158–64.

84. Strater R, Kurnik K, Heller C, et al. Aspirin versus low-dose low-molecular-weight heparin: antithrombotic therapy in pediatric ischemic stroke patients: a prospective follow-up study. Stroke 2001;32: 2554–8.

85. Burak CR, Bowen MD, Barron TF. The use of enoxaparin in children with acute, nonhemorrhagic ischemic stroke. Pediatr Neurol 2003;29:295–8.

86. Bernard TJ, Goldenberg NA, Tripputi M, et al. Anticoagulation in childhood-onset arterial ischemic stroke with non-moyamoya arteriopathy: findings from the Colorado and German (COAG) collaboration. Stroke 2009;40:2869–71.

87. Monagle P, Chalmers E, Chan A, et al. Antithrombotic therapy in neonates and children: American College of Chest Physicians Evidence-Based Clinical Practice Guidelines (8th Edition). Chest 2008; 133:887S–968S.

88. Pediatric Stroke Working Group. Stroke in childhood: Clinical guidelines for diagnosis, management, and rehabilitation. Royal College of Physicians; 2004. Available at: http://bookshop.replondon.ac.uk/contents/f98c6540-a541-4bed-837d-ef293ac458bf.pdf. Accessed January 31, 2012.

89. Georgiadis D, Arnold M, von Buedingen HC, et al. Aspirin vs anticoagulation in carotid artery dissection: a study of 298 patients. Neurology 2009;72: 1810–5.

90. Lyrer P, Engelter S. Antithrombotic drugs for carotid artery dissection. Cochrane Database Syst Rev 2010;(10):CD000255.

91. Lee MC, Frank JI, Kahana M, et al. Decompressive hemicraniectomy in a 6-year-old male after unilateral hemispheric stroke. Case report and review. Pediatr Neurosurg 2003;38:181–5.

92. Soman T, Rafay MF, Hune S, et al. The risks and safety of clopidogrel in pediatric arterial ischemic stroke. Stroke 2006;37:1120–2.

93. Shellhaas RA, Smith SE, O'Tool E, et al. Mimics of childhood stroke: characteristics of a prospective cohort. Pediatrics 2006;118:704–9.

94. Fathallah H, Atweh GF. Induction of fetal hemoglobin in the treatment of sickle cell disease. Hematology Am Soc Hematol Educ Program 2006;58–62.

95. Monagle P, Barnes C, Ignjatovic V, et al. Developmental haemostasis. Impact for clinical haemostasis laboratories. Thromb Haemost 2006;95:362–72.

96. Pegelow CH, Adams RJ, McKie V, et al. Risk of recurrent stroke in patients with sickle cell disease treated with erythrocyte transfusions. J Pediatr 1995;126:896–9.

97. Ware RE, Zimmerman SA, Sylvestre PB, et al. Prevention of secondary stroke and resolution of transfusional iron overload in children with sickle cell anemia using hydroxyurea and phlebotomy. J Pediatr 2004;145:346–52.

98. Vichinsky E, Onyekwere O, Porter J, et al. A randomised comparison of deferasirox versus deferoxamine for the treatment of transfusional iron overload in sickle cell disease. Br J Haematol 2007;136:501–8.

99. Stumpf JL. Deferasirox. Am J Health Syst Pharm 2007;64:606–16.

100. Adams RJ, McKie VC, Hsu L, et al. Prevention of a first stroke by transfusions in children with sickle cell anemia and abnormal results on transcranial Doppler ultrasonography. N Engl J Med 1998;339:5–11.

101. Adams RJ, Brambilla D. Discontinuing prophylactic transfusions used to prevent stroke in sickle cell disease. N Engl J Med 2005;353:2769–78.

102. Zimmerman SA, Schultz WH, Burgett S, et al. Hydroxyurea therapy lowers transcranial Doppler flow velocities in children with sickle cell anemia. Blood 2007;110:1043–7.

103. Zimmerman SA, Schultz WH, Davis JS, et al. Sustained long-term hematologic efficacy of hydroxyurea at maximum tolerated dose in children with sickle cell disease. Blood 2004;103:2039–45.

104. Adams RJ. Stroke prevention and treatment in sickle cell disease. Arch Neurol 2001;58:565–8.

105. Panepinto JA, Walters MC, Carreras J, et al. Matched-related donor transplantation for sickle cell disease: report from the Center for International Blood and Transplant Research. Br J Haematol 2007;137:479–85.

106. Hoppe CC, Walters MC. Bone marrow transplantation in sickle cell anemia. Curr Opin Oncol 2001;13:85–90.

107. Kirkham FJ, Hogan AM. Risk factors for arterial ischemic stroke in childhood. CNS Spectr 2004;9:451–64.

108. Kim CY, Wang KC, Kim SK, et al. Encephaloduroarteriosynangiosis with bifrontal encephalogaleo(periosteal)synangiosis in the pediatric moyamoya disease: the surgical technique and its outcomes. Childs Nerv Syst 2003;19:316–24.

109. Yoshida Y, Yoshimoto T, Shirane R, et al. Clinical course, surgical management, and long-term outcome of moyamoya patients with rebleeding after an episode of intracerebral hemorrhage: an extensive follow-Up study. Stroke 1999;30:2272–6.

110. Chiu D, Shedden P, Bratina P, et al. Clinical features of moyamoya disease in the United States. Stroke 1998;29:1347–51.

111. Smith ER, Scott RM. Surgical management of moyamoya syndrome. Skull Base 2005;15:15–26.

112. deVeber GA, MacGregor D, Curtis R, et al. Neurologic outcome in survivors of childhood arterial ischemic stroke and sinovenous thrombosis. J Child Neurol 2000;15:316–24.

113. Jordan LC, van Beek JG, Gottesman RF, et al. Ischemic stroke in children with critical illness: a poor prognostic sign. Pediatr Neurol 2007;36:244–6.

114. Lee YY, Lin KL, Wang HS, et al. Risk factors and outcomes of childhood ischemic stroke in Taiwan. Brain Dev 2008;30:14–9.

115. Hogan AM, Kirkham FJ, Isaacs EB. Intelligence after stroke in childhood: review of the literature and suggestions for future research. J Child Neurol 2000;15:325–32.

116. Gout A, Seibel N, Rouviere C, et al. Aphasia owing to subcortical brain infarcts in childhood. J Child Neurol 2005;20:1003–8.

117. Max JE, Mathews K, Manes FF, et al. Attention deficit hyperactivity disorder and neurocognitive correlates after childhood stroke. J Int Neuropsychol Soc 2003;9:815–29.

118. Lansing AE, Max JE, Delis DC, et al. Verbal learning and memory after childhood stroke. J Int Neuropsychol Soc 2004;10:742–52.

119. Everts R, Pavlovic J, Kaufmann F, et al. Cognitive functioning, behavior, and quality of life after stroke in childhood. Child Neuropsychol 2008;14:323–38.

120. Pavlovic J, Kaufmann F, Boltshauser E, et al. Neuropsychological problems after paediatric stroke: two year follow-up of Swiss children. Neuropediatrics 2006;37:13–9.

121. Gordon AL, Ganesan V, Towell A, et al. Functional outcome following stroke in children. J Child Neurol 2002;17:429–34.

122. Lopez-Vicente M, Ortega-Gutierrez S, Amlie-Lefond C, et al. Diagnosis and management of pediatric arterial ischemic stroke. J Stroke Cerebrovasc Dis 2010;19:175–83.

Index

Note: Page numbers of article titles are in **boldface** type.

A

Aneurysms. See specific sites and types.

Arterial dissection(s), as risk factor for arterial ischemic stroke in children, 785–788
  cerebral, and cervical arterial dissections, spontaneous, **661–671**
  cerebral angiography in, 664
  cerebral arterial, epidemiology of, 662
    pathophysiology of, 662
  cervical, and cerebral arterial dissections, spontaneous, **661–671**
  cervical cerebral, treatment of, 665–668
    endovascular, 666–668
    medical, 665–666
    surgical, 668
  cervicocranial, natural history of, 662
  craniocervical, clinical presentation of, 662–663
  CT in, 664
  diagnostic imaging of, 663–664
  MRI in, 664

Arteriopathy, focal cerebral, as risk factor for arterial ischemic stroke in children, 787–788, 789
  inflammatory, as risk factor for arterial ischemic stroke in children, 788–790

Arteriovenous fistula(s), cerebral dural, 625–631
    and pial, endovascular treatment of, **625–636**
    clinical presentation and assessment of, 626–627
    imaging studies and classification of, 627–628
    Jefferson Hospital for Neuroscience experience with, 630–631
    natural history of, 626
    treatment of, and follow-up of, 628–629
      endovascular neurosurgical techniques in, 629–630
  cerebral pial, 631–633, 732–734, 737, 739–740
    and dural, endovascular treatment of, **625–636**
    clinical presentation of, 632
    endovascular treatment of, 632–633
    in children, 752–753
    natural history of, 631–632
  epidural, 735, 738, 743
  high-flow pial, in children, 766–767
  infantile, and dural sinus malformations, 767–768
  of childhood, 760
  paraspinal, in children, 753, 754
  spinal dural, 734–735, 737–738, 740–742
    in children, 753

Arteriovenous lesions, spinal, adult, diagnostic spinal angiography in, 738–739
    endovascular treatment of, **729–747**
      studies reporting, 742
    epidemiology, clinical presentation, and natural history of, 732–735
    imaging findings in, 737–739
    pathophysiology of, 735–737
    treatment of, 739–743
      follow-up, 741
    classification of, 731–732

Arteriovenous malformation syndromes, alcohol for embolization in, 713–714
  clinical presentation of, 712
  diagnostic imaging in, 713
  ethylene vinyl alcohol (Onyx) in, 716, 717
  gamma knife in, 716
  n-BCA in, 714–716
  natural history/epidemiology of, 712–713
  surgery in, 717
  treatment of, 713–717

Arteriovenous malformation(s), cerebral, coils in, 613–614
    curative therapy in, 610–611
    cyanoacrylate in, 611–612
    embolizates in, 611
    endovascular treatment of, **605–624**
      complications of, 619–621
      formulating strategy for, 606
      indications for, 606–611
      postoperative care in, 619
    EtOH in, 612–613
    EVOH copolymer-DMSO solvent in, 612
    liquid embolics in, 611
    palliative therapy in, 611
    preoperative embolization in, 607
      technique of, 614–619
    preradiopsurgery in, 608–610
    PVA/embospheres in, 613
    targeted therapy in, 607–608
  of spinal cord, 732, 733, 737, 739
    pial, in children, 751–752, 762
  pial, in children, cause of, 757
    diagnosis of, 758–759
    natural history of, 758
    outcome of, 760
    presentation of, 758
    treatment of, 759–760

http://dx.doi.org/10.1016/S1052-5149(13)00086-5
1052-5149/13/$ – see front matter © 2013 Elsevier Inc. All rights reserved.

United States Postal Service

Statement of Ownership, Management, and Circulation
(All Periodicals Publications Except Requestor Publications)

1. Publication Title
Neuroimaging Clinics of North America

2. Publication Number
0 1 0 - 5 4 8 8

3. Filing Date
9/14/13

4. Issue Frequency
Feb, May, Aug, Nov

5. Number of Issues Published Annually
4

6. Annual Subscription Price
$342.00

7. Complete Mailing Address of Known Office of Publication (Not printer) (Street, city, county, state, and ZIP+4®)
Elsevier Inc.
360 Park Avenue South
New York, NY 10010-1710

Contact Person
Stephen R. Bushing

Telephone (Include area code)
215-239-3688

8. Complete Mailing Address of Headquarters or General Business Office of Publisher (Not printer)
Elsevier Inc., 360 Park Avenue South, New York, NY 10010-1710

9. Full Names and Complete Mailing Addresses of Publisher, Editor, and Managing Editor (Do not leave blank)
Publisher (Name and complete mailing address)
Linda Belfus, Elsevier, Inc., 1600 John F. Kennedy Blvd. Suite 1800, Philadelphia, PA 19103-2899

Editor (Name and complete mailing address)
Pamela Hetherington, Elsevier, Inc., 1600 John F. Kennedy Blvd. Suite 1800, Philadelphia, PA 19103-2899

Managing Editor (Name and complete mailing address)
Adrianne Brigido, Elsevier, Inc., 1600 John F. Kennedy Blvd. Suite 1800, Philadelphia, PA 19103-2899

10. Owner (Do not leave blank. If the publication is owned by a corporation, give the name and address of the corporation immediately followed by the names and addresses of all stockholders owning or holding 1 percent or more of the total amount of stock. If not owned by a corporation, give the names and addresses of the individual owners. If owned by a partnership or other unincorporated firm, give its name and address as well as those of each individual owner. If the publication is published by a nonprofit organization, give its name and address.)

Full Name	Complete Mailing Address
Wholly owned subsidiary of	1600 John F. Kennedy Blvd., Ste. 1800
Reed/Elsevier, US holdings	Philadelphia, PA 19103-2899

11. Known Bondholders, Mortgagees, and Other Security Holders Owning or Holding 1 Percent or More of Total Amount of Bonds, Mortgages, or Other Securities. If none, check box → ☐ None

Full Name	Complete Mailing Address
N/A	

12. Tax Status (For completion by nonprofit organizations authorized to mail at nonprofit rates) (Check one)
The purpose, function, and nonprofit status of this organization and the exempt status for federal income tax purposes:
☐ Has Not Changed During Preceding 12 Months
☐ Has Changed During Preceding 12 Months (Publisher must submit explanation of change with this statement)

PS Form **3526**, September 2007 (Page 1 of 3 (Instructions Page 3)) PSN 7530-01-000-9931 **PRIVACY NOTICE:** See our Privacy policy in www.usps.com

---

13. Publication Title
Neuroimaging Clinics of North America

14. Issue Date for Circulation Data Below
May 2013

15. Extent and Nature of Circulation		Average No. Copies Each Issue During Preceding 12 Months	No. Copies of Single Issue Published Nearest to Filing Date
a. Total Number of Copies (Net press run)		1113	1021
b. Paid Circulation (By Mail and Outside the Mail)	(1) Mailed Outside-County Paid Subscriptions Stated on PS Form 3541. (Include paid distribution above nominal rate, advertiser's proof copies, and exchange copies)	736	670
	(2) Mailed In-County Paid Subscriptions Stated on PS Form 3541 (Include paid distribution above nominal rate, advertiser's proof copies, and exchange copies)		
	(3) Paid Distribution Outside the Mails Including Sales Through Dealers and Carriers, Street Vendors, Counter Sales, and Other Paid Distribution Outside USPS®	154	116
	(4) Paid Distribution by Other Classes Mailed Through the USPS (e.g. First-Class Mail®)		
c. Total Paid Distribution (Sum of 15b (1), (2), (3), and (4))	▲	890	786
d. Free or Nominal Rate Distribution (By Mail and Outside the Mail)	(1) Free or Nominal Rate Outside-County Copies Included on PS Form 3541	52	35
	(2) Free or Nominal Rate In-County Copies Included on PS Form 3541		
	(3) Free or Nominal Rate Copies Mailed at Other Classes Through the USPS (e.g. First-Class Mail)		
	(4) Free or Nominal Rate Distribution Outside the Mail (Carriers or other means)		
e. Total Free or Nominal Rate Distribution (Sum of 15d (1), (2), (3) and (4))	▲	52	35
f. Total Distribution (Sum of 15c and 15e)	▲	942	821
g. Copies not Distributed (See instructions to publishers #4 (page #3))	▲	171	200
h. Total (Sum of 15f and g)		1113	1021
i. Percent Paid (15c divided by 15f times 100)		94.48%	95.74%

16. Publication of Statement of Ownership
If the publication is a general publication, publication of this statement is required. Will be printed
in the **November 2013** issue of this publication.
☐ Publication not required

17. Signature and Title of Editor, Publisher, Business Manager, or Owner

Stephen R. Bushing
Stephen R. Bushing – Inventory Distribution Coordinator

Date
September 14, 2013

I certify that all information furnished on this form is true and complete. I understand that anyone who furnishes false or misleading information on this form or who omits material or information requested on the form may be subject to criminal sanctions (including fines and imprisonment) and/or civil sanctions (including civil penalties).

PS Form **3526**, September 2007 (Page 2 of 3)

Moving?

Make sure your subscription moves with you!

To notify us of your new address, find your **Clinics Account Number** (located on your mailing label above your name), and contact customer service at:

Email: journalscustomerservice-usa@elsevier.com

800-654-2452 (subscribers in the U.S. & Canada)
314-447-8871 (subscribers outside of the U.S. & Canada)

Fax number: 314-447-8029

Elsevier Health Sciences Division
Subscription Customer Service
3251 Riverport Lane
Maryland Heights, MO 63043

*To ensure uninterrupted delivery of your subscription, please notify us at least 4 weeks in advance of move.

Printed and bound by CPI Group (UK) Ltd, Croydon, CR0 4YY

03/10/2024

01040309-0006